COPING WITH COVID-19

THE MEDICAL, MENTAL, AND SOCIAL CONSEQUENCES OF THE PANDEMIC

COPING WITH COVID-19

THE MEDICAL, MENTAL, AND SOCIAL CONSEQUENCES OF THE PANDEMIC

Samoon Ahmad, MD

Clinical Professor
Department of Psychiatry
NYU Grossman School of Medicine
New York, New York

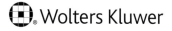 Wolters Kluwer

Philadelphia • Baltimore • New York • London
Buenos Aires • Hong Kong • Sydney • Tokyo

Acquisitions Editor: Chris Teja
Development Editor: Ariel S. Winter
Editorial Assistant: Victoria Giansante
Marketing Manager: Kirsten Watrud
Production Project Manager: Barton Dudlick
Design Coordinator: Stephen Druding
Manufacturing Coordinator: Beth Welsh
Prepress Vendor: TNQ Technologies

9 8 7 6 5 4 3 2 1

Printed in Mexico

Library of Congress Cataloging-in-Publication Data

ISBN-13: 978-1-975188-99-3

Cataloging in Publication data available on request from publisher.

shop.lww.com

Dedication

To all those who perished, suffered,
and lost their loved ones.

To all health care workers who worked selflessly
to save so many.

And in loving memory of my father who I lost
during the pandemic.

S.A.

Foreword

COVID-19 has fundamentally altered our way of life. We are now beginning to look beyond the immediate pandemic to understand more fully the profound effects of COVID-19 on our society; emotionally, politically, socially, and economically. Not in recent memory have we experienced such collective trauma and grief, and the pandemic is far from over.

Dr. Ahmad's international experience studying the prevalence of posttraumatic stress disorders after disasters places him well to write a sweeping analysis of how COVID-19 has affected medicine, public health, and our national psyche. Dr. Ahmad's work is a valuable and insightful contribution.

Dr. Ahmad has used his own experience as a frontline medical worker in a psychiatric inpatient unit, who contracted COVID-19 in the early days of the pandemic as a starting point for the book. He describes a desperate need to make sense of the pandemic for others, a feeling familiar to me not only from this current pandemic but also from the HIV/AIDS epidemic and long ago my memory of the polio pandemic.

Dr. Ahmad explores complex issues such as difficult ethics issues, psychosocial impacts, and how to prepare our physicians for future pandemics. While intended for a clinical audience, the work is accessible to anyone who is looking to deepen their understanding of how the pandemic will shape our future.

Dr. Ahmad also shares my frustration about how infectious disease control and pandemic planning has been treated as a low priority for decades, a casualty of the bottom line. His book examines the lessons we've learned and presents a path forward for the future. It is my profound hope with the contribution that Dr. Ahmad and others will make to the literature, that even though future pandemics may occur, future generations will never have to endure such a tragedy as we have.

William A. Haseltine, PhD
Chair and President, ACCESS Health International

Prologue

As you glance through this book, the natural question to ask is, "Why should I read this?" The simple answer is that it is not just yours and mine, but our story. We have lived through an historical time with nothing in recent history that mirrors this era, and the end is still yet to be determined. I am sure we are all searching for the truth in terms of science, and to discover policies that dictate mandates in accordance with what we desire and, most importantly, mitigate the impact of the virus on our collective suffering. I decided to write this book with these facts in mind and hope that I am able to present an objective view of what led us here and where we might go.

The morning of March 23, 2020, was like any other day—or so I thought. I woke up as usual to get ready and make my way to the hospital, but as soon as my foot hit the ground, I realized that I was not myself. I felt nauseous, bloated, and needed to make my way to the restroom. After a shower and getting ready, I felt a bit better and decided to make my way to work. Once there, I fell into my routine but felt weak, dizzy, and tired. I checked my temperature, but I was within normal range, so I attributed my symptoms to having eaten something bad or most likely some stomach bug.

In hindsight, these were some of the telltale signs of COVID-19, but at the time it was still considered to be a respiratory illness. I work on a psychiatric inpatient unit and was just beginning to deal with the emergence of the disease and the newly established guidelines that were being updated daily. Looking back, it is astounding how little we knew about the SARS-CoV-2 virus at that time, that we were still not mandated to wear masks, and that we were not testing patients who were admitted to the hospital unless they showed any clear signs or symptoms of COVID-19.

By that afternoon, I was coughing and feverish, so I contacted the occupational health services (OHS) who recommended that I go home and regularly update them about my condition, especially if my fever reached above 100.4° F. That evening it did climb to 101° F, and after communicating with OHS I was asked to stay home until I was cleared to return, though exactly when or how I would be cleared to come back to work had yet to be determined. Though it was frustrating, as a clinician I understood the reason for the lack of clarity but still understand the frustration felt by millions of Americans who struggled to understand this constant shift in recommendations. This is an important point and something that may have added to a lot of the confusion and skepticism among the general public who are not aware of how the rapidly evolving landscape of infectious diseases necessitates changes in recommendations as more clinical data emerge, and we improve our understanding about the pathology and route of transmission of a disease. This is especially important, as a lack of clear and appropriate messaging about the need for constant revision and updating of guidelines led many to be doubtful and suspicious of the accuracy of the information and guidelines issued by state and federal agencies.

For the next 2 weeks I remained quarantined at home. Though I luckily did not experience high fever or require any other acute interventions, the disease did take a toll on the body, and it took weeks to recover from a lingering cough and fatigue. However, eventually I was able to make a full recovery and to return to work.

Despite being a physician and trained as a psychiatrist, it was hard to be objective about my symptoms and overall health, since listening to the nonstop news about this mysterious virus causing thousands of daily deaths was anything but settling. Every day I would find something new about this virus, which seemed to affect every organ in the body and people of all ages, though the worst impact was among the elderly and medically compromised individuals. It was not reassuring to hear that having a good immune system is not a guarantee of recovery since cytokine storm, which is an aberrant and hyperactive immune reaction that can damage one's organs and lead to a fatal outcome, can happen even in otherwise healthy individuals. All in all, the subtle and not so subtle drum of headlines about the virus starts to affect you emotionally and can be a source of psychological distress, especially when you are in recovery. A lot has been written on this subject, though from a personal experience nothing can relieve the anxiety and dread of the unknown impact of the virus or what tomorrow will bring in terms of its short- and long-term effects. It is during these times that one recognizes the value of companionship and social support, especially family and friends.

Even before I had fully recovered, I began delving into the origin, source, pathology, and transmission of the virus, but soon realized it was like going down a rabbit hole. There was no end to it and, strangely, the holes kept on branching off in new directions as I dug deeper. Moreover, I started to realize just how dramatic the psychological impact of the pandemic was going to be as the physical toll of the virus was subsiding. I recognized that it was not just the disease, but the secondary effects like quarantine, social isolation, loss of jobs, empty streets, and virtual everything (shopping, conferencing, dating) were going to send shockwaves throughout the world, and they were going to have lingering economic, psychological, and psychosocial impacts for years to come. I can recall the days walking from home to the hospital and being one of a handful or at times the only one on the street. It was like being Will Smith in *I am Legend*. I could stand in the middle of First Avenue and not see a car in sight. "Doomsday," "post-apocalyptic," or any other words would not do justice to this sight or the emotional impact of seeing the city that never sleeps suddenly go silent. Perhaps this feeling of desolation would have been less impactful in a suburban setting but standing in the middle of the avenue at rush hour in Manhattan and not seeing another soul around you is an eerie feeling.

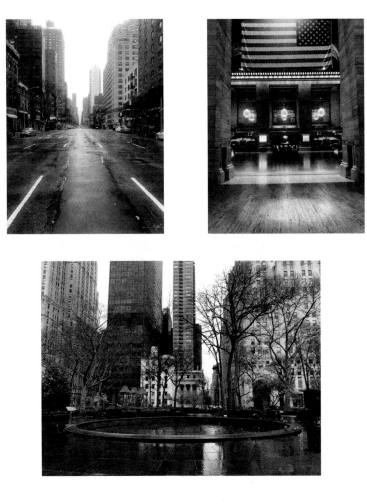

As I continued to research and come to understand the numerous aspects of this novel virus and its myriad effects on our physical and psychological health, I soon realized that it is impossible for an individual to find up-to-date information in one place that is easily accessible, palatable in terms of understanding the science, and more importantly open to discussing the neuropsychiatric implications of the disease, like long COVID. Moreover, I felt that there needed to be a single source that also addressed the psychological, social, and economic effects of the virus, and lastly the ethics of saving lives on the one hand and saving the economy and millions of jobs on the other. These issues were the driving force behind my research, and they motivated me to bring this information together in a scientific manner that is independent of any political rhetoric or bias and is presented in a concise and simple way for the reader to gain some perspective on what happened, what is happening, and how to navigate moving forward. I hope this journey into the science, ethics, medical, and psychological effects of COVID-19 will not only be a source of information, but transformative as well.

As we continue to learn and search for answers, there is no doubt that we will need to rethink and revise how we mount an international response to pathogens that have the potential to become global public health threats. However, I think one of the other lessons that became apparent during the COVID-19 pandemic was that we need an all-hands-on-deck approach. There is no question that epidemiology should be given primacy as we develop plans for future public health crises and pour more resources into preventing these events from happening. At the same time, it is equally important that we incorporate perspectives from a multitude of disciplines, including economists, physicists, and medical professionals from a variety of specialties who can recognize the psychosocial consequences of public health policies should we once again face a cataclysm of this magnitude. My hope is to give readers a broad and clear perspective on these matters since policy changes at the state and federal level can only be resolved by the voice of the people. We owe it to the nearly 200 million who have suffered from COVID-19 and the close to 4 million who have perished so far to come to some agreement on a global as well as national levels. We have the expertise and the resources; we only need a greater willingness to work together to make certain future generations never have to undergo this kind of experience again.

Acknowledgments

My deepest thanks go to my mentor and colleague Benjamin J. Sadock, MD, Menas S. Gregory Professor of Psychiatry, NYU Grossman School of Medicine. His guidance and support remain unparalleled. His encouragement has paved the way for me to step outside of my comfort zone and take on bigger challenges. I am immensely thankful to Ben and his wife Virginia for their lifelong friendship.

Maryanne Badaracco, MD, Director and Chief of Psychiatry, Bellevue Hospital, has been a constant source of support in my pursuit of academic excellence. I additionally extend my gratitude to Charles Marmar, MD, Lucius R. Littauer Professor and Chair of the Department of Psychiatry, NYU Grossman School of Medicine, for his encouragement and leadership.

Immeasurable thanks go to Jay Fox, my research and editorial assistant. His diligence, dedication, and critical eye for detail are second to none. Considering the time constraints and rapid pace of evolving information on the topic, his contributions were crucial to the preparation of this book.

I would also like to thank all my colleagues at Bellevue Hospital for their tireless work and dedication, which inspire me to be a better clinician and human being.

Additionally, I would like to acknowledge my publisher Wolters Kluwer for their contribution to advancing highly relevant and important topics, and special thanks to Chris Teja for making this project possible.

Last but not least, my utmost gratitude and innumerable thanks to my wife Kim and our son Daniel for their tremendous support for me to take time away and write this book. And, above all, I thank my mother Riffat whose own career and dedication as a physician, a healer, and an altruist, inspired me to follow in her footsteps.

Samoon Ahmad, MD
Clinical Professor
Department of Psychiatry
NYU Grossman School of Medicine
New York, New York

Disclaimer

*C*oping *With COVID-19: Medical, Mental, and Social Consequences of the Pandemic* was researched, written, and prepared by Dr. Samoon Ahmad in his personal capacity. The opinions and views expressed in this publication are those of the author and do not reflect the opinions or views of the author's affiliated hospital systems or academic institution.

Contents

PART

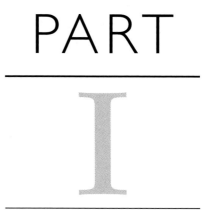

I

Pandemics are natural disasters, and an individual's ability to cope with such epic, horrific phenomena is partly dependent on cultural norms, faith, spiritual and religious beliefs, and last but not least, social support systems. Within the past century, industrialized countries have developed and established increasingly sophisticated response systems that include intervention and aid by federal and local governments, fire and police departments, medical personnel, and, more recently, mental health professionals.

History has taught us that the need for mental health professionals is essential after the initial burden of physical trauma or ailment has ended and necessary medical care has been provided. This is true in cases where an individual is affected by a traumatic experience, and it no doubt holds true when larger populations are impacted.

Part of what has made the COVID-19 pandemic so unique has been the worldwide scope of its impact and that its psychological effects are not limited to only those afflicted by the virus. The suffering and trauma extend to the hundreds of millions worldwide who have endured months of lockdowns and the tens of millions who have been forced to remain in isolation due to social distancing guidelines. While this can be justified and characterized as necessary to "flatten the curve," this still constitutes solitary confinement, which is well-known to have severe psychological sequela over the long term. We are slowly moving away from the peak of the pandemic, and though there are glimmers of hope that seem to be shining a little bit brighter by the day, there will still be pockets of outbreaks, especially among the unvaccinated. Therefore, it is imperative to have increased vigilance even among those who are vaccinated for the foreseeable future. Though we would like a full return to normalcy, it will remain frustratingly elusive for months if not years to come. Even after this, COVID-19 will continue to cast a long shadow. For many people throughout the world, successfully leaving the COVID Era behind will require an extended recovery phase, and we need to keep in mind that not everyone's timeline will be the same.

The first four chapters contained within the first part of this book are meant to present the basic facts and science of the virus. The first chapter covers its origin, spread, containment efforts, and the virology of SARS-CoV-2. The second chapter focuses on transmission. The third and fourth chapters examine the acute pathogenesis of COVID-19 and the long-term symptoms associated with so-called "long COVID," respectively. Like the rest of the book, my hope is to dispel any myths and eliminate misinformation. This requires a thorough examination of available evidence as it becomes available and an open mind, as well as recognition that policies, our understanding of the virus, and data on everything from vaccine efficacy to mortality rates have rapidly been evolving since the virus emerged and will likely continue to change as we fight to bring this pandemic to an end. While this book has been written with clinicians in mind, I also anticipate a wider audience due to the interest in the subject matter. Consequently, I have included brief primers on a variety of subjects throughout the first few chapters. Those with research and medical backgrounds will no doubt be familiar with the material and may choose to scan over these sections or use them as brief refreshers.

At the time of writing this book, there has been considerable debate on the origins of the pandemic as researchers have tried to establish if it was a natural or manmade disaster. Arguments in favor of both will be presented. Irrespective of the source of the virus, the physical and mental health toll and magnitude of human suffering is immeasurable and continues to ravage a large part of the planet, and if we are to move on from this cataclysm, we will need to focus less on where it came from and more on the direction in which it would benefit the society.

1

History, Origin, Spread, and Virology of SARS-CoV-2

Severe acute respiratory syndrome coronavirus 2 (SARS-CoV-2) first emerged in China's Hubei Province at the end of 2019. It quickly spread throughout the province's largest city, Wuhan, before escaping into other parts of China, Southeast Asia, and then the rest of the world. The virus is responsible for coronavirus disease of 2019 (COVID-19), which is now recognized to not only cause acute respiratory disease but also have a system-wide effect throughout the body. This chapter examines the historical context in which the outbreak took place by looking at previous pandemics and outbreaks involving other coronaviruses; follows the timeline between the first emergence of the virus until March 2020, when COVID-19 was declared a pandemic by the World Health Organization (WHO); and the basic virology of SARS-CoV-2.

The Dawn of the COVID Era

As 2019 came to an end, hospitals in Wuhan, a city in China's Hubei Province, reported that they were seeing an alarming rise in cases of atypical pneumonia. Several days later, the genome of SARS-CoV-2 was sequenced, and the WHO announced that the novel coronavirus was the pathogen behind the wave of illness.[1] On January 9, 2020, the first fatality due to coronavirus disease 2019 (COVID-19) was recorded.[2] In the weeks that followed, the virus spread throughout the world, infecting thousands.

It was finally declared a pandemic by the WHO on March 11, 2020. In the months that followed, the virus brought world commerce grinding to a halt as the number of infections rose exponentially due to multiple concurrent surges.

By the dawn of 2021, the pandemic had gone through at least three distinct waves of infections across the globe, and as of the summer of 2021, the pandemic was still not under control and many now believe that COVID-19 may become endemic, particularly in areas where vaccination efforts have lagged. However, various preventative measures had likely saved at least hundreds of thousands of lives and many national health care systems from collapse, while the herculean effort to create and test both the efficacy and the safety of multiple vaccines in record time had yielded several viable results that were approved for emergency use by governments around the world. Since that time, challenges have persisted in manufacturing and distributing the vaccines on an international basis, numerous variants of concern have emerged, and surges in the Americas, Europe, and Southeast Asia have caused innumerable deaths, but the worst of the initial phases of the pandemic appear to be behind us as we enter the autumn of 2021. It should be noted that this is cautious optimism based on emerging evidence rather than a prediction, and that we are by no means out of the woods yet, especially in regions where there is limited access to vaccines or where medical resources are scarce.

In the coming years, we will likely struggle to fully grasp the horrific impact of the pandemic between 2020 and 2021, even if SARS-CoV-2 continues to persist as an endemic illness. Beyond the immediate emotional and financial turmoil that the pandemic left in its wake, millions of people will grapple with long-term psychological problems due to an array of stressors that were directly and indirectly related to the pandemic, and these will likely be compounded by political and economic repercussions that will continue to evolve for months or years to come. For an unfathomably large number of individuals across the globe, recovery will require rethinking how they approach their mental health and coming to terms with the fact that a return to normalcy, as defined by routines from the prepandemic period, may not be possible. This includes not only those who have since been diagnosed with posttraumatic stress disorder (PTSD) due to the experience of being stricken ill by the virus or those who have struggled with cognitive issues (eg, "brain fog," memory lapses, migraine) following a less severe or asymptomatic case of COVID-19. It also concerns those who remained in isolation for months and emerged to find themselves incapable of simply resuming "normal" activities as if nothing had changed.

Before delving into these issues, however, we must first understand the scope of the pandemic and the science of the SARS-CoV-2 virus. In this chapter, as well as the three subsequent chapters, I will explore multiple aspects of the virus, including historic precedent, the timeline of the pandemic, and the virology and epidemiology of SARS-CoV-2. This is by no means an exhaustive review of all the material on the coronavirus or COVID-19, and it is certainly not to be taken as the final word but merely a summation of the best information that is available at the time of this writing.[i]

Pandemics

When an infectious disease suddenly and rapidly spreads throughout a community, it is known as an epidemic (a combination of the Greek words *epi* and *demos*, meaning "among" and "people," respectively). When an infectious disease rapidly spreads between and affects multiple communities across countries or continents, it is known as a pandemic (*pan-* coming from the Greek for "all"). When an infectious disease has become common within a population, it is known as being endemic (*en* is Greek for "in"). It means it is literally part of the community. As Devi Sridhar, chair of global public health at the University of Edinburgh, told the *Washington Post* in an article published in June 2021, "Throughout history, pandemics have ended when the disease ceases to dominate daily life and retreats into the background like other health challenges."[3] As of early 2021, a majority of epidemiologists interviewed by *Nature* said this is the most likely outcome for the SARS-CoV-2 virus.[4]

Those of us who have lived through the events of 2020 and early 2021 will likely shudder at the very mention of the word "pandemic" for years to come. The word will be associated with quarantine, social distancing measures, rolling death counts on the nightly news, and specific personal tragedies and traumas. However, most pandemics, while no doubt deadly, do not elicit the kind of global response that has been necessary to reduce the spread of SARS-CoV-2. When one uses the classical definition of a pandemic, "an epidemic occurring worldwide, over a very wide area crossing international boundaries and usually affecting a large

---

[i] It is important to stress that researchers are still uncovering new information about the SARS-CoV-2 virus—its origins, how it spreads, and how it mutates. Similarly, many questions persist about COVID-19, especially why only in a certain number of cases does it set off a series of events ranging from severe immune system responses (cytokine storms) to symptoms in others that continue to linger even after the primary infection has been resolved ("long COVID"). I encourage anyone who wants to explore any subject within this book deeper to read the sources cited throughout this book. Throughout 2020 and into 2021, most publications have made all COVID-related articles free to the public to encourage the spread of information that could potentially be used to advance research, stamp out misinformation, and ultimately save lives.

number of people,"[5] these events turn out to be surprisingly common given our globalized world. This will likely continue to be the case so long as communities remain economically and culturally interconnected, and so long as worldwide travel remains quick, easy, and affordable. As Mark Harrison concluded in *Contagion*, his seminal work on the subject, "Commerce has been a major factor in the redistribution of diseases, allowing pathogens and their vectors to circulate more widely than before, often with catastrophic results."[6]

Given the above definition and the fact that increasing commercial activity has allowed for pathogens to spread across the globe more easily, it should not be surprising that most people had already lived through at least one pandemic by the time SARS-CoV-2 emerged in Wuhan. Just over a decade before, in 2009, the "swine flu," which was caused by the influenza A (H5N1) pdm09 virus, jumped from a pig to a human in a Mexican village and proceeded to rapidly spread around the world.[7] By June of that year, the WHO declared that it was a pandemic. By the end of 2010, the virus had infected tens of millions of people and led to the deaths of an estimated 284,500 individuals.[8]

While this is no doubt an enormous tragedy, most of us have but a hazy recollection of a very bad flu season between fall 2009 and spring 2010. A similar thing can be said for those who remember the influenza pandemics of 1957 or 1968.[9] Worldwide, the two pandemics caused between 500,000 and 2 million and between 1 million and 2 million deaths, respectively, but they did not lead to widespread closures of public institutions or even modest changes to the lives of most people.[10] The only somewhat recent influenza pandemic to rival the response of the COVID-19 pandemic occurred between 1918 and 1919. In those two years, three distinct waves of infection spread around the world and caused the deaths of between 45 and 100 million people.[11,12] The Great War, which ranged from 1914 to 1919, is estimated to have only killed around 20 million people.

Beyond the extremely high number of deaths, the 1918-1919 flu (known as "the Spanish flu") and the COVID-19 pandemic share a number of unfortunate similarities according to historical records and the testimonies of the handful of people who lived to see both.[13] Like the COVID-19 pandemic, the influenza pandemic's rapacity was only matched by its scope. It was a truly global phenomenon because the introduction of modern means of travel had made it possible to reach even the most remote locations on Earth. Public health measures were also taken during the influenza pandemic to stop the spread, including closing schools, churches, theaters, and other public spaces. It was also found that cities that took proactive steps to stop the spread of disease and mandated social distancing measures typically fared better than those that did not, and that reopening too early often proved to be disastrous. For example, New York City, which reacted quicker than other cities in the United States by requiring quarantines and staggering business hours, experienced one of the lowest death rates in the Northeast.[12] Philadelphia, unfortunately, waited to implement similar measures. To make matters worse, the city infamously held a parade to support the war effort even though cases of the virus had been reported in the area. An estimated 200,000 people attended the parade, and the effects were both swift and nothing short of cataclysmic.[14] Every bed in all 31 area hospitals was filled within 72 hours. The city ultimately saw the sharpest spike and highest peak death rate of any American city.[12]

As was the case in 2020, masks also became a common part of everyday life and mandatory face mask laws went into effect in a myriad of cities (see Figure 1.1). They also became a symbol of division. While it does not seem as though resistance was nearly as partisan or widespread as it was in 2020 or 2021, there were some organized efforts to fight mandatory face coverings as being either ineffective or unconstitutional. The most notable example of the latter was the Anti-Mask League in San Francisco.[15] An example of the former can be found in a statement issued by the U.S. Navy in 1919, which read: "Masks of improper design, made of wide-mesh gauze, which rest against the mouth and nose, become wet with saliva, soiled with fingers, and are changed infrequently, may lead to infection rather than prevent it, especially when worn by persons who have not even a rudimentary knowledge of the mode of transmission of the causative agents of communicable diseases."[16] This condescending remark occurred more than a decade before influenza A was isolated and identified as a virus.[17]

In addition to the discord between those who demanded the public take part in efforts to stem the spread of the disease and those who

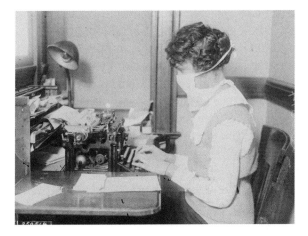

Figure 1.1 Woman in mask while working in an office circa. 1919. (Image used with the permission of the National Archives [local identifier: 165-WW-269B-16].)

believed that such demands were examples of governmental overreach, there was yet another similarity between the viruses that led to the pandemic of 1918 and the COVID-19 pandemic. Part of what made the 1918 flu so deadly was the novelty of the influenza strain (H5N1), particularly among communities of individuals who had experienced limited or no exposure to most "Old World" diseases (measles, smallpox, cholera, influenza, etc). Indigenous peoples in the United States, New Zealand, and Australia were found to have fatality rates of four times that of surrounding populations, which were predominately comprised of individuals of European descent.[18] Among the Māori of New Zealand, the death rate was calculated to be 4230 per 100,000—7.3 times higher than the European rate.[19] Virtually every Pacific island affected by the virus saw at least 5% of their population perish. In Western Samoa, 22% (approximately 38,000 individuals) of the population died in a matter of weeks.[18] The novelty of SARS-CoV-2 has also been one of the reasons why it is so deadly; there does not appear to be any group of people who possess a comparable form of immunity.

Beyond the dangers of novel viruses, there are three takeaways to be gathered from the comparisons between the H1N1 flu of 1918 and the SARS-CoV-2 virus that first emerged in 2019.

First, the COVID-19 pandemic was not unprecedented. Precedents for pandemics have been set multiple times, perhaps no more explicitly than 100 years before the SARS-CoV-2 virus emerged in Wuhan. The only thing that was unprecedented was how much we chose to ignore the lessons learned from experience. As Wendy Parmet and Mark Rothstein wrote in an introductory segment to the *American Journal of Public Health*'s centennial on the 1918 influenza pandemic, which was published in November 2018: "Today, three of the leading threats to global public health are attitudinal: hubris, isolationism, and distrust. As to hubris, it is true that we live in the age of genomics, vaccines, antibiotics, mechanical ventilators, and other features of high-technology medicine that were unavailable in 1918. Nevertheless, our technology remains woefully ineffective in preventing influenza." They continued, "As to the second threat, isolationism, some world leaders erroneously believe that they can seal off their nation's borders after a public health threat emerges and thus escape the ravages of epidemics in other parts of the world. Public health experts universally reject this naive approach. More than ever, a public health event in any part of the world can create a public health threat everywhere." Rather presciently, they concluded, "A third problem is distrust. In our era of political polarization, 'fake news,' and tribal politics, trust in the media, government officials, and even science is fading. This can be catastrophic if an influenza or another type of pandemic arises. Under such circumstances, the public's failure to trust the guidance offered by public health officials may well make a bad situation worse."[20]

The second takeaway is that the classical definition of a pandemic refers to scope rather than mortality rate. Consequently, the number of fatalities associated with even a seemingly minor pandemic (which certainly sounds oxymoronic) becomes astronomical because of the sheer number of individuals who become infected. Even if an outbreak that hits pandemic levels seems relatively mild in hindsight, millions of people may be made severely ill or perish.[ii,21] For example, a 1.0% mortality rate may sound like no big deal, but it could amount to 10 million deaths if 1 billion people are infected with the disease.

Third, pandemics are relatively common. This does not mean that they are events that can be ignored or that one does not need to take them seriously. Just the opposite. We should view this information as a reminder that we have enjoyed a relatively tranquil window free of pestilence for a long time, and that this is not the normal state of affairs. There have been several near misses that raised alarm bells when they occurred, but then relatively quickly faded from public memory. Ebola is but one example. Far more worrisome was the H5N1 "bird flu" that emerged in Vietnam in January 2005. Human-to-human transmission did not ever appear to occur, but the virus was extremely transmissible among chickens, ducks, geese, and other fowl raised for human consumption, and hundreds of humans who interacted with infected birds became sick over the course of that year. Had it mutated in a way to make human-to-human transmission possible, there is no telling how deadly it could have been.

Writing just before the SARS-CoV-2 pandemic, the esteemed Czech-Canadian scientist Vaclav Smil observed that, "The typical frequency of influenza pandemics was once every 50 to 60 years between 1700 and 1889

[ii] One of the most frustrating pieces of misinformation to be spread during 2020 was that the novel coronavirus was "no different than the flu" or that the average flu season kills tens of thousands of Americans. This simply is not accurate. Dr. Jeremy Samuel Faust, who practices emergency medicine at Brigham and Women's Hospital in Boston, wrote an excellent opinion piece in *Scientific American* on this subject in April 2020, noting that he had almost never seen anyone pass away because of the flu in his four years of emergency medicine residency and three and a half years as an attending physician. If the flu killed tens of thousands of Americans every year, however, it would make sense for them to be as common as deaths by gunshot wounds, opioids, or traffic accidents—causes of death that he, unfortunately, regularly observed. However, they were not. The same was true for his colleagues. They regularly treated individuals who had been shot or who had overdosed on opioids, but few had seen more than, at most, a handful of flu mortalities. Why? The answer is twofold: The first is that the Centers for Disease Control and Prevention (CDC) estimates the number of influenza deaths each year and tends to add significant padding to the number, only to lower it when a more accurate count is available later. The second is that the CDC's flu numbers include pneumonia deaths. Faust concludes, "If we compare...the number of people who died in the United States from COVID-19 in the second full week of April to the number of people who died from influenza during the worst week of the past seven flu seasons (as reported to the CDC), we find that the novel coronavirus killed between 9.5 and 44 times more people than the seasonal flu."

... and only once every 10 to 40 years since 1889. The recurrence interval, calculated simply as the mean time elapsed between the last six known pandemics, is about 28 years, with the extremes of 6 and 53 years."[22] In other words, Smil's calculations reveal that, at present, influenza pandemics occur roughly every 28 years and may occur as little as six years apart.

What is perhaps most concerning is that Smil's figures are for just one virus: Influenza A. We have discovered more than 200 other species of virus that have demonstrated the ability to infect humans.[23] There are an untold number of other novel viruses on this Earth that we have yet to discover, and the number of outbreaks and the number of emerging and novel pathogens has been increasing since 1980.[24] These figures will continue to increase as long as human population growth continues, the globalization of goods and travel continues, deforestation continues, and humans continue to practice intensive animal farming where cramped conditions make the spread of disease extremely easy.[25]

The writing is on the wall. Outbreaks are likely to become more common, and these diseases will have a better chance of reaching pandemic levels if we do not take steps to prepare ourselves. We ignore the lessons that we have learned from the past and the COVID-19 pandemic at our own peril.

Previous Coronavirus Outbreaks

Previous coronavirus outbreaks were far less widespread than the COVID-19 pandemic. This was extremely fortunate, as severe acute respiratory syndrome (SARS) and Middle Eastern respiratory syndrome (MERS) both have terrifyingly high mortality rates—9.56% and approximately 34.5%, respectively.[26] As is the case with many coronaviruses, both the SARS and the MERS viruses appear to have come originally from bats. As of late May 2021, the theory on the origin of SARS suggests that a single population of horseshoe bat from China's Yunnan province appears to be the natural reservoir of the virus. Research has shown that the virus was passed from bats to masked palm civets (*Paguma larvata*) at an animal market in Guangdong, and then to humans, and subsequently led to human-to-human transmission that then fueled the epidemic.[27] Raccoon dogs (*Nyctereutes procyonoides*) may have also served as intermediaries.[28] In the case of MERS, the reservoir bat species appears to be based in Africa, and dromedary camels are believed to be the source of zoonotic infection.[29] MERS appears to be endemic among these beasts of burden in Africa but reports of MERS infections have all been tied to the Arabian Peninsula. It is not clear if this is due to extreme underreporting in Africa, some form of natural immunity, or if it is because MERS strains on the continent are less virulent than those found on the Arabian Peninsula.[30]

SARS (2002-2004)

The SARS-CoV virus was the first known coronavirus to cause severe illness in humans. The most common clinical features include persistent fever, nonproductive cough, myalgia, chills/rigor, headache, and shortness of breath. Symptoms may also include joint pain, sore throat, rhinorrhea, dizziness, nausea, vomiting, and diarrhea. Diarrhea was reported in 60% of patients and appears to have played a role in virus transmission.[31] Renal failure was also reported, with 6.6% of patients developing acute renal failure at a median time of 20 days following symptom onset.[31]

Though SARS was assumed to be spread via close contact or respiratory droplets when an infected individual coughed or sneezed, strong evidence of a fecal-oral route also emerged.[32] This suggests that the virus can be aerosolized and that airborne transmission is possible (see *Chapter 2: Transmission of SARS-CoV-2*). The high rate of infection among health care workers lends additional credence to the possibility of airborne transmission, since aerosols are generated by procedures like endotracheal intubation and bronchoscopy.[33] These were common procedures used to manage patients critically ill with SARS.[34]

SARS was first observed in China's Guangdong Province on November 16, 2002. It was initially referred to as a case of atypical pneumonia. Officially, 305 cases were reported in the province between November and February 9, 2003, many of whom were health care workers. Later that month, on February 22, a doctor from Guangdong arrived in Hong Kong, stayed at Metropole Hotel, and spread the virus to 10 other people after either coughing or vomiting in the hallway of his floor. From these 10 individuals, the virus then spread to 29 countries.[35] The outbreak peaked in May and ultimately lasted through July 2003, infecting 8098 and causing the deaths of 774 people.[36] Following the primary outbreak, a few additional cases of SARS were reported at the end of 2003 and early 2004 and were linked to zoonotic transmission involving civet cats from live animal markets in Guangdong.[35]

A disproportionate number of health care workers were infected around the world and represented as many as 20% of worldwide cases of SARS.[37] This is due to several factors, including workers' close contact with patients, but infections may have also occurred following procedures that created aerosolized particles laden with viable viruses.

The latter seems possible because secondary illness rates in households were reportedly only 15% in Hong Kong and 6% in Singapore, while total household secondary attack rates were reportedly 7.5%.[35,38] Another peculiarity concerned transmission rates on airplanes, with at least 40 known flights carrying symptomatic cases on board, yet only 29 secondary cases have been linked to these flights. Furthermore, 22 of these cases can be linked to a single flight. Even then, only 22 of 119 (18%) passengers became ill.[35]

Clearly, SARS was a very contagious virus, but we did not witness the kind of spread that has taken place with SARS-CoV-2. One of the primary reasons for the lack of widespread transmission was due to the symptoms associated with SARS. Individuals infected with SARS were acutely aware of the illness and were able to differentiate symptoms from seasonal allergies or a common cold, and more importantly, asymptomatic cases were exceptionally rare. Also, contrary to SARS-CoV-2, symptom onset was relatively quick—occurring within a few days so individuals knew relatively early whether or not they had been infected. This made contact tracing and quarantining far easier and helped to prevent community spread (when the source of the infection comes from somewhere in the community rather than a specific source or person).

Another important reason behind the successful containment of SARS was due to the relatively early identification of the outbreak. This allowed for some logistical advantages since WHO coordinators, pathologists, and epidemiologists arrived in affected locations before the number of infected patients had swelled, and, consequently, teams could concentrate their efforts and not stretch resources too thin.[39] They were able to quarantine those who had been infected and focus on treating those who were sick. As a result of early identification and appropriate distribution of resources, they were able to contain the outbreak and bring it to an end more effectively.

Though the timely global response and collective action that quickly snuffed out the SARS outbreak was praised worldwide, the WHO recognized the need for a more organized response to outbreaks and issued new International Health Regulations that went into force in 2007.[6] Despite a positive outcome, many organizations and governments also recognized that the outbreak could have been contained far sooner had the Chinese government been more forthcoming. Consequently, the Chinese government faced a great deal of international criticism not only because of their failure to inform the WHO of the outbreak, but for their decision to wait for more than two months to tell Chinese citizens about the cases of atypical pneumonia in Guangdong.[40]

MERS (2012-Ongoing)

The first case of MERS appears to have occurred in Zarqa, Jordan, in April 2012.[10] It was identified initially only as an acute respiratory illness at a public hospital, and those infected included three civilians and eight health care workers. One of the nurses later died.[41] An individual in Saudi Arabia reported similar symptoms in June 2012 and died after being admitted to the hospital. After testing sputum from the patient, it was determined that the cause of death was a novel form of coronavirus—Middle Eastern respiratory syndrome coronavirus (MERS-CoV).[10]

From 2012 until December 2019, sporadic outbreaks of MERS have occurred around the Arabian Peninsula, with the highest number of cases occurring in Saudi Arabia, and all cases can be traced back to this part of the world. This includes the 2015 outbreak in South Korea, as well as the handful of cases reported in Europe, the United Kingdom, and the United States. As of late May 2021, the WHO reports that there have been 2574 laboratory-confirmed cases in 27 countries with 886 reported deaths.[42]

Similar to SARS, the clinical presentation of MERS may include flulike symptoms (cough, fever, chills, rhinorrhea, myalgia, fatigue, joint pain, etc) or may include more severe symptoms like shortness of breath and respiratory failure, which may require intubation and ventilation. Gastrointestinal symptoms (nausea, vomiting, diarrhea, abdominal pain, etc) have also been reported.[43] Acute renal damage has occurred in more than half of patients, and the majority of cases have required renal replacement therapy.[31]

Infections originating in a hospital setting (nosocomial) are very common with MERS. The basic reproduction (R0) number for the virus is estimated to be below 1, but it has been calculated to be in the range of 2 to 5 in a hospital setting.[44] Like SARS, this suggests that there is a possibility of aerosolization following certain medical procedures (ie, endotracheal intubation, bronchoscopy), which could allow for airborne transmission even if close contact with infected individuals and droplet transmission are believed to be the most common routes of infection.[45]

The most notable differences between MERS and SARS are that MERS is far deadlier, having a 34.4% mortality rate, and that it appears to jump from dromedary camel to humans relatively easily.[42] The incidence of MERS in camel shepherds and slaughterhouse workers is 15 and 23 times higher, respectively, compared to the general population.[43]

H5N1 (2005)

The 2005 H1N1 "bird flu" outbreak occurred following the outbreak of SARS and prior to the first case of MERS. Though the threat of human-to-human transmission did not materialize, the high probability that a similar flu variant might do so in the future led the United States to ramp up their biodefense and biosurveillance capabilities and to devise strategies to quickly respond to pandemic scenarios.

One positive outcome of this interest in biodefense was a program called Global Argus, which monitored open-source information to detect and track early indications of foreign biological events that may represent threats to global health and national security. The general idea was that indirect and public information could be far more valuable to epidemiologists than waiting for confirmation of an outbreak from a government that may lack the resources for effective biomonitoring or may actively seek to suppress information that would clearly indicate that an epidemic or pandemic was brewing. An individual who worked on the program explained to *The Atlantic*'s James Fallows that the indicators could be something that would seem insignificant to the untrained eye. Take, for example, a sudden fall in the price of chicken in a village in Thailand. Fluctuations in price are extremely common and a momentary crash in price may be due to a variety of reasons that have nothing to do with disease. Conversely, a sudden drop in price may mean that a novel form of avian flu has entered into circulation in the region and that several farmers have slaughtered their entire flock at once and sent them to market on the same day.[46] It may not be a telltale sign of an outbreak on its own, but if enough of pieces like this come together in a region where new strains of avian flus frequently materialize, it could spell trouble.

Ultimately, the project was capable of processing quarter million pieces of news per day. In the waning days of the Obama administration, the Pandemic Prediction and Forecasting Science Technology Working Group released a report showcasing the advances in prediction technology since the early days of Global Argus and described an even more sophisticated biosurveillance system that had been supercharged by faster processing speeds and advances in artificial intelligences systems.[47] It did not go into details, but given that Global Argus predated the release of the first iPhone, there is good reason to believe that the capabilities of the new monitoring systems are exponentially more advanced.

These open-source monitoring programs were enhanced by teams of epidemiological observers who were stationed around the world, including in China, under the United States Agency for International Development's PREDICT program. The program was created in 2009 in a response to the H5N1 outbreak as a way to improve detection of new disease threats, improve preparedness, and promote ways to minimize practices that trigger spillover (zoonotic) events.[48] Unfortunately, fieldwork ended in September 2019 after the program's funding was eliminated.[49]

These two biosurveillance programs were buttressed by playbooks created by the Bush and Obama administrations—the "National Strategy for Pandemic Influenza" and "Playbook for Early Response to High-Consequence Emerging Infectious Disease Threats and Biological Incidents," respectively. Though the technologies referred to in the guidebooks were vastly different because they are separated by 10 years, and though the Bush and Obama administrations differed in several crucial respects, their recommendations and their strategies for monitoring, containing, and (in the worst-case scenario) responding to outbreaks of transmissible and potentially deadly pathogens were very similar.[46]

Emergence of SARS-CoV-2 (Fall 2019-January 2020)

It is unclear exactly when or where the first human was infected with SARS-CoV-2. There have been numerous stories about different individuals playing the part of "patient zero," as well as attempts to use indirect means to trace the virus back to an origin point, but no definitive answer has been produced yet. The consensus at this point in time seems to be that the virus began circulating in Wuhan in October or November 2019.

There is no shortage of theories that question this timeline, and in the United States alone hundreds, perhaps even thousands, of people claim that they had COVID-19 in November or December of 2019. This assumption is based on their perception that their symptoms were more severe than the typical seasonal illnesses that most people suffer from at that time of the year.[50] As sick as many of these people became, it is extremely unlikely that the illness was COVID-19. All available evidence suggests that SARS-CoV-2 did not arrive in the United States until December 2019 at the earliest, which means extensive community spread in 2019 would not have been possible. An unrelated program that collected blood specimens on patients from January 2, 2020, through March 18, 2020, found that 9 out of 24,079 (0.037%) participants tested positive for SARS-CoV-2 antibodies, and that the earliest positive sample was taken on January 7, 2020, in Illinois, and January 8, 2020, in Massachusetts.[51] Since it takes approximately 14 days from the time of infection for the body to develop enough antibodies to be detectable, this means infection may have occurred around December 24, 2019, or a little earlier.

Some evidence presents more significant aberrations from the generally accepted timeline. Several teams of researchers, not all of whom were searching for the origins of the pandemic, have found indications of SARS-CoV-2 circulation dating back to months before the virus was believed to have arrived in their respective regions. Brazilian researchers found evidence of the virus in a sample of wastewater from the southern city of Florianópolis dating back to November 27, 2019.[52] An Italian team screening patients for lung cancer found evidence of SARS-CoV-2 antibodies in samples dating back to September 2019.[53] Finally, Spanish researchers found traces of the virus in Barcelona wastewater samples taken all the way back in March 2019.[54] If any of these findings are confirmed, it would radically disrupt our understanding of how events unfolded, but contamination or false positives cannot not be ruled out at this time.

A more unconventional attempt to reconstruct a timeline of the outbreak examined satellite images of traffic in Wuhan. These researchers found that there was increased traffic around the city's hospitals from late August through December 2019. They also found increased online searches for symptoms associated with COVID-19, including "cough" and "diarrhea."[55] The researchers behind this claim conclude that the virus could have entered circulation in late summer 2019.

One of the more promising means of searching for an origin point was performed by researchers based at the University of California San Diego School of Medicine, the University of Arizona, and Illumina, Inc. They used epidemiological simulations and retrospective molecular clock inference to answer how long the virus had been circulating in China before it was discovered and combined three important pieces of information: a detailed understanding of how SARS-CoV-2 spread in Wuhan prior to the lockdown, the genetic diversity of the virus in China, and reports documenting the earliest cases of COVID-19 in Hubei. "By combining these disparate lines of evidence, we were able to put an upper limit of mid-October," the authors wrote in a report that was published in *Science* in March 2021.[56] They also found that the virus fizzled out without starting a pandemic in approximately 67% of simulations.

One of the most frequently cited accounts of a patient zero story stems from a March 2020 report from the *South China Morning Post*, which claimed that a 55-year-old from Hubei province was the first known person to be infected with the virus. She reportedly became ill on November 17, 2020, and while this story cannot be corroborated, and though there is no indication that this woman was the first to be infected, it does suggest that community spread could have already been occurring in Hubei as early as November 2020.[40]

The murkiness of the early timeline of the virus is exacerbated by the fact that the origin of the virus also continues to be an open question as of this writing. There are more theories about where the virus came from than can be addressed here, but the vast majority of them fall into one of two camps that can be generalized as coming from (1) a spillover event (zoonosis) or (2) a laboratory. Unfortunately, hard evidence to support either is simply not available, so each must be treated as viable, even if the implications of the latter are difficult to accept. In May 2021, the nation's top security agencies began an investigation to delve deep into the origins of the virus as more information has given more credibility to the hypothesis of a laboratory accident and a cover-up. Unfortunately, the final report was unable to conclude whether the virus emerged from a laboratory or if it was a spillover event that occurred outside of a research facility.[57]

The zoonosis model claims that the SARS-CoV-2 virus was transmitted from a bat to a human, possibly at a wet market in Wuhan, in either November or very early December 2019. Based on prior pandemics, it is possible that an intermediary species may have been involved. Some have posited that the intermediary species was a Malayan pangolin, *Manis javanica*, and there is some evidence to support this claim. The receptor-binding domain (see *Viruses* below) of pangolin coronaviruses is similar to the receptor-binding domain of SARS-CoV-2. Moreover, pangolin coronaviruses have shown strong binding affinities to the human proteins that the SARS-CoV-2 virus uses to break into cells, at least one group of pangolins that was smuggled into China have tested positive for coronaviruses closely related to SARS-CoV-2, and pangolins are sold in Chinese wet markets, but there are inherent problems with this evidence, too. For one, the smuggled pangolins found to be infected with the coronavirus similar to SARS-CoV-2 may have been infected by their abductors.[58] Secondly, pangolin coronaviruses do not appear to be well adapted to pangolins, suggesting limited natural intraspecies spread.[59] Finally, pangolins are largely solitary animals, which would also have impeded intraspecies spread. These critiques do not discount the theory, but they do make it unlikely. Direct transmission to a human, most likely from a horseshoe bat that was captured in a relatively remote part of southern China, seems far more plausible even if direct evidence is currently lacking.[60] A more detailed examination of routes of transmission will be explored in *Chapter 2: Transmission of SARS-CoV-2*.

The second group of origin stories support the far more controversial claim that the virus escaped from a laboratory, most likely the Wuhan Institute of Virology. This was once a third rail belief, but it is not as farfetched as many of the theories that have arisen in the wake of the COVID-19 pandemic. To discount it because it has been supported by individuals who have proposed more incoherent ideas about the virus is a case of guilt by association.

None of the central tenets of the laboratory theory are particularly outlandish. The SARS outbreak did emerge from bat populations that were traced back to southern China, and there was a legitimate concern that another coronavirus outbreak could turn into a very deadly pandemic if a particularly rapacious virus were to jump to a human host following a spillover event. It was no secret that the Wuhan Institute of Virology was studying coronaviruses precisely for this reason. In some cases, researchers were traveling to remote parts of China to retrieve samples of bat coronaviruses that were known to be dangerous. For example, the RaTG13 coronavirus (which shares 96.2% of its genetic identity with SARS-CoV-2) was recovered from the Tongguan mineshaft in Mojiang in 2013, a year after six miners who had been working in the same tunnel cleaning guano developed a severe, pneumonia-like illness that proved fatal to three of those affected.[61] Researchers working at the laboratory even wrote in a 2017 paper published in *PLOS Pathogens* that their work "provides new insights into the origin and evolution of SARS-CoV and highlights the necessity of preparedness for future emergence of SARS-like diseases."[62]

The Wuhan Institute of Virology was not a minor research facility. It was extremely sophisticated and the first laboratory in China to achieve the highest level of international bioresearch safety (BSL-4) when it opened in 2017,[63] but, unfortunately, it did not seem to be operated in a safe manner. Between 2017 and 2018 diplomats from the United States repeatedly visited the institute and reported back to Washington their worries about the facility. In a *Politico* article adapted from his book, *Chaos Under Heaven*, *Washington Post* columnist Josh Rogin noted that the two most concerning findings were that the researchers "didn't have enough properly trained technicians to safely operate their BSL-4 lab" and that they "had found new bat coronaviruses that could easily infect human cells."[64]

This would be deeply concerning on its own, but US intelligence reports have come to light claiming that three researchers from the Wuhan Institute of Virology sought hospital care in November 2019 for an illness with symptoms consistent with "both COVID-19 and common seasonal illnesses."[65] This would fall within the bounds of the generally accepted belief about when the virus was introduced to the community, but Chinese officials have denied the veracity of the report, as it would make the theory that the virus was introduced to the community via laboratory escape entirely possible. The US intelligence report has yet to be corroborated, and as of this writing, agents are actively searching for evidence to either support or disprove this hypothesis. As of September 2021, whether or not the virus escaped from a laboratory continues to be a thoroughly debated issue as facts about its origins are still coming to light.

While these two theories are vastly dissimilar, they do agree that the city of Wuhan, the sprawling capital of central China's Hubei province, is the site of the first major outbreak of the virus, and that it was the hub from which the virus began its spread within China, and then to the rest of the world. Evidence of the spread from late December 2019 forward is relatively well documented and will be reviewed. For those who would like a more precise version of the early months of the outbreak, it is recommended that they consult the unclassified timeline complied by the Congressional Research Service, which is freely available online.[40]

December 2019

In December 2019, hospitals in the city of Wuhan began seeing cases of atypical pneumonia that were caused by an unknown pathogen. According to the WHO, the earliest that any patient reported symptom onset was December 8, 2019.[66] Contrary to this timeline, Huang and colleagues published an online article in *The Lancet* at the end of January 2020 on the clinical features of patients infected with the virus claiming, "The symptom onset date of the first patient identified was December 1, 2019."[67] These two accounts indicate that the first infections were taking place in mid- to late-November 2019. Interestingly, the account from Huang and colleagues notes that none of the first patient's family members became ill and that an epidemiological link could not be established between this patient and the others, 66% of whom had a connection to the Huanan Seafood Wholesale Market. This would suggest that the market was but one of the many locations that played a role in the beginnings of the outbreak.

Physicians from hospitals around Wuhan began taking samples from patients and sending them to commercial companies for analysis in late December 2019. At least eight patient samples were sent out to different genomics companies.[68] The first completed genomic sequencing of the virus is believed to have been performed by BGI Genomics on December 29, 2019, based on a sample that was sent out on December 26, 2019. This was several days before the Wuhan Institute of Virology successfully sequenced the genome.[68]

Meanwhile, the earliest sample that later confirmed infection appears to have been taken on December 24, 2019, from a 65-year-old deliveryman who worked at the Huanan Seafood Wholesale Market. This patient had been admitted to the Central Hospital of Wuhan on December 18, 2019, with pneumonia and later died. The patient's samples were sent to Guangzhou-based Vision Medicals on December 27, 2019, and a representative from the company made the unusual move of calling the hospital and speaking with the head of respiratory medicine, Dr. Zhao Su. The representative said that the company had sequenced most of the virus's genome and they recognized that it appeared to be a novel coronavirus closely related to SARS. Several representatives from the company later visited the city of Wuhan in person and spoke directly to both hospital officials and disease control authorities.[68]

A separate sample, also from the Central Hospital of Wuhan, was taken from a 41-year-old patient on December 27, 2019, and sent to Beijing-based CapitalBio MedLab. Though this patient had no history of contact with the Huanan Seafood Wholesale Market, his test results, which became available on December 30, 2019, would show a false positive for SARS.[68] Dr. Ai Fen, head of emergency medicine at Wuhan Central Hospital, circled the word SARS, took a photograph of the report, and shared the document with colleagues and a former classmate from Tongji Hospital.[40] Earlier in the day, Ai had also recorded an 11-second clip of a CT scan of the patient and sent it to the colleague from Tongji Hospital, who had read online that the Wuhan Municipal Health Commission had issued "urgent notices" to area hospitals earlier in the day about cases of pneumonia said to be linked to the Huanan Seafood Wholesale Market. The 11-second clip and the image of the report showing a false positive for SARS quickly began spreading around the medical community in Wuhan.

A few hours later, the image and the video were sent to Ai via WeChat by an ophthalmologist colleague who also worked at Wuhan Center Hospital, but with whom she has no personal relationship. The sender, Dr. Li Wenliang, included several other recipients in the chat and encouraged them to take precautions against any potential outbreak. Li's messages were circulated widely online, sparking uproar among average citizens who demanded to know more information about the virus. Both Ai and Li were reprimanded by senior officials, and Li was later summoned to the Public Security Bureau to sign a statement agreeing to stop "spreading rumors" or face punishment but he continued to speak out despite the danger of doing so. He was hospitalized with COVID-19 symptoms on January 12, 2020, and died on February 7, 2020, at the age of 33 years.[69]

The Wuhan Municipal Health Commission issued a second "urgent notice" later that day after the exchange between Ai and Li. It was leaked online, and a day later the outbreak was reported in the Chinese media, where it was referred to as "pneumonia of unknown cause."[40] The story was picked up by a user of the US-based Program for Monitoring Emerging Diseases (ProMED), which describes itself as "the largest publicly available system conducting global reporting of infection diseases outbreaks." A contributor published the story just before midnight on December 30, 2019.[70]

On the last day of 2019, there were 59 patients suspected of having COVID-19 and they were all transferred to the infectious disease unit at Wuhan Jinyintan Hospital. The patients, as well as medical staff, were kept in quarantine and under the surveillance of security guards.[71] At that time, there may have been less than 1000 people infected with the virus, and it seems likely that almost all of them were confined to the city of Wuhan.[46]

January 2020

The WHO China Country Office officially made the request for the Chinese government to provide verification of the outbreak of pneumonia cases on January 1, 2020, which Chinese officials apparently did on January 3, 2020. China officially began reporting to WHO about the outbreak on this day.[40]

The first public statement from WHO about COVID-19 was released via tweet on January 4, 2020, which read, "China has reported to WHO a cluster of pneumonia cases—with no deaths—in Wuhan, Hubei Province. Investigations are underway to identify the cause of this illness."[72] The first formal public statement was issued by WHO the following day. "Based on the preliminary information from the Chinese investigation team," the notice read, "no evidence of significant human-to-human transmission and no health care worker infections have been reported."[73]

On January 9, 2020, the WHO issued a statement identifying the pathogen behind the pneumonia cases as a novel coronavirus, but added a comment stating that it "does not recommend any specific measures for travelers."[1] The following day, the WHO's *Advice for International Travel and Trade in Relation to the Outbreak of Pneumonia Caused by a New Coronavirus in China* recommended against entry screening because it requires "considerable resources" and claimed "preliminary investigation suggests that there is no significant human-to-human transmission, and no infections among health care workers have occurred."[74] As late as January 14, 2020, WHO headquarters was still stating that there was no evidence of human-to-human transmission, even if Dr. Maria Van Kerkove, acting head of WHO's emerging diseases unit, noted that *"it is certainly possible that there is limited human-to-human transmission"* while at a press conference in Geneva.[40]

Meanwhile, on January 12, 2020, Chinese officials began referring to the virus as "novel coronavirus infection pneumonia" (it had been referred to as "viral pneumonia" since January 1, 2020). However, it should be noted that the China Centers for Disease Control and Prevention (CDC) is believed to have completed sequencing the virus genome on January 3, 2020, even if the official timeline claims January 7, 2020.[40] They only shared the genomic sequence of the virus with the WHO on January 12, 2020.[40] In addition to the China CDC having sequenced the genome by that point in time, the virus had already been sequenced by at least two private companies and the Wuhan Institute of Virology.[40] Testing kits were developed by the institute as early as January 10, 2020.[40]

The first reported COVID-19 death was recorded on January 9, 2020. The patient, a 61-year-old man, was reportedly a regular customer at the Huanan Seafood Wholesale Market and news of his death was announced on January 11, 2020.[2] The same day, the Wuhan Municipal Health Commission claimed that no new infections had occurred since January 3, 2020, and that the number of active cases had actually declined to 41—down from 59, as had been reported on January 5, 2020. Once again, the commission claimed that there was no evidence of person-to-person transmission or infection among health care workers.[40] On January 15, 2020, China reported a total of zero new cases, while the Wuhan Municipal Health Commission responded to a question about transmission with the following: "Existing investigative results indicate no clear evidence of person-to-person transmission. We cannot rule out the possibility of limited person-to-person transmission, but the risk of sustained person-to-person transmission is low."[40]

On January 20, 2020, it was revealed to the Chinese people and the world that the risk of person-to-person transmission was more significant than had been indicated when Dr. Zhong Nanshan, head of the National Health Commission's high-level exert group and one of the most highly respected members of the medical community in China, publicly disclosed this information for the first time. Nanshan also admitted that many medical workers acted without due caution or the necessary personal protective equipment (PPE) they would have donned had they known the potential dangers of the virus. One of the most salient examples was of a neurosurgery that was conducted at Wuhan Union Hospital on January 7, 2020. Though the patient had not yet started to show symptoms of COVID-19, the procedure was believed to have caused 14 medical workers to become infected, making the patient the first definitive "superspreader."[40]

This superspreading event was paltry by comparison to a January 18, 2020, potluck in Wuhan held in anticipation of the coming Lunar New Year, and it involved an estimated 40,000 households.[40] Assuming the risk of person-to-person transmission to be low due to official statements, Wuhan Mayor Zhou Xianwang decided not to cancel the annual banquet. Consequently, tens of thousands of people may have been infected by attendees who were presymptomatic, asymptomatic, or perhaps even symptomatic but acting under the belief that their illness was nothing serious.

Five days later, on January 23, 2020, the city's transportation systems were shut down and interprovince travel was suspended between Hubei Province and the rest of China. Unfortunately, an estimated 5 million people had already left Wuhan to celebrate the Lunar New Year with friends and families throughout China and the rest of the world.[75] Had there been any hope of containing the virus, it was officially lost by this time.

Meanwhile, the WHO's diffident approach continued. On January 22, 2020, an Emergency Committee under the International Health

Regulations, which was created in the wake of the SARS epidemic, was convened. It was extended into the next day but failed to reach a consensus on whether or not the outbreak was a Public Health Emergency of International Concern (PHEIC). The committee announced plans to revisit the emerging crisis 10 days later but reconvened in only one week because the number of confirmed cases had risen from 571 with 17 deaths and 10 cases in seven countries or territories outside of China to 7736 confirmed cases with 179 deaths and 107 cases in 21 countries by January 30, 2020. Only then did the committee declare the novel coronavirus to be a PHEIC.[76]

In the coming weeks, China would implement restrictions nationwide, but the lockdown would be the most extreme in Wuhan.[77] What initially seemed draconian and excessive to the rest of the world quickly became normalized as other countries went into shutdown to "flatten the curve."

Criticism of China's Early Handling of the Outbreak

While eventually cooperative with international efforts, the initial response by Chinese officials appears to have been to try to cover up the outbreak, to censor those who spoke up, and to suppress information that could tarnish the government's image internationally and domestically. At least one employee from an unnamed genomics firm received a threatening phone call on January 1, 2020, from an official at the Hubei Provincial Health Commission, who ordered the firm to stop testing samples believed to be related to what was then being called the "viral pneumonia" that had recently emerged in Wuhan, to destroy existing samples, to stop releasing test results, and to report any future test results to the authorities.[68] Two days later, China's National Health Commission said all samples needed to be moved to approved testing facilities or destroyed.[68] Despite this, on January 5, 2020, Prof. Zhang Yongzhen of Fudan University in Shanghai sequenced the genome of the virus and promptly shared their findings with the Shanghai Municipal Health Commission, China's National Health Commission, and the U.S. National Institutes of Health's GenBank—a public database. A paper on the sequencing work was submitted to the journal *Nature* on January 7, 2020.[78] The paper was also uploaded to Virological.org in its prepublished form on January 11, 2020, by one of Zhang's long-time collaborators, Edward Holmes, who is based in Australia.[79] Zhang's laboratory mysteriously closed for "rectification" the day after the paper appeared on the website.

In addition to punishing researchers and reprimanding potential whistleblowers like Drs. Ai and Li, the Chinese government was also extremely slow to respond and did not inform the public about the dangers posed by the virus, which meant fewer precautions on the part of Chinese citizens and more vulnerable hosts for the virus. While there were reports that the Huanan Seafood Wholesale Market was being disinfected at night for at least two nights before it was finally shuttered on January 1, 2020, there was what seemed like wishful thinking that the virus would prove to only spread to humans from an undetermined animal source rather than human-to-human, and this blind optimism seemed to override the capacity for lucid policymaking.[40] The WHO cautiously acknowledged that the virus was spread human-to-human as early as January 14, 2020, but China's health ministry only confirmed this information on January 20, 2020.[80] Without question, preventative measures should have been taken earlier, especially in the city's hospital where the infected were concentrated. Hundreds of medical workers were not wearing the kind of PPE they would have had they been told that human-to-human transmission was at the very least possible, which led many to become ill or worse.

As noted above, it was not until January 9, 2020, that Chinese authorities announced that a novel coronavirus was behind the outbreak in Wuhan, and they did not share the genomic sequence with the WHO until January 12, 2020, even though the China CDC sequenced the virus on either January 3 or January 7, 2020, and failed to notify the WHO of the outbreak in a timely manner. While the Chinese government became far more open about sharing information relating to the virus as the outbreak turned into an epidemic, they still had not shared any viral or clinical samples as late as April 25, 2020.[40]

Knowing what we know now, there is no doubt that China took several critical missteps in the earliest days of the outbreak and, contrary to glowing reports from media outlets and the WHO, repeated almost verbatim the same mistakes that allowed SARS to go from a provincial outbreak into a global epidemic.

Criticism of the World Health Organization

The WHO has been criticized for being far too credulous when dealing with the Chinese government. *The Atlantic*'s Kathy Gilsinan summed up this position in an April 12, 2020, article, writing: "The WHO...was getting its information from the same Chinese authorities who were misinforming their own public, and then offering it to the world with its own imprimatur."[81]

Ultimately, the WHO was not designed to be the world's lie detector. It is structurally incapable of resolving issues of veracity when regimes wish to shape the definition of reality to their whims. Short of accusing a member state of lying or actively spying on them, there is nothing a nongovernment organization can do to force a member's hand and make them tell the truth.

Unfortunately, this suggests that the WHO simply is not designed to respond to outbreaks that occur in countries living under repressive regimes.

As a corollary, criticism has also been levied against the organization and director-general Adhanom Ghebreyesus for waiting until January 30, 2020, to declare the outbreak a PHEIC.[82] Had the PHEIC declaration been issued 12 days beforehand, prior to most of the Lunar New Year celebrations, there is a chance the virus could have been contained. Had it been issued 7 days before, the opportunity to prevent the spread may have already been lost, but it still could have had an impact. Then again, the declaration would have only been as effective as state agencies allowed. If the PHEIC declaration encouraged them to take steps to combat the virus, it could have made a tremendous difference. Conversely, if the PHEIC declaration fell on deaf ears, it would not have prevented the pandemic.

Unfortunately, it seems as though the second possibility seems more likely. As Amy Maxmen wrote in *Nature*, "Several reports note that politicians and the public mainly ignored the PHEIC declaration and Tedros's corresponding recommendations in January 2020 but started listening when the organization used the unofficial term 'pandemic' to describe COVID-19 in March, once it was spreading in multiple continents."[83]

Spread of SARS-CoV-2 Outside of China (January 2020-March 2020)

By January 20, 2020, the virus had spread well beyond Hubei Province. The first confirmed case was reported in Thailand on January 13, 2020; Japan on January 16, 2020; Guangdong on January 19, 2020; and South Korea on January 20, 2020. On January 21, 2020, new cases were announced in several major cities across China, including Beijing, Shanghai, and Shenzhen, and the first cases were reported in Taiwan, Hong Kong, and the United States. By the end of the month, the list of countries reporting cases had grown to include Singapore, Malaysia, Vietnam, Nepal, France, Australia, Canada, Germany, Sri Lanka, Cambodia, Finland, the United Arab Emirates, the Philippines, India, the United Kingdom, Italy, and Russia. In addition, North Korea, Mongolia, and Russia closed their borders with China; Japan and the United States begin evacuating their nationals from the Wuhan area; and several airlines suspended flights to China from North America, Europe, and other parts of Asia.[84] Most of these events occurred before the WHO declared the outbreak to be a PHEIC.

By February 2020, community spread was beginning to take place in Iran, Europe, and North America. Other milestones include the WHO's February 11, 2020, decision to name the disease caused by the virus "COVID-19" to avoid stigmatizing a place or group of people; the first death in Europe (in France) on February 14, 2020; the first reported case in Latin America (in Brazil) on February 26, 2020; and the first US death of a patient due to COVID-19, which occurred in Washington state on February 29, 2020.[85]

Outbreaks in Iran and Italy seemed to happen one after the other in late February 2020. In Iran, the epidemic took many by surprise because the first official statement referring to the virus came from a report about two deaths in the city of Qom on February 19, 2020. In other words, Iran reported deaths before infections. Sources familiar with Iranian politics claim that many officials did not want to acknowledge the outbreak because it coincided with the anniversary of the 1979 revolution on February 11 and parliamentary elections on February 21, 2020.[86] Even with news of the outbreak downplayed, turnout for the election was the lowest since the revolution. The Iranian leadership blamed the Western media's attempts to "dissuade Iranian voters and resorting to the excuse of disease and the virus."[87]

By February 28, 2020, the country was experiencing the worst outbreak outside of China and putatively had the highest mortality rate in the world, though it seems as though undercounting the total number of cases likely skewed this figure.[86] In response to the surge in cases, the country imposed some lockdown measures and established screening stations at transit hubs in February, but cases continued to climb. The virus spread rapidly as millions of people traveled to take part in Persian New Year celebrations lasting from March 19 through the beginning of April 2020.[88]

Shortly after the wave of cases in Iran began to overwhelm the Islamic Republic, Italy also saw a surge in cases. The outbreak was centered in the northern part of the country, particularly the Lombardy region. The first secondary infection case was confirmed on February 20, 2020, in the town of Codogno.[89] Less than three weeks later, on March 8, 2020, Italy's health care system was straining under the pressure caused by COVID-19. There were 399 patients in the ICU, 2616 hospitalized patients, and 3372 confirmed cases of COVID-19. The reported parity between hospitalized patients and confirmed patients was an anomaly due to a lack of adequate testing equipment, and it has been estimated that the actual number of infected individuals was 15 times that amount (ie, over 50,000 cases or a rate of 82.9 per 100,000).[90]

Given the severity of the situation, Italy was turned into a "red zone," meaning that public gatherings were canceled, schools were closed, and restrictions on movement were put in place. These restrictions would become even stricter between March 20 and April 30, 2020, and ultimately remain in effect until May 4, 2020.[90] Similar lockdowns would be imposed in Spain, France, Germany, and other parts of the European Union later in March 2020, and individual US states would begin issuing shelter-in-place orders or similar directives shortly thereafter. By early April 2020, 95% of the US population lived in an area where people were under instructions to stay home.[91]

While it does seem as though SARS-CoV-2 managed to take hold in every country where it was introduced, there is evidence that sustained transmission only occurred part of the time. The first outbreak to be reported in Germany involved an employee of an automobile supplier who had traveled from Shanghai to the company headquarters in Bavaria on January 20, 2020, and subsequently infected more than a dozen employees. Evidence suggests that Germany managed to contain this outbreak with rapid testing and quarantining. Similarly, the first person in the United States to test positive for the virus, after flying back to the Seattle area from Wuhan on January 15, 2020, does not appear to have caused the initial outbreak on the West Coast. Two subsequent outbreaks in California in the month of February also appear to have been contained.[92] Sadly, the outbreak on the East Coast of the United States, which phylogenic research shows arrived by way of Europe, was not.[93]

This brings up the elephant in the room. The US response under the administration in power as of early 2020 has been litigated in the press and on social media *ad nauseam* for the past year and will likely be the subject of numerous books that will focus exclusively on the history of the pandemic and the performance of said administration. There will be no shortage of opinions on the matter. While it is beyond the scope of this book to offer an analysis of this administration's response to the crisis, it would also be a dereliction of duty to sidestep the issue altogether.

What is clear is that biosurveillance systems were in place and the playbooks to address the crisis did exist. Previous administrations had created plans to keep an outbreak from becoming an epidemic, an epidemic from becoming a pandemic, and a pandemic from bringing the world grinding to a halt. It is also clear that several individuals within the administration and at the State Department tried to sound the alarm about the dangers posed by the virus. As early as January 3, 2020, the Director of the US CDC, Robert Redfield, first spoke with the head of the China CDC, Director-General Gao Fu, about the outbreak. Redfield relayed what he heard from Director-General Fu to US Health and Human Services (HHS) Secretary Alex M. Azar II, who then passed the message on to the National Security Council at the White House.[40] While it is possible that information about the outbreak was being shared among high-ranking US officials before January 3, 2020, what is certain is that this information began circulating among senior-level officials shortly after Director Redfield's conversation with Director-General Fu. Concerns of a pandemic were being discussed within HHS as early as January 18, 2020.[40] What is unclear is why a more urgent response was not initiated.[94] The former president's first open discussion of the outbreak and the potential danger it posed was on January 22, 2020, when he acknowledged that one person in the United States had tested positive for COVID-19, but expressed optimism that the situation was under control.[94]

The administration finally restricted travel between the United States and China on January 31, 2020, but by then it was logistically unworkable and too late to be effectual. The travel restrictions included numerous exclusions and pushed the onus of monitoring and tracking those who had returned from China onto state agencies that were ill-prepared to handle the responsibility. In addition, the states were allowed to opt out of the program.[95] Due to these exclusions, an estimated 40,000 people arrived in the United States from China between the months of February and March 2020,[96] and since coordination between state and federal agencies was unworkable, no one has any idea how many of them were screened.

Meanwhile, the restrictions on travel from Mainland China (but not territories like Hong Kong or Macau) occurred far too late to prevent the spread of the virus. It had already established itself in Southeast Asia, Europe, and even North America. Closing off access to China may have plugged up the largest hole in the figurative dam, but it ignored the others. It did nothing to stop the deluge of infected individuals from entering the United States from other places that started seeing community spread in February 2020. The East Coast was hit especially hard by an early variant of the virus that had already become dominant in Europe, especially Italy, suggesting that the spread in the United States came from there instead of directly from China.[92]

The decision to implement a travel ban on 26 nations in Europe was criticized for similar reasons. It came far too late (on March 11, 2020), and due to the two-day grace period before restrictions were put into place, it ensured that airports throughout the United States and Europe would be overrun with people scrambling to return home.[97] There is no way of knowing how many of them were COVID positive.

It is well documented and was reported by various media outlets that poor coordination and planning between various departments and agencies in early 2020 prevented an effective response to the pandemic. Had there been a robust US response from the start of the outbreak, it could have significantly reduced the global spread of the virus and possibly prevented the virus from being more than an epidemic.

On March 11, 2020, COVID-19 was declared a pandemic.[98]

The Politics of Naming a Virus

Though this should go without saying, the reason we no longer refer to viruses by the location from which they originate is because there is a danger that individuals will then associate the ethnicity from that region with disease and discriminate against them. Worse, some may seek to avenge the sick by participating in random acts of violence against individuals who can trace their ancestors back to the areas close to where the pathogen originated.

Many of those who have had their lives turned upside down by the pandemic may be looking for someone to blame and associating the virus with a region or an ethnicity provides them an easy scapegoat, and unfortunately, this seems to have happened repeatedly. Evidence of hate crimes against people of East Asian ancestry have skyrocketed since the virus emerged, and this served as the impetus to pass the COVID-19 Hate Crimes Act on May 20, 2021.[99]

To avoid negative connotations associated with variants of the virus (see *SARS-CoV-2* below), the WHO has devised a new naming system utilizing the Greek alphabet so that one can refer to them by a letter rather than from where they arose (see Table 1.1).[100] So far, the names for the variants have been issued in the order in which they have emerged. This includes the Alpha variant (previously known as the B.1.1.7 variant, which first appeared in the United Kingdom), the Beta variant (previously known as the B.1.351 variant, which first appeared in South Africa), the Gamma variant (previously known as the P.1 variant, which first appeared in Brazil), and the Delta variant (previously known as the B.1.617 variant, which first appeared in India).[101] Given that the WHO believes that SARS-CoV-2 will continue to mutate and circulate around the world, and that the disease is here to stay with us, it is likely that variants will continue to emerge.[102]

TABLE 1.1 Variants of Concern and Variants of Interest as of September 2021[100]

WHO Label	Pango Lineage[a]	Earliest Samples	Date of Designation
Variants of Concern			
Alpha	B.1.1.7	United Kingdom—September 2020	December 18, 2020
Beta	B.1.351	South Africa—May 2020	December 18, 2020
Gamma	P.1	Brazil—November 2020	January 11, 2021
Delta	B.1.617.2	India—October 2020	May 11, 2021
Variants of Interest			
Epsilon[b]	B.1.427/B.1.429	United States—March 2020	March 5, 2021
Zeta[c]	P.2	Brazil—April 2020	March 17, 2021
Eta	B.1.525	Multiple sites—December 2020	March 17, 2021
Theta[d]	P.3	Philippines—January 2021	March 24, 2021
Iota	B.1.526	United States—November 2020	March 24, 2021
Kappa	B.1.617.1	India—October 2020	April 4, 2021
Lambda	C.37	Peru—December 2020	June 14, 2021
Mu	B.1.621	Colombia—January 2021	August 30, 2021

[a]Pango is an acronym for phylogenic assignment of named global outbreak lineages. The Pango team maintains a site with daily updated information about circulating lineages here at cov-lineages.org.
[b]Epsilon had ceased to be a variant of interest by July 2021.
[c]Zeta had ceased to be a variant of interest by July 2021.
[d]Theta had ceased to be a variant of interest by July 2021.

Viruses

To fully appreciate the complexity of fighting a disease caused by a virus and the extraordinary difficulties associated with containment, an examination of the science of viruses is necessary. Even those who only want to understand the history and psychological effects of the COVID Era are encouraged to read through this section, though you should not get frustrated if some of the material gets too hairy and you walk away without understanding 100% of the material. After all, researchers spend their entire lives trying to unlock the secrets of viruses and cell biology.

At their most basic, viruses are particles that are made of the most elementary building blocks of life: nucleic acids and proteins. Though viruses contain distinct genetic material, viruses do not meet the criteria for life because a virus cannot make new viruses on its own, they lack metabolic functions, and they remain inert until they encounter a host cell that they are capable of infecting. This precludes them from being considered life, but many biologists are hesitant to say that they are inanimate because viruses are composed of organic molecules and show characteristics that are more in line with cellular organisms than minerals.

One of the characteristics that makes viruses both most lifelike and most troublesome is that viruses are capable of replication. Viruses replicate by attaching to a susceptible host cell and inserting genetic material into that cell. The virus's genetic material then hijacks the cell's machinery in order to make more viruses. Because viruses cannot complete their life cycle without exploiting the machinery of a viable host, viruses are known as *obligate parasites*.

Virus Composition

Nucleic acids make up viruses' genetic material—the basic instructions for viral replication—and can come in the form of deoxyribonucleic acid or ribonucleic acid (more familiarly known as DNA and RNA, respectively). RNA viruses can then be broken down into two groups: positive-sense RNA (also known as plus-strand) and negative-sense RNA (also known as minus-strand).

The remainder of the virus is comprised mostly of proteins. Some proteins, known as nucleoproteins, are bound to the viral RNA or DNA and assist with replication. Other proteins form a shell that protects the genetic material and nucleoproteins. This shell is known as a capsid. The combined unit—capsid proteins, nucleic acids, and nucleoproteins—is known as the nucleocapsid.

In some cases, the viral genome may be protected by yet another layer that is known as an envelope. Envelopes are comprised of a lipid bilayer derived from host cell membranes and contain a myriad of glycoproteins—including spike (S), envelope (E), and membrane (M) proteins—that help the virus avoid the host's immune system or bind to receptor proteins on the host's cell membrane.

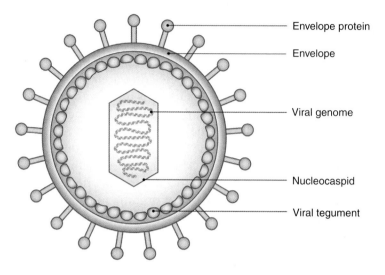

Envelope protein

Envelope

Viral genome

Nucleocaspid

Viral tegument

Figure 1.2 Structurally, viruses are nothing more than tiny packages of genetic material (ribonucleic acid [RNA] or deoxyribonucleic acid [DNA]) that are protected by proteins. In the more colorful words of Sir Peter Medawar, viruses are "a piece of bad news wrapped up in protein." (Illustration courtesy of Ben Taylor.)

The entire infective virus structure, which includes the nucleocapsid and (if present) the envelope, is known as a virion (see Figure 1.2).

Cells and Cellular Signaling

Cells are the most fundamental units of life, and single-cell organisms are the most simplistic forms of life on the planet. Larger, multicellular organisms, meanwhile, can be made up of thousands, millions, billions, or even trillions of cells. This includes the larger world of plants and animals with which we interact on a day-to-day basis. Figure 1.3 shows the basic components of animal cells.

Multicellular organisms are not comprised of the same types of cells. The cells in our eyes, for example, are distinct from the cells that make up our kidneys. There is an extremely vast number of differentiated cell types, and they each serve a specific function. This function is dictated in part by a cell's genome, which is contained in its DNA. The cell's function is also determined by its ancestor cells or cues that it receives through extracellular signaling. Extracellular signaling occurs when cells exchange information via chemical messengers. Signaling can occur between cells that are very close to one another or over long distances. For example, many of the chemicals that are vital to brain function, known as neurotransmitters, are

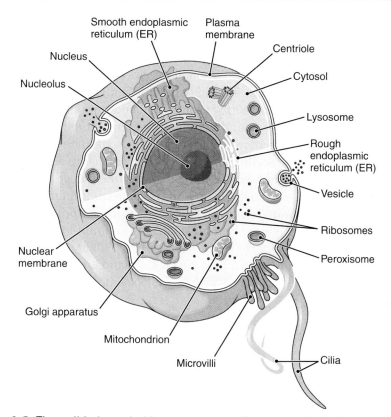

Figure 1.3 The cell is bounded by a membrane that is studded with protein receptors. Within the cell are thousands of structural elements built out of proteins and membrane-bound bodies known as organelles that perform specific functions ranging from producing the cell's energy (mitochondria in animal cells) to assembling proteins (ribosomes) to regulating and maintaining genetic expression (nucleus). The contents of the cell are suspended in cytoplasm. (Cohen, B. *Medical Terminology: An Illustrated Guide*. Wolters Kluwer/Lippincott Williams & Wilkins; 2011.)

released from organs or glands outside of the central nervous system (CNS), and then travel to the brain.

When one cell sends a signaling molecule to another, it is referred to as a *signal cell*. The cell that receives the molecule is referred to as the *target cell*. For a target cell to receive the message, it must have a *receptor protein* on its plasma membrane that recognizes the signal molecule. To better visualize this, think of sending a text message to your friend. In this analogy, you are the signal cell, the text message you send is the signaling molecule, your friend is the target cell, and your friend's phone is the receptor protein.

In general, extracellular signal molecules fall in one of two types.

The first type binds with the receptor and passes its message to signal molecules inside the cell (intracellular signal molecules), but the molecule does not pass through the plasma membrane. As yet another analogy, think of these kinds of signal molecules like keys and the receptors like locked doors. If the key fits, then the lock opens. If the key does not fit, then nothing happens. Furthermore, locks tend to be specific. You cannot open any lock with any key. The key must be the right shape to fit into the lock. The same is true of signaling molecules and receptor proteins: They tend to be highly selective.

A second type of extracellular signal molecule is smaller and is therefore capable of binding to the receptor and then crossing the plasma membrane. Rather than relaying its message through intermediaries, it interacts with organelles (ribosomes, mitochondria, cell nuclei) inside the cell directly.

Viral Replication

To successfully replicate, a virus must go through seven stages:

1. *Attachment*
2. *Penetration*
3. *Uncoating*
4. *Replication*
5. *Assembly*
6. *Maturation*
7. *Release*

Viral infection occurs when a virus attaches to a susceptible cell and delivers the viral genome and any necessary proteins needed for replication into the host's cytoplasm. This is accomplished by attaching to the same receptor proteins that cells use to communicate with one another. For nonenveloped viruses, the capsid attaches to specific receptors and utilize these receptors to mediate viral entry events. For enveloped viruses, spike proteins allow the virus to attach to the receptor, and then deliver the viral genome after fusing with the cellular membrane via endocytosis (see Figure 1.4).[104]

Viral attachment proteins are extremely varied, and different types of viruses can attach to different receptors. This affects host range and what tissues are susceptible to the virus. For example, the human immunodeficiency virus (HIV) binds with the cluster of differentiation 4 (CD4) receptor, so only cells that contain these receptor proteins are susceptible to the virus. If a virus cannot bind to a receptor, attach to a cell surface, puncture a cell's membrane, or gain entry by fusing with the host cell's membrane, it cannot infect the host.

Once a virus has penetrated the host cell membrane, the nucleocapsid enters the cell's cytoplasm. Uncoating occurs when the capsid reacts

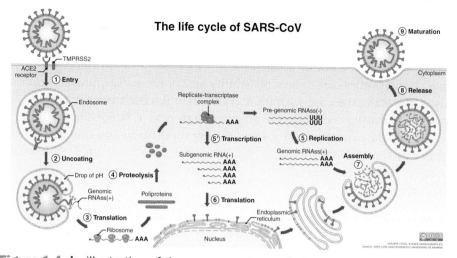

Figure 1.4 An illustration of the severe acute respiratory syndrome coronavirus 2 (SARS-CoV-2) attaching to a human angiotensin-converting enzyme 2 (ACE2) receptor and the life cycle of the virus.[103] (Vega Asensio, 2020. *This file is licensed under the Creative Commons Attribution-Share Alike 4.0 International license.* https://commons.wikimedia.org/wiki/File:SARS-CoV-2_cycle.png)

with cellular enzymes in the cell, thereby exposing the viral genome and any nucleoproteins that assist with the transcription and/or translation of viral proteins. The viral genome then hijacks the cell's machinery to make copies of the virus's genetic material, proteins, and any other viral components. Once replication is complete, the virion is assembled within the cell's cytoplasm and then goes through a maturation process whereby it goes from a noninfectious bundle of proteins and nucleic acids to a fully infectious virion. The virion then makes its exit through the cell membrane. In some cases, the new virion may leave quietly via viral budding or exocytosis. In other cases, the virions may burst from the cell via viral lysis.

A single infected cell may produce thousands of new virions and hundreds of thousands or even millions of cells may be infected over the course of an illness. Consequently, there are oftentimes billions of virions produced during an infection (a preprint article estimates the number of for SARS-CoV-2 virions at peak infection to be in the range of 10^9-10^{11}).[105] A viral outbreak may produce millions of infections. Consequently, a virus is almost certain to experience mutations over the course of a pandemic, even if these events are relatively rare on paper. If a specific mutation gives a virus an advantage, there is a better chance that that particular virus will proliferate. The most concerning advantages include changes in virulence, improved ability to evade our immune defenses, and increased transmissibility.[106]

When the number of occurrences is high enough, even the most unlikely of events (say, something that is assumed to have a probability of occurrence in the vicinity of 1 in 1 trillion) become not only likely, they become inevitable. In other words, the more people a virus infects, the more a mutation ceases to be a possibility and becomes an inevitability. This is especially the case with RNA viruses. Unlike DNA viruses, which "proofread" during replication to ensure a high rate of fidelity, most RNA viruses lack the capacity to proofread during replication and mutate at a far higher rate than DNA viruses.

Coronaviruses

Coronaviruses are enveloped positive-sense RNA viruses classified under the subfamily *Coronavirinae* (see Figure 1.5) and are widespread among birds, humans, and other mammals. They typically cause relatively minor infections in the lower respiratory tract and gastrointestinal tract, but can also result in more severe respiratory, enteric, neurologic, and hepatic

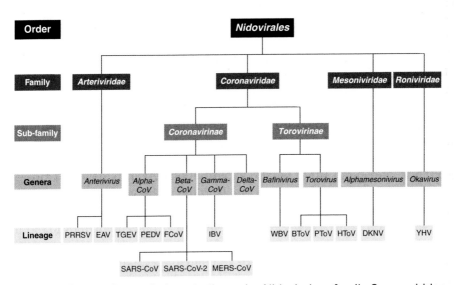

Figure 1.5 Coronaviruses belong to the order Nidovirales, family Coronaviridae, and subfamilies Coronavirinae. Coronavirinae fall into four genera: *Alphacoronavirus*, *Betacoronavirus*, *Gammacoronavirus*, and *Deltacoronavirus*. Subgenera of *Betacoronavirus* include *Embecovirus* (formerly known as lineage A), *Sarbecovirus* (formerly known as lineage B), *Merbecovirus* (formerly known as lineage C), and *Nobecovirus* (formerly known as lineage D). Severe acute respiratory syndrome coronavirus 1 and 2 (SARS-CoV-1 and SARS-CoV-2) belong to the subgenus *Sarbecovirus*, while Middle Eastern respiratory syndrome coronavirus (MERS-CoV) belongs to the *Merbecovirus* subgenus.

diseases.[26] Coronaviruses can be stored at temperatures of −80 °C for years and remain infective when removed from cold storage, while exposure to steady ultraviolet light or heat will result in inactivation. The process of inactivation occurs in 3 minutes after exposure to temperatures of 75 °C or more, approximately 5 minutes after exposure to temperatures of 65 °C, and 20 minutes after exposure to temperatures above 60 °C.[107] They can also be deactivated by disinfectants that contain chlorine, peracetic acid, and solutions with 75% or more ethanol.[10]

More than 200 coronaviruses have been identified in bats, and more than one-third of the bat virome (the genomes of all viruses that inhabit bats) that has been sequenced is composed of coronaviruses.[108] Of the coronaviruses thus far discovered, the majority fall within the genus *Betacoronavirus*.[109]

In the 1960s, it was discovered that coronaviruses can cause human infections. Since that time, seven coronaviruses capable of infecting humans have been isolated.[10] The four that were isolated prior to 2002 caused only minor respiratory and enteric infections, and it was believed that coronaviruses were not capable of causing severe illnesses in humans. Since 2002, three novel coronavirus outbreaks have occurred that contradict that assumption. Outbreaks include two epidemics—SARS-CoV (SARS) in 2002 and MERS-CoV (MERS) in 2012—and the SARS-CoV-2 pandemic that is the subject of this book. All three belong to the *Betacoronavirus* genus. SARS and SARS-CoV-2 belong to the *Sarbecovirus* subgenus; MERS belongs to the *Merbecovirus* genus.[10]

Examination of the coronavirus under an electron microscope reveals numerous features, the most prominent being the club-shaped spike (S) proteins that originate on the surface of the virus. After observing these protrusions for the first time in the mid-1960s, June Almeida (née Hart) and David Tyrell believed that they resembled a halo or a crown, and therefore called them coronaviruses—the word *corona* being Latin for the word "crown."[110] Beyond the crown, the most distinctive feature of the viral family is genome size. Coronaviruses have some of the largest known genomes of any RNA viruses. SARS-CoV, SARS-CoV-2, and MERS-CoV have genome lengths of 27.9, 29.9, and 30.1 kilobases, respectively.[26] The structural proteins (including the S, M, and E proteins) make up one-third of the viral coding capacity, while the remaining two-thirds encode the nonstructural, nucleocapsid proteins.

In coronaviruses, the S protein can be broken down into two subunits, S1 and S2. The receptor-binding domain is contained in S1 and is responsible for attaching to and engaging with host receptors. S2 subsequently mediates membrane fusion, which then allows the viral genome to enter host cytoplasm. Following binding, the S protein is cleaved and activated by host cell-surface proteases while cleavages occur at two sites.[111] The first is at the boundary between the S1 and S2 subunits. The cleaving event effectively separates S1 from S2, while a second cleavage site becomes exposed within the S2 domain, which is known as the S2′ site.[112] This second cleavage at the S2′ site contains the fusion peptides that, when activated, primes the S protein for fusion with the host cell membrane.[111] (Because of the distinctive shape of the S protein, it is targeted by the body's immune system and was recognized as a strong target for the development of vaccines and therapeutics.)[113] Following fusion, the viral RNA and accompanying proteins are released into the cytoplasm and hijack the cell's machinery to replicate. The virus's envelope proteins (E), membrane proteins (M), and nucleoproteins (N) are responsible for virus assembly, morphogenesis, and budding.[31]

This general strategy is used by all coronaviruses, though the individual targeted receptors and proteases are unique to each virus. Moreover, several proteases may mediate cleavages in a coronaviruses' S protein, including TMPRSS2, cathepsin CTSL, trypsin, and furin.[114]

Though RNA viruses are prone to mutating more often than DNA viruses, coronaviruses appear to be the sole RNA viruses with the capacity to proofread.[115] This is due to nonstructural gene *nsp14*.[116] Consequently, coronaviruses mutate far slower than other RNA viruses. SARS-CoV-2 has been estimated to evolve at a rate of $<1 \times 10^{-3}$ substitutions per site per year or approximately 2 substitutions per genome per month.[92] However, viral recombination (the naturally occurring recombination of at least two viral genomes that takes place when a cell is infected by more than one strain of a virus) occurs relatively frequently in coronaviruses.[117] Recombination may even play a significant role in the evolution of individual coronaviruses, possibly even SARS-CoV-2.[118] Specifically, it may play a role in cross-species transmission and host range expansion.[119]

SARS-Cov-2

SARS-CoV-2 (see Figure 1.6) belongs to the *Sarbecovirus* subgenus. The closest known relative of the SARS-CoV-2 virus is BatCoV RaTG13, which was detected in *Rhinolophus affinis* in the southern part of Yunnan Providence and just north of China's border with both Laos and Vietnam.[120] RaTG13 shares 96.2% of its genetic identity with SARS-CoV-2, while SARS-CoV-2 shares less than 80% nucleotide identity with SARS, and only about 50% with MERS.[120] It has been suggested that a relative of *Rhinolophus affinis*, *Rhinolophus malayanus* (a type of horseshoe bat native to Southeast Asia), could be a natural host of SARS-CoV-2.[121] This remains conjecture at this time.

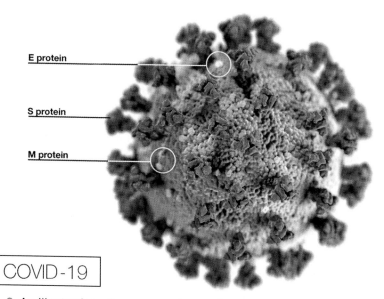

E protein

S protein

M protein

COVID-19

Figure 1.6 An illustration of severe acute respiratory syndrome coronavirus 2 (SARS-CoV-2). (Courtesy of the Centers for Disease Control and Prevention; Alissa Eckert, MSMI; Dan Higgins, MAMS.)

Both SARS and SARS-CoV-2 bind to angiotensin-converting enzyme 2 (ACE2) receptors with their S protein. (The primary binding receptor for MERS is dipeptidyl peptidase 4 [DPP4].) The receptor-binding domain of SARS-CoV-2 has been found to have a 10- to 20-fold higher binding affinity to ACE2 when compared to SARS-CoV.[111] Like SARS-CoV, TMPRSS2 is responsible for the priming of the S protein at the S2′ cleavage site. Unlike SARS-CoV, which is cleaved by serine proteases or cathepsins at the S1/S2 junction, the S1/S2 junction for SARS-CoV-2 contains a furin cleavage site. This distinction is not an anomaly for coronaviruses, as MERS also contains a furin cleavage site at the S1/S2 junction.[122] However, SARS-CoV-2 is more closely related to SARS than MERS. This does not preclude insertion of a furin cleavage site via a natural recombination event, but it has raised eyebrows, especially because *Sarbecoviruses* have not demonstrated an ability to recombine with viruses from other genera. That said, there are probably scores of *Sarbecoviruses* that have yet to be discovered in the bat-infested caves of Yunnan, and a recombination event with one such virus after SARS-CoV-2 and RaTG13 diverged is entirely possible. Furthermore, it should be noted that Papa et al has found, "although furin is a highly important cofactor, it is not absolutely essential for SARS-CoV-2 infection and replication will occur even in its absence."[123] There is also evidence to suggest that SARS-CoV-2 can bind to neuropilin-1 (NRP1) receptors, which are widely expressed throughout the body, including in lung and neural tissue, and may be a potential route of CNS infection.[124]

The first major mutation of the SARS-CoV-2 virus was followed in real time and occurred in Europe in early 2020, when amino acid 614 (of 1273[125]) changed from an aspartic acid (D) to a glycine (G). The G614 mutation did not make cases of COVID-19 more severe, but it did appear to make the virus more transmissible because it created a stronger bond between subunits S1 and S2, and it ensures that S1 does not break off prematurely, thereby exposing the S2′ site before binding to ACE2 occurs. Consequently, it quickly became the dominant strain wherever it was in circulation.[126]

More recently, several variants have arisen that appear to have augmented transmissibility and have gone on to become the dominant strains in their respective regions. Some appear to have increased the severity of infection, and for this reason, they are regarded as variants of concern. This includes the Alpha variant (previously known as the B.1.1.7 variant), the Beta variant (previously known as the B.1.351 variant), the Gamma variant (previously known as the P.1 variant), and the Delta variant (previously known as the B.1.617 variant).[101] There are also several variants of interest and more than a dozen variants under monitoring as of September 2021. Some of these strains appear to be more transmissible or capable of evading the protections provided by vaccination, though real world data are still lacking.

The most concerning variant as of this writing is the Delta variant, which has become the dominant strain wherever it has taken root. This is largely because it is believed to be approximately twice as transmissible as previous variants, with Liu and Rocklöv finding a mean R0 of 5.08 compared to 2.79 observed in ancestral strains of the virus.[127] Others have reported even higher R0 values, 6 to 7, which would mean it is less transmissible than chickenpox (R0 = 9-10) or the measles (R0 = 18), but far more transmissible than ancestral strains of SARS-CoV-2 or influenza A (R0 = 2).[128] Evidence suggests that it is more transmissible because individuals become contagious almost two days before developing symptoms, whereas this window only lasted less than 1 day in previous strains.[129] Additionally, the Delta variant appears to be both more transmissible and more severe in both children and adults than ancestral strains. Though the underlying reason for this remains unclear, there has been a clear rise in the number of pediatric COVID-19 cases requiring hospitalization since the Delta variant became the dominant strain in the United States.[130] In England, Twohig and colleagues analyzed data from more than 43,300 COVID-19 cases that occurred among all age groups between March 29, 2021, and May 23, 2021, and found that unvaccinated adults who are infected with the Delta variant were 2.26 more likely to be hospitalized with severe COVID-19 symptoms within 2 weeks of a positive test than unvaccinated adults who were infected with the Alpha variant.[131]

The Delta variant also presents a greater risk of symptomatic infection to vaccinated individuals than previous strains. The Israeli government reported in early July that the efficacy of the Pfizer/BioNTech vaccine (BNT162b2) fell from 94% to 64% once the Delta became the dominant strain in the country, and then later updated their estimate of the vaccine's efficacy to 39% in late July.[132] Public Health Scotland reported a similar decline in protection against symptomatic infection as the Alpha variant was supplanted by the Delta variant for both the Pfizer/BioNTech and Oxford AstraZeneca (AZD1222) vaccines—from 92% to 79% and from 73% to 60%, respectively.[133] Bernal and colleagues, meanwhile, reported that a single dose of either the Oxford AstraZeneca or Pfizer/BioNTech vaccines was 30.7% effective at preventing symptomatic disease, while two doses offered effectiveness against the Delta variant of 67% and 88%, respectively.[134] Despite a decreased immunity from symptomatic infection, vaccines still offer very strong protection against severe illness, hospitalization, and death. An examination of cases, hospitalizations, and deaths among Americans 18 years of age or older across 13 states between April 4 and July 17, 2021, found that unvaccinated individuals, when compared to fully vaccinated individuals, were 4.5 times more likely to become infected with SARS-CoV-2, approximately 10 times more likely to be hospitalized with COVID-19, and had 10 times the mortality risk.[135]

Unlike other coronaviruses, a significant number of SARS-CoV-2 cases remain asymptomatic—especially among younger individuals. Studies have found that asymptomatic individuals account for 59% of all transmission (24% from individuals who never develop symptoms and 35% from individuals who later become symptomatic).[136] Preliminary evidence suggests that presymptomatic transmission is significantly higher among individuals infected with the Delta variant and that 74% of Delta variant infections take place during the presymptomatic phase.[129] Theories abound as to why this is the case, but a definitive answer continues to elude researchers.

A brief overview of the differences between MERS, SARS, and SARS-CoV-2 can be found in Table 1.2. Subsequent chapters will explore more of the characteristics of SARS-CoV-2 and COVID-19 in greater depth.

TABLE 1.2 General Epidemiological and Clinical Characteristics of SARS, MERS, and COVID-19[26]

Virus	SARS	MERS	COVID-19
Origin date	November 2002	June 2012	Late 2019
Location of original outbreak	Guangdong, China	Jeddah, Saudi Arabia	Wuhan, China
Confirmed cases	8098	2574[42]	+254 million[a]
Confirmed deaths	774	886[42]	+5.1 million[a]
Case fatality rate	9.56%	34.4%[42]	2.06%[a]
Genus	Beta-CoV lineage B (*Sarbecovirus*)	Beta-CoV lineage C (*Merbecovirus*)	Beta-CoV lineage B (*Sarbecovirus*)
Genome length	27.9 kb	30.1 kb	29.9 kb
Incubation period	2-10 d	2-14 d	1-14 d
Reproduction number (R0)	2-3	<1	2.79-7 (depends on variant)[128]
Cell receptor target	ACE2	DPP4 (CD26)	ACE2
Common signs and symptoms	Fever, fatigue, headache, diarrhea, cough, shortness of breath	Fever, fatigue, diarrhea, cough, shortness of breath	Fever, fatigue, dry cough, shortness of breath
Major complications	Pneumonia, severe ARDS, death	Pneumonia, severe ARDS, death	Pneumonia, severe ARDS, death

ARDS, acute respiratory distress syndrome; COVID-19, coronavirus disease of 2019; MERS, Middle Eastern respiratory syndrome; SARS, Severe acute respiratory syndrome.
[a]These figures are still preliminary. As of November 18, 2021, the WHO Coronavirus dashboard has confirmed 254,256,432 cases and 5,112,461 deaths globally (https://covid19.who.int/).

Conclusion

Many questions still remain about the genesis of SARS-CoV-2. While this is extremely frustrating because of how much the virus has impacted the lives of nearly everyone on the planet, there is hope that daylight will eventually shine on the origins of the virus.

What is less frustrating is the amount of knowledge that has been accumulated over the course of the approximately two years since the virus emerged. In this time, the global scientific community banded together to study the SARS-CoV-2 genome, unlock its secrets, and devise vaccines that have proven extremely effective at preventing viral transmission and severe COVID-19. Never before have so many scientists and researchers been dedicated to the same cause. This gives me hope that we can continue to work together to solve many of the problems that will persist even after the pandemic has ended.

REFERENCES

1. World Health Organization. *WHO Statement Regarding Cluster of Pneumonia Cases in Wuhan, China*. January 9, 2020. Accessed May 21, 2021. https://www.who.int/china/news/detail/09-01-2020-who-statement-regarding-cluster-of-pneumonia-cases-in-wuhan-china
2. Qin A, Hernández JC. China reports first death from new virus. *New York Times*. Updated January 21, 2020. Accessed May 22, 2021. https://www.nytimes.com/2020/01/10/world/asia/china-virus-wuhan-death.html
3. Tharoor I. The pandemic is getting worse, even when it seems like it's getting better. *Washington Post*. Published June 2, 2021. Accessed June 2, 2021. https://www.washingtonpost.com/world/2021/06/02/global-pandemic-worsening/
4. Phillips N. The coronavirus is here to stay—here's what that means. *Nature*. 2021;590(7846):382-384. doi:10.1038/d41586-021-00396-2
5. Last JM, ed. *A Dictionary of Epidemiology*. 4th ed. Oxford University Press; 2001. Quoted in Kelly H. The classical definition of a pandemic is not elusive. *Bull World Health Organ*. 2011;89:540-541. doi:10.2471/BLT.11.088815
6. Harrison M. *Contagion: How Commerce Has Spread Disease*. Yale University Press; 2012.
7. Mena I, Nelson MI, Quezada-Monroy F, et al. Origins of the 2009 H1N1 influenza pandemic in swine in Mexico. *ELife*. 2016;5:e16777. doi:10.7554/eLife.16777
8. Dawood FS, Iuliano AD, Reed C, et al. Estimated global mortality associated with the first 12 months of 2009 pandemic influenza A H1N1 virus circulation: a modeling study. *Lancet Infect Dis*. 2012;12(9):687-695. doi:10.1016/S1473-3099(12)70121-4
9. Honigsbaum M. Revisiting the 1957 and 1968 influenza pandemics. *Lancet*. 2020;395(10240):1824-1826. doi:10.1016/S0140-6736(20)31201-0
10. Khan M, Adil SF, Alkhathlan HZ, et al. COVID-19: a global challenge with an old history, epidemiology and progress so far. *Molecules*. 2021;26(1):39. doi:10.3390/molecules26010039
11. Al Hajjar S, McIntosh K. The first influenza pandemic of the 21st century. *Ann Saudi Med*. 2010;30(1):1-10. doi:10.4103/0256-4947.59365
12. Strochlic N, Champine RD. How some cities 'flattened the curve' during the 1918 flu pandemic. *National Geographic*. Published March 27, 2020. Accessed May 19, 2021. https://www.nationalgeographic.com/history/article/how-cities-flattened-curve-1918-spanish-flu-pandemic-coronavirus

13. CBC Radio. *This 107-year-old remembers the 1918 Spanish flu, and sees the similarities with COVID-19*. Published April 10, 2020. Accessed May 17, 2021. https://www.cbc.ca/radio/thecurrent/the-current-for-april-10-2020-1.5529055/this-107-year-old-remembers-the-1918-spanish-flu-and-sees-the-similarities-with-covid-19-1.5529264

14. Davis KC. Philadelphia threw a WWI parade that gave thousands of onlookers the flu. *Smithsonian Magazine*. Published September 21, 2018. Accessed May 19, 2021. https://www.smithsonianmag.com/history/philadelphia-threw-wwi-parade-gave-thousands-onlookers-flu-180970372/

15. Hauser C. The mask slackers of 1918. *New York Times*. Updated December 10, 2021. Accessed May 19, 2021. https://www.nytimes.com/2020/08/03/us/mask-protests-1918.html

16. Dolan B. Unmasking history: who was behind the Anti-Mask League protests during the 1918 influenza epidemic in San Francisco? *Perspect Med Humanities*. Published May 19, 2020;5(5):1-28. doi:10.34947/M7QP4M. Accessed May 19, 2021. https://escholarship.org/uc/item/5q91q53r

17. Van Epps HL. Influenza: exposing the true killer. *J Exp Med*. 2006;203(4):803. doi:10.1084/jem.2034.fta

18. McMillen CW. *Pandemics: A Very Short Introduction*. Oxford University Press; 2016.

19. Wilson N, Barnard LT, Summers JA, Shanks GD, Baker MG. Differential mortality rates by ethnicity in 3 influenza pandemics over a century, New Zealand. *Emerg Infect Dis*. 2012;18(1):71-77. doi:10.3201/eid1801.110035

20. Parmet WE, Rothstein MA. The 1918 influence pandemic: lessons learned and not—introduction to the special section. *Am J Public Health*. 2018;108(11):1435-1436. doi:10.2105/AJPH.2018.304695

21. Faust JS. Comparing COVID-19 deaths to flu deaths is like comparing apples to oranges. *Scientific American*. Published April 28, 2020. Accessed May 17, 2021. https://blogs.scientificamerican.com/observations/comparing-covid-19-deaths-to-flu-deaths-is-like-comparing-apples-to-oranges/

22. Smil V. *A Complete History of Pandemics*. The MIT Press Reader website; March 30, 2020. Accessed May 14, 2021. https://thereader.mitpress.mit.edu/a-complete-history-of-pandemics/

23. Woolhouse M, Scott F, Hudson Z, Howey R, Chase-Topping M. Human viruses: discovery and emergence. *Philos Trans R Soc Lond B Biol Sci*. 2012;367(1604):2864-2871. doi:10.1098/rstb.2011.0354

24. Smith KF, Goldberg M, Rosenthal S, et al. Global rise in human infectious disease outbreaks. *J R Soc Interface*. 2014;11(101):20140950. doi:10.1098/rsif.2014.0950

25. Hui EKW. Reasons for the increase in emerging and re-emerging viral infectious diseases. *Mocrobes Infect*. 2006;8(3):905-916. doi:10.1016/j.micinf.2005.06.032

26. Ganesh B, Rajakumar T, Malathi M, et al. Epidemiology and pathobiology of SARS-CoV-2 (COVID-19) in comparison with SARS, MERS: an updated overview of current knowledge and future perspectives. *Clin Epidemiol Glob Health*. 2021;10:100694. doi:10.1016/j.cegh.2020.100694

27. Cyranoski D. Bat cave solves mystery of deadly SARS virus—and suggests new outbreak could occur. *Nature*. 2017;552:15-16. doi:10.1038/d41586-017-07766-9

28. Guan Y, Zheng BJ, He YQ, et al. Isolation and characterization of viruses related to the SARS coronavirus from animals in southern China. *Science*. 2003;302(5643):276-278. doi:10.1126/science.1087139

29. El-Kafrawy SA, Corman VM, Tolah AM, et al. Enzootic patterns of Middle East respiratory syndrome coronavirus in imported African and local Arabian dromedary camels: a prospective genomic study. *Lancet Planet Health*. 2019;3(1):E521-E528. doi:10.1016/S2542-5196(19)30243-8

30. Mok CKP, Zhu A, Zhao J, et al. T-cell responses to MERS coronavirus infection in people with occupational exposure to dromedary camels in Nigeria: an observational cohort study. *Lancet Infect Dis*. 2021;21(3):385-395. doi:10.1016/S1473-3099(20)30599-5

31. Hu T, Liu Y, Zhao M, Zhuang Q, Xu L, He Q. A comparison of COVID-19, SARS, and MERS. *Peer J*. 2020;8:e9725. doi:10.7717/peerj.9725

32. Kang M, Wei J, Yuan J, et al. Probable evidence of fecal aerosol transmission of SARS-CoV-2 in a high-rise building. *Ann Intern Med*. 2020;173(12):974-980. doi:10.7326/M20-0928

33. La Rosa G, Fratini M, Della Libera S, Iaconelli M, Muscillo M. Viral infections acquired indoors through airborne, droplet or contact transmission. *Ann Ist Super Sanita*. 2013;49(2):124-132. doi:10.4415/ANN_13_02_03

34. Lau AC, Yam YK, So LK. Management of critically ill patients with severe acute respiratory syndrome (SARS). *Int J Med Sci*. 2004;1(1):1-10. doi:10.7150/ijms.1.1

35. Cherry JD, Krogstad P. SARS: the first pandemic of the 21st century. *Pediatr Res*. 2004;56(1):1-5. doi:10.1203/01.PDR.0000129184.87042.FC

36. Centers for Disease Control and Prevention. *SARS Basic Fact Sheet*. Updated December 6, 2017. Accessed May 22, 2021. https://www.cdc.gov/sars/about/fs-sars.html

37. Hugonnet S, Pittet D. Transmission of severe acute respiratory syndrome in critical care: do we need a change? *Am J Respir Crit Care Med*. 2004;169(11):1177-1178. doi:10.1164/rccm.2403004

38. Madewell ZJ, Yang Y, Longini IM Jr, Halloran ME, Dean NE. Household transmission of SARS-CoV-2: a systematic review and meta-analysis. *JAMA Netw Open*. 2020;3(12):e2031756. doi:10.1001/jamanetworkopen.2003.31756

39. Nakashima E. Vietnam took lead in containing SARS. *The Washington Post*. Published May 5, 2003. Accessed May 23, 2021. https://www.washingtonpost.com/archive/politics/2003/05/05/vietnam-took-lead-in-containing-sars/b9b97e91-b325-42f9-98ef-e23da9f257a0/

40. Lawrence SV. *COVID-19 and China: A Chronology of Events (December 2019-January 2020)*. Congressional Research Service. Updated May 13, 2020. Accessed May 21, 2021. https://crsreports.congress.gov/product/pdf/r/r46354

41. Lucey DR. Editorial commentary: still learning from the earliest known MERS outbreak, Zarqa, Jordan, April 2021. *Clin Infect Dis*. 2014;59(9):1234-1236. doi:10.1093/cid/ciu638

42. Middle East respiratory syndrome. World Health Organization Regional Office for the Eastern Mediterranean. Accessed May 23, 2021. http://www.emro.who.int/health-topics/mers-cov/mers-outbreaks.html

43. Al-Osail AM, Al-Wazzah MJ. The history and epidemiology of Middle East respiratory syndrome coronavirus. *Multidiscip Respir Med*. 2017;12:20. doi:10.1186/s40248-017-0101-8

44. Choi S, Jung E, Choi BY, Hur YJ, Ki M. High reproduction number of Middle East respiratory syndrome coronavirus in nosocomial outbreaks: mathematical modeling in Saudi Arabia and South Korea. *J Hosp Infect*. 2018;99(2):162-168. doi:10.1016/j.jhin.2017.09.017

45. Tellier R, Li Y, Cowling BJ, Tang JW. Recognition of aerosol transmission of infectious agents: a commentary. *BMC Infect Dis*. 2019;19:101. doi:10.1186/s12879-019-3707-y

46. Fallows J. The 3 weeks that changed everything. *The Atlantic*. Published June 29, 2020. Accessed May 21, 2021. https://www.theatlantic.com/politics/archive/2020/06/how-white-house-coronavirus-response-went-wrong/613591/

47. Pandemic Prediction and Forecasting Science and Technology Working Group of the National Science and Technology Council. *Towards Epidemic Prediction: Federal Efforts and Opportunities in Outbreak Modeling*. December 2016. Accessed May 21, 2021. https://obamawhitehouse.archives.gov/sites/default/files/microsites/ostp/NSTC/towards_epidemic_prediction-federal_efforts_and_opportunities.pdf

48. USAID. *Emerging Pandemic Threats Program*. Updated November 25, 2014. Accessed May 26, 2021. https://www.usaid.gov/ept2

49. McNeil DG Jr. Scientists were hunting for the next Ebola. Now the U.S. has cut off their funding. *New York Times*. Published October 25, 2019. Accessed May 23, 2021. https://www.nytimes.com/2019/10/25/health/predict-usaid-viruses.html

50. Judkis M. So many people are convinced that they had COVID-19 already. *Washington Post*. Published May 6, 2020. Accessed May 21, 2021. https://www.washingtonpost. com/lifestyle/style/why-everyone-you-know-is-convinced-that-they-had-covid-19-already/2020/05/05/aef406ac-8a38-11ea-8ac1-bfb250876b7a_story.html

51. Roy M. Five U.S. states had coronavirus infections even before the first reported cases—study. *Reuters*. Published June 15, 2021. Accessed June 18, 2021. https://www.reuters. com/business/healthcare-pharmaceuticals/five-us-states-had-coronavirus-infections-even-before-first-reported-cases-study-2021-06-15/

52. Fongaro G, Stoco PH, Souza DS, et al. The presence of SARS-CoV-2 RNA in human sewage in Santa Catarina, Brazil, November 2019. *Sci Total Environ*. 2021;778:146198. doi:10.1016/j.scitotenv.2021.146198

53. Vagnoni G. Researchers find coronavirus was circulating in Italy earlier than thought. *Reuters*. Published November 16, 2020. Accessed May 21, 2021. https://www.reuters.com/ article/health-coronavirus-italy-timing/researchers-find-coronavirus-was-circulating-in-italy-earlier-than-thought-idUSKBN27W1J2

54. Allen N, Landauro I. Coronavirus traces found in March 2019 sewage sample, Spanish study shows. *Reuters*. Published June 26, 2020. Accessed May 21, 2021. https://www. reuters.com/article/us-health-coronavirus-spain-science/coronavirus-traces-found-in-march-2019-sewage-sample-spanish-study-shows-idUSKBN23X2HQ

55. Folmer K, Margolin J. Satellite data suggests coronavirus may have hit China earlier: researchers. *ABC News*. Published June 8, 2020. Accessed May 21, 2021. https://abcnews. go.com/International/satellite-data-suggests-coronavirus-hit-china-earlier-researchers/ story?id=71123270

56. Pekar J, Worobey M, Moshiri N, Scheffler K, Wertheim JO. Timing the SARS-CoV-2 index case in Hubei province. *Science*. 2021;372(6540):412-417. doi:10.1126/science.abf8003

57. Nakashima E, Abutaleb Y, Achenbach J. Biden receives inconclusive intelligence report on covid origins. *Washington Post*. Published August 24, 2021. Accessed August 30, 2021. https://www.washingtonpost.com/politics/2021/08/24/ covid-origins-biden-intelligence-review/

58. Frutos R, Serra-Cobo J, Chen T, Devaux CA. COVID-19: time to exonerate the pangolin from the transmission of SARS-CoV-2 to humans. *Infect Genet Evol*. 2020;84:104493. doi:10.1016/j.meegid.2020.104493

59. Segreto R, Deigin Y, McCairn K, et al. Should we discount the laboratory origin of COVID-19? *Environ Chem Lett*. 2021;1-15. Accessed May 21, 2021. doi:10.1007/ s10311-021-01211-0

60. Boni MF, Lemey P, Jiang X, et al. Evolutionary origins of the SARS-CoV-2 sarbecovirus lineage responsible for the COVID-19 pandemic. *Nature Microbiol*. 2020;5:1408-1417. doi:10.1038/s41564-020-0771-4

61. Rahalkar MC, Bahulikar RA. Lethal pneumonia in Mojiang miners (2012) and the mineshaft could provide important clues to the origin of SARS-CoV-2. *Front Public Health*. 2020;8:581569. doi:10.3389/fpubh.2020.581569

62. Hu B, Zeng LP, Yang XL, et al. Discovery of a rich gene pool of bat SARS-related coronaviruses provides new insights into the origin of SARS coronavirus. *PLoS Pathog*. 2017;13(11):e1006698. doi:10.1371/journal.ppat.1006698

63. Cyranoski D. Inside the Chinese lab poised to study world's most dangerous pathogens. *Nature*. 2017;542(7642):399-400. doi:10.1038/nature.2017.21487

64. Rogin J. In 2018, diplomats warned of risky coronavirus experiments in a Wuhan lab. No one listened. *Politico*. Published March 8, 2021. Accessed May 24, 2021. https://www.politico.com/news/magazine/2021/03/08/ josh-rogin-chaos-under-heaven-wuhan-lab-book-excerpt-474322

65. Reuters. Wuhan staff sought hospital care before COVID-19 outbreak disclosed—WSJ. Published May 24, 2021. Accessed May 24, 2021. https://www.reuters.com/business/ healthcare-pharmaceuticals/wuhan-lab-staff-sought-hospital-care-before-covid-19-outbreak-disclosed-wsj-2021-05-23/

66. World Health Organization disease outbreak news. *Novel coronavirus –
China*. January 12, 2020. Accessed May 21, 2021. https://www.who.int/csr/
don/12-january-2020-novel-coronavirus-china/en/

67. Huang C, Wang Y, Li X, et al. Clinical features of patients infected with 2019 novel
coronavirus in Wuhan, China. *Lancet*. 2020;395(10223):497-506. doi:10.1016/
S0140-6736(20)30183-5

68. Yu G, Yanfeng P, Rui Y, et al. In depth: how early signs of a SARS-like virus were spotted,
spread, and throttled. *Caixin Global*. Published February 29, 2020. Accessed May 21, 2021.
https://www.caixinglobal.com/2020-02-29/in-depth-how-early-signs-of-a-sars-like-virus-
were-spotted-spread-and-throttled-101521745.html

69. Green A. Li Wenliang. *Lancet*. 2020;395(10225);682. doi:10.1016/S0140-6736(20)
30382-2

70. McKenna M. How ProMED crowdsourced the arrival of COVID-19 and SARS. *Wired*.
Published March 23, 2020. Accessed May 26, 2021. https://www.wired.com/story/
how-promed-crowdsourced-the-arrival-of-covid-19-and-sars/

71. Sparrow A. The Chinese government's cover-up killed health care workers worldwide.
Foreign Policy. Published March 18, 2021. Accessed May 21, 2021. https://foreignpolicy.
com/2021/03/18/china-covid-19-killed-health-care-workers-worldwide/

72. Tweet by World Health Organization. January 4, 2020. Accessed May 21, 2021. https://
twitter.com/WHO/status/1213523866703814656?s=20

73. World Health Organization. *Pneumonia of Unknown Cause – China*.
January 5, 2020. Accessed May 21, 2021. https://www.who.int/csr/
don/05-january-2020-pneumonia-of-unkown-cause-china/en/

74. World Health Organization. *WHO Advice for International Travel and Trade in Relation
to the Outbreak of Pneumonia Caused by a New Coronavirus in China*. January 10, 2020.
Accessed May 22, 2021. https://www.who.int/news-room/articles-detail/who-advice-for-
international-travel-and-trade-in-relation-to-the-outbreak-of-pneumonia-caused-by-a-new-
coronavirus-in-china

75. Chen S, Yang J, Yang W, Wang C, Bärnighausen T. COVID-19 control in China during
mass population movements at New Year. *Lancet*. 2020;395(10226):764-766. doi:10.1016/
S0140-6736(20)30421-9

76. Durrheim DN, Gostin LO, Moodley K. When does a major outbreak become a Public
Health Emergency of International Concern? *Lancet Infect Dis*. 2020;20(8):887-888.
doi:10.1016/S1473-3099(20)30401-1

77. Feng E, Cheng A. Restrictions and rewards: how China is locking down half a billion
citizens. *NPR*. Published February 21, 2020. Accessed May 25, 2021. https://www.npr.
org/sections/goatsandsoda/2020/02/21/806958341/restrictions-and-rewards-how-china-is-
locking-down-half-a-billion-citizens

78. Wu F, Zhao S, Yu B, et al. A new coronavirus associated with human respiratory disease
in China. *Nature*. 2020;579;265-269. doi:10.1038/s41586-020-2008-3

79. Virological.org. *Novel 2019 Coronavirus Genome*. January 10, 2020. Accessed May 21,
2021. https://virological.org/t/novel-2019-coronavirus-genome/319

80. Kuo L. China confirms human-to-human transmission of coronavirus. *The Guardian*.
January 20, 2020. Accessed May 14, 2021. https://www.theguardian.com/world/2020/
jan/20/coronavirus-spreads-to-beijing-as-china-confirms-new-cases

81. Gilsinan K. How China deceived the WHO. *The Atlantic*. April 12, 2020.
Accessed May 23, 2021. https://www.theatlantic.com/politics/archive/2020/04/
world-health-organization-blame-pandemic-coronavirus/609820/

82. World Health Organization (WHO). *Archived: WHO Timeline – COVID-19*.
April 27, 2020. Accessed May 14, 2021. https://www.who.int/news/
item/27-04-2020-who-timeline---covid-19

83. Maxmen A. Why did the world's pandemic warning system fail when COVID hit? *Nature*.
Published January 23, 2021. Accessed May 23, 2021. https://www.nature.com/articles/
d41586-021-00162-4

84. Kantis C, Keirnan S, Bardi JS. Updated: timeline of the Coronavirus. Published March 26, 2021. Accessed May 25, 2021. https://www.thinkglobalhealth.org/article/updated-timeline-coronavirus

85. Taylor DB. A timeline of the coronavirus pandemic. *New York Times*. Published March 17, 2021. Accessed May 24, 2021. https://www.nytimes.com/article/coronavirus-timeline.html

86. Wright R. How Iran became a new epicenter for the coronavirus outbreak. *The New Yorker*. Published February 28, 2020. Accessed May 25, 2021. https://www.newyorker.com/news/our-columnists/how-iran-became-a-new-epicenter-of-the-coronavirus-outbreak

87. Nada G. 2020 Parliamentary election results. *The Iran Primer*. Published February 24, 2020. Accessed May 25, 2021. https://iranprimer.usip.org/blog/2020/feb/24/2020-parliamentary-election-results

88. Kaffashi A, Jahani F. Nowruz travelers and the COVID-19 pandemic in Iran. *Infect Control Hosp Epidemiol*. 2020;41(9):1121. doi:10.1017/ice.2020.152

89. Malara A. *Diagnosing the First COVID-19 Patient in Italy – Codogno, Italy*. European Society of Cardiology. Published March 25, 2020. Accessed May 25, 2021. https://www.escardio.org/Education/COVID-19-and-Cardiology/diagnosing-the-first-covid-19-patient-in-italy-codogno

90. Russo L, Anastassopoulou C, Tsakris A, et al. Tracing day-zero and forecasting the COVID-19 outbreak in Lombardy, Italy: a compartmental modelling and numerical optimization approach. *PLoS One*. 2020;15(10):e0240649. doi:10.1371/journal.pone.0240649

91. Mervosh S, Lu D, Swales V. See which states and cities have told residents to stay home. *New York Times*. Updated April 20, 2020. Accessed May 25, 2021. https://www.nytimes.com/interactive/2020/us/coronavirus-stay-at-home-order.html

92. Worobey M, Pekar J, Larsen BB, et al. The emergence of SARS-CoV-2 in Europe and North America. *Science*. 2020;370(6516):564-570. doi:10.1126/science.abc8169

93. Korber B, Fischer WM, Gnanakaran S, et al. Tracking changes in SARS-CoV-2 spike: evidence that D614G increases infectivity of the COVID-19 virus. *Cell*. 2020;182:812-827. doi:10.1016/j.cell.2020.06.043

94. Lipton E, Sanger DE, Haberman M, Shear MD, Mazzetti M, Barnes JE. He could have seen what was coming; behind Trump's failure on the virus. *New York Times*. Updated April 26, 2021. Accessed May 21, 2021. https://www.nytimes.com/2020/04/11/us/politics/coronavirus-trump-response.html

95. Braun S, Dearen J. Trump's 'strong wall' to block COVID-19 from China had holes. *AP News*. Published July 4, 2020. Accessed May 25, 2021. https://apnews.com/article/donald-trump-us-news-ap-top-news-macau-virus-outbreak-355a58005d4f7c57978f6b7cba5dbd82

96. Eder S, Fountain H, Keller MH, Xiao M, Stevenson A. 430,000 people have traveled from China to U.S. since coronavirus surfaced. *New York Times*. Updated April 15, 2020. Accessed May 25, 2021. https://www.nytimes.com/2020/04/04/us/coronavirus-china-travel-restrictions.html

97. Beaubien J. Public health experts question Trump's ban on most travelers from Europe. *NPR*. Published March 12, 2020. Accessed May 25, 2021. https://www.npr.org/sections/health-shots/2020/03/12/815146007/public-health-experts-question-trumps-ban-on-most-travelers-from-europe

98. World Health Organization. *WHO Director-General's Opening Remarks at the Media Briefing on COVID-19 – March 11, 2020*. March 11, 2020. Accessed May 25, 2021. https://www.who.int/director-general/speeches/detail/who-director-general-s-opening-remarks-at-the-media-briefing-on-covid-19---11-march-2020

99. Sprunt B. Here's what the new hate crimes law aims to do as attacks on Asian Americans rise. *NRP*. Published May 20, 2021. Accessed May 25, 2021. https://www.npr.org/2021/05/20/998599775/biden-to-sign-the-covid-19-hate-crimes-bill-as-anti-asian-american-attacks-rise

100. World Health Organization. *Tracking SARS-CoV-2 variants*. Updated September 2, 2021. Accessed September 10, 2021. https://www.who.int/en/activities/tracking-SARS-CoV-2-variants/

101. World Health Organization. *Tracking SARS-CoV-2 variants*. Updated May 31, 2021. Accessed June 1, 2021. https://www.who.int/en/activities/tracking-SARS-CoV-2-variants/

102. Mendez R. WHO says COVID will mutate like the flu and is likely here to stay. *CNBC*. Updated September 7, 2021. Accessed September 14, 2021. https://www.cnbc.com/2021/09/07/who-says-covid-is-here-to-stay-as-hopes-for-eradicating-the-virus-diminish.html

103. de Wit E, van Doremalen N, Falzarano D, Munster VJ. SARS and MERS: recent insights into emerging coronaviruses. *Nat Rev Microbiol*. 2016;14(8):523-534. doi:10.1038/nrmicro.2016.81

104. Maginnis MS. Virus-receptor interactions: the key to cellular invasion. *J Mol Biol*. 2018;430(17):2590-2611. doi:10.1016/j.jmb.2018.6.024

105. Sender R, Bar-On YM, Gleizer S, et al. The total number and mass of SARS-CoV-2 virions. Preprint. November 17, 2020. Revised April 5, 2021. medRxiv. doi:10.1101/2020.11.16.20232009.

106. Hackenthal V. Tracking the evolution of SARS-CoV-2. *Medpage Today*. Published May 6, 2021. Accessed May 21, 2021. https://www.medpagetoday.com/special-reports/exclusives/92454

107. Abraham JP, Plourde BD, Cheng L. Using heat to kill SARS-CoV-2. *Rev Med Virol*. 2020;30:e2115. doi:10.1002/rmv.2115

108. Banerjee A, Kulcsar K, Misra V, Frieman M, Mossman K. Bats and coronaviruses. *Viruses*. 2019;11(1):41. doi:10.3390/v11010041

109. Payne S. Family Coronaviridae. *Viruses*. 2017;149-158. doi:10.1016/B978-0-12-803109-4.00017-9

110. Chorba T. The concept of the crown and its potential role in the downfall of coronavirus. *Emerg Infect Dis*. 2020;26(9):2302-2305. doi:10.3201/eid2609.ac2609

111. Hartenian E, Nandakumar D, Lari A, Ly M, Tucker JM, Glaunsinger BA. The molecular virology of coronaviruses. *J Biol Chem*. 2020;295(37):12910-12934. doi:10.1074/jbc.REV120.013930

112. Peacock TP, Goldhill DH, Zhou J, et al. The furin cleavage site in the SARS-CoV-2 spike protein is required for transmission to ferrets. *Nat Microbiol*. 2021;6(7):899-909. doi:10.1038/s41564-021-00908-w

113. Du L, He Y, Zhou Y, Liu S, Zheng BJ, Jiang S. The spike protein of SARS-CoV – a target for vaccine and therapeutic development. *Nat Rev Microbiol*. 2009;7(3):226-236. doi:10.1038/nrmicro2090

114. Wu Y, Zhao S. Furin cleavage sites naturally occur in coronaviruses. *Stem Cell Res*. 2020;50:102115. doi:10.1016/j.scr.2020.102115

115. Smith EC, Sexton NR, Denison MR. Thinking outside the triangle: replication fidelity of the largest RNA viruses. *Annu Rev Virol*. 2014;1(1):111-132. doi:10.1146/annurev-virology-031413-085507

116. Minskaia E, Hertzig T, Gorbalenya AE, et al. Discovery of an RNA virus 3'->5' exoribonuclease that is critically involved in coronavirus RNA synthesis. *Proc Natl Acad Sci U S A*. 2006;103(13):5108-5113. doi:10.1073/pnas.0508200103

117. Simon-Loriere E, Holmes EC. Why do RNA viruses recombine? *Nat Rev Microbiol*. 2011;9:617-626. doi:10.1038/nrmicro2614

118. Li X, Giorgi EE, Marichannegowda MH, et al. Emergence of SARS-CoV-2 through recombination and strong purifying selection. *Sci Adv*. 2020;6(27):eabb9153. doi:10.1126/sciadv.abb9153

119. Graham RL, Baric RS. Recombination, reservoirs, and the modular spike: mechanisms of coronavirus cross-species transmission. *J Virol*. 2010;84(7):3134-3146. doi:10.1128/JVI.01394-09

120. Zhou P, Yang XL, Wang XG, et al. A pneumonia outbreak associated with a new coronavirus of probable bat origin. *Nature*. 2020;(579):270-273. doi:10.1038/s41586-020-2012-7

121. Wong G, Bi YH, Wang QH, Chen XW, Zhang ZG, Yao YG. Zoonotic origins of human coronavirus 2019 (HCoV-19/SARS-CoV-2): why is this work important? *Zool Res*. 2020;41(3):213-219. doi:10.24272/j.issn.2095-8137.2020.031

122. Tang T, Jaimes JA, Bidon MK, Straus MR, Daniel S, Whittaker GR. Proteolytic activation of SARS-CoV-2 spike at the S1/S2 boundary: potential role of proteases beyond furin. *ACS Infect Dis*. 2021;7(2):264-272. doi:10.1021/acsinfecdis.0C00701

123. Papa G, Mallery DL, Alebcka A, et al. Furin cleavage of SARS-CoV-2 spike promotes but is not essential for infection and cell-cell fusion. *PLoS Pathog*. 2021;17(1):e1009246. doi:10.1371/journal.ppat.1009246

124. Kyrou I, Randeva HS, Spandidos DA, Karteris E. Not only ACE2—the quest for additional host cell mediators of SARS-CoV-2 infection: neuropilin-1 (NPR1) as a novel SARS-CoV-2 host cell mediator implicated in COVID-19. *Signal Transduct Target Ther*. 2021;6(1):21. doi:10.1038/s41392-020-00460-9

125. Huang Y, Yang C, Xu XF, Xu W, Liu SW. Structural and functional properties of SARS-CoV-2 spike protein: potential antiviral drug development for COVID-19. *Acta Pharmacol Sin*. 2020;41:1141-1149. doi:10.1038/s41401-020-0485-4

126. Choe H, Farzan M. How SARS-CoV-2 first adapted in humans. *Science*. 2021;372(6541):466-467. doi:10.1126/science.abi4711

127. Liu Y, Rocklöv J. The reproductive number of the Delta variant of SARS-CoV-2 is far higher compared to the ancestral SARS-CoV-2 virus. *J Travel Med*. 2021;28(7):taab124. Accessed August 19, 2021. doi:10.1093/jtm/taab124

128. Doucleff M. The Delta variant isn't as contagious as chickenpox, but it's still highly contagious. *NPR*. Published August 11, 2011. Accessed August 20, 2011. https://www.npr.org/sections/goatsandsoda/2021/08/11/1026190062/covid-delta-variant-transmission-cdc-chickenpox

129. Mallapaty S. Delta's rise is fueled by rampant spread from people who feel fine. *Nature*. Published August 19, 2021. Accessed August 20, 2021. https://www.nature.com/articles/d41586-021-02259-2

130. Cha AE. 'This is real': fear and hope in an Arkansas pediatric ICU. *Washington Post*. Posted August 13, 2021. Accessed August 20, 2021. https://www.washingtonpost.com/health/2021/08/13/children-hospitalizations-covid-delta/

131. Twohig KA, Nyberg T, Zaidi A, et al. Hospital admission and emergency care attendance risk for SARS-CoV-2 delta (B.1.617.2) compared with alpha (B.1.1.7) variants of concern: a cohort study. *Lancet Infect Dis*. Published August 27, 2021. doi:10.1016/S1473-3099(21)00475-8. Accessed August 31, 2021. https://www.thelancet.com/journals/laninf/article/PIIS1473-3099(21)00475-8/fulltext

132. Lovelace B Jr. Israel says Pfizer COVID vaccine is just 39% effective as Delta spreads, but still prevents severe illness. *CNBC*. Updated July 23, 2021. Accessed August 19, 2021. https://www.cnbc.com/2021/07/23/delta-variant-pfizer-covid-vaccine-39percent-effective-in-israel-prevents-severe-illness.html

133. Sheikh A, McMenamin J, Taylor B, Robertson C, Public Health Scotland and the EAVE II Collaborators. SARS-CoV-2 Delta VOC in Scotland: demographics, risk of hospital admission, and vaccine effectiveness. *Lancet*. 2021;397(10293):2461-2462. doi:10.1016/S0140-6736(21)01358-1

134. Bernal JL, Andrews N, Gower C, et al. Effectiveness of COVID-19 vaccines against the B.1.617.2 (Delta) variant. *N Eng J Med*. 2021;385(7):585-594. doi:10.1056/NEJMoa2108891

135. Scobie HM, Johnson AG, Suthar AB, et al. Monitoring incidence of COVID-19 cases, hospitalizations, and deaths, by vaccination status—13 U.S. Jurisdictions, April 4-July 17, 2021. *MMWR Morb Mortal Wkly Rep*. 2021;70(37):1284-1290. doi:10.15585/mmwr.mm7037e1

136. Johansson MA, Quandelacy TM, Kada S, et al. SARS-CoV-2 transmission from people without COVID-19 symptoms. *JAMA Netw Open*. 2021;4(1):e2035057. doi:10.1001/jamanetworkopen.2020.35057

2

Transmission of SARS-CoV-2

This chapter includes an overview of the viral transmission and the phases of infection before providing specifics about SARS-CoV-2. Following the description of SARS-CoV-2 transmission dynamics, the next section will focus on the subject of masks, a topic that has been ubiquitous within COVID-19 discourse. Transmission follows the chain of infection, which begins with a pathogenic agent being released from a *reservoir* that eventually travels through a *portal of exit*. The pathogen is then conveyed by a *mode of transmission* before it infects a *susceptible host* via a *portal of entry* (see Figure 2.1). Laypersons and clinicians who would like a brief refresher will benefit from reviewing sections Reservoirs and Hosts, Routes of Transmission, Portals, and Phases of Infection.

Reservoirs and Hosts

A viral reservoir is an organism in which a virus lives, grows, and multiples. In some cases, a reservoir may harbor a virus and be clinically affected by the infection. In other cases, a reservoir may harbor a virus and be capable of transmitting it even if it may not show symptoms of infection. This may be because symptoms have yet to appear or because the individual has an asymptomatic infection, in which case that individual is known as a carrier. Entire species may harbor a virus and only develop limited clinical disease when infected. When this occurs, the organism is known as a reservoir host. Bats, for example, frequently serve as reservoir hosts and have been associated with more zoonotic viruses than any other mammalian order.[1]

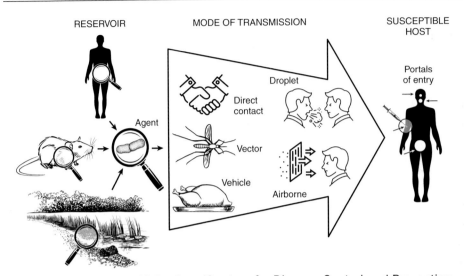

Figure 2.1 The chain of infection. (Centers for Disease Control and Prevention. *Principles of epidemiology*. 2nd ed. Atlanta: U.S. Department of Health and Human Services;1992. Reference to specific commercial products, manufacturers, companies, or trademarks does not constitute its endorsement or recommendation by the U.S. Government, Department of Health and Human Services, or Centers for Disease Control and Prevention.)

There are potentially trillions of virus species and an estimated 10^{31} individual virions on Earth. Luckily, only an infinitesimally small percentage of them pose any threat to humans.[2] Most viruses have a limited host range, meaning they have adapted to infect only a handful of species very well. Hosts are only susceptible to infection if the virus can access cells that express receptors to which the virus can bind (see Chapter 1, Section Viruses). Cells must also be permissive to infection, meaning they contain the intercellular mechanisms necessary to allow for viral replication and assembly. Tissue tropism refers to the cell types within an organism that a virus targets and uses for replication. Some viruses have demonstrated a broad tropism and can infect many kinds of cell tissues in multiple organs, while other viruses are more specific and only attack a narrow range of tissue types.

When a virus does manage to make the jump between an animal and a human, this is known as a spillover event. A disease that infects people by way of animals is known as zoonosis. Spillover events appear to be relatively common, but most cross-species infections are either transient or abortive.[3] In other words, individual spillover events may lead to an infection and even a disease within a human host, but the virus is often incapable of then spreading to other humans. When a virus jumps from an animal reservoir to a human host on several separate occasions without resulting in human-to-human transmission, it is known as viral chatter.[4]

There have been at least two instances of limited viral chatter involving coronaviruses in the past 5 years. Surprisingly, neither has received a great deal of attention in the media. One was a canine-feline recombinant alphacoronavirus that infected at least eight individuals in Malaysia and caused cases of pneumonia from which all patients recovered.[5] The other, described in a preprint article, was a deltacoronavirus that appears to have jumped from pigs to three children in Haiti and caused acute undifferentiated febrile illness.[6]

Routes of Transmission

Viruses can be spread through direct or indirect means and often through multiple routes (or modes) of transmission. Direct transmission includes person-to-person contact and large droplet spread. Indirect transmission occurs when there is an intermediary in the chain of infection and intermediaries can include dust or aerosolized particles that are smaller than droplets. It can also include vehicles (objects like food, water, or surfaces [fomites]) or vectors, which are organisms that carry and transmit pathogens into another organism (mosquitos, ticks, fleas, etc).

It should be noted that the distinction between droplets and aerosols (see Figure 2.2) is not categorical, but rather determined by particle size (typically 5 microns [μm]), and that there is some debate about the cutoff mark between the two. However, droplets are usually defined as large particles and greater than 5 μm. Moreover, particles that fall in the twilight

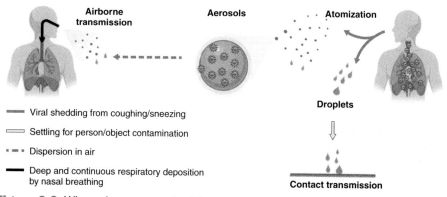

Figure 2.2 When viruses are shed from the respiratory tract of an infected individual, they may be transmitted by multiple routes. This illustration shows how the virus may be spread via aerosolized particles and larger droplets that tend to be quickly pulled down by gravity. (Illustration courtesy of Zhang R, Li Y, Zhang AL, Wang Y, Molina MJ. Identifying airborne transmission as the dominant route for the spread of COVID-19. *PNAS*. 2020;117(26):14857-14863. doi:10.1073/pnas.2009637117)

between aerosol and droplet can behave a bit like both. To elaborate, particles in the range of 5 to 20 μm are not only capable of lingering in the air for longer than their larger counterparts; they have also demonstrated some ability to penetrate deep into the alveolar tissues of the lower respiratory tract.[7] Despite these concerns, the World Health Organization (WHO) and the Centers for Disease Control and Prevention (CDC) have both maintained that the lower limit for droplet size is 5 μm.[7]

Person-to-Person Contact

Person-to-person transmission occurs when a pathogen is spread from one person to another. Person-to-person contact is when an infection occurs following physical contact with an infected person. Transmission may occur when body fluids are exchanged or through skin-to-skin contact. Sexually transmitted diseases represent the most notorious examples of pathogen spread through person-to-person contact but are by no means the only ones. Human rhinoviruses, for example, have been shown to spread very efficiently following hand-to-hand contact.[8]

Droplet

Droplet spread occurs when an individual has a respiratory infection and expels virions while talking, coughing, sneezing, or singing.[9] These virions travel within large droplets (>≈5 μm), and the distance and length of time they remain in the air depends on several factors, particularly relative humidity and temperature. Larger particles from the respiratory tract have been shown to travel farthest in environments with low temperatures and high levels of relative humidity.[10]

When an individual coughs or sneezes, very large droplets (measured in millimeters instead of microns) rarely travel more than 2 m. Consequently, many social distancing guidelines that were put in place recommended that people remain 2 m or 6 ft apart to prevent the spread of the coronavirus, which was initially believed to be transmitted primarily via large respiratory droplets.

Smaller droplets (ranging from 5 to 1000 μm) are capable of traveling beyond this range and in cool and humid conditions may travel up to 4.5 m (14.7 ft) or 8 m (26 ft) when an infected individual either coughs or sneezes, respectively.[7] It should be noted, however, that approximately 95% of virions carried by respiratory droplets travel 1.4 m (4.5 ft) or less even in extremely cool and humid conditions and that ventilation matters.[10] In outdoor settings, droplets dissipate relatively quickly, thereby making the risk of infection via this mode of transmission relatively low, particularly if individuals are more than 2 m apart. Risk is significantly higher when indoors, especially if the area is not well ventilated and is cool and damp. A preprint study found the odds of a primary case transmitting SARS-CoV-2 in a closed environment to be 18.7 times higher than in an open-air environment.[11] (In addition to dispersing the virus, being outdoors in the sunlight may be safer than the indoors because simulated sunlight has been found to inactivate SARS-CoV-2 in a matter of minutes.[12])

Infection occurs when virions are inhaled or make direct contact with mucous membranes (see Portal of Entry). In some cases, droplets from an infected individual may contaminate another individual's hands, and then cause infection if that person touches their eyes, nose, or mouth (hence the reason why good hand hygiene is so important). Droplets may also land on and contaminate surfaces. These contaminated surfaces are referred to as fomites.

Viruses typically do not survive on skin for very long. A sample of influenza A virus was found to survive for approximately 1.82 hours on a sample of human skin, while the same study showed that the SARS-CoV-2 virus survived on human skin for an average of 9 hours.[13] SARS-CoV-2 and influenza A virions have been shown to remain viable on stainless steel for upward of 72 hours.[14,15]

Airborne

Like droplet spread, airborne spread occurs when an infected individual expels virions while talking, singing, coughing, or sneezing, but this is not the sole manner in which aerosols are released. Certain medical procedures and fast-running water (particularly after toilet flushes) can produce aerosols, and these aerosols can provide a means of conveyance for virions. According to a scientific brief published by the WHO, medical procedures that can produce aerosols include "endotracheal intubation, bronchoscopy, open suctioning, administration of nebulized treatment, manual ventilation before intubation, turning the patient to the prone position, disconnecting the patient from the ventilator, noninvasive positive-pressure ventilation, tracheostomy, and cardiopulmonary resuscitation."[16]

As is the case with droplet transmission, the range of smaller, virus-laden particles is also affected by environmental conditions, but conversely, they spread farthest when temperatures are high and humidity levels are low.[10] They can also linger in the air for a matter of hours. SARS-CoV-2, for example, was found to remain viable in the air for 3 hours and to have a half-life as an aerosol of 1.1 hour.[15]

Like droplet spread, infection occurs when virus-laden aerosols are inhaled or make direct contact with mucous membranes.

Vehicles and Vectors

Vehicles refer to nonliving substances that can harbor virions or bacteria and indirectly spread disease. Some examples include contaminated surfaces (fomites), water, blood, and food. Vectors are living intermediaries that transmit bacteria or viruses. Bloodsucking insects, especially mosquitoes, ticks, and fleas, are some of the most common vectors and are responsible for the spread of the Zika virus, Lyme disease, and bubonic plague, respectively.

Portals

Portals refer to the point of entry and point of exit of a virus. They include the skin, the respiratory tract, the gastrointestinal tract, the genital tract, or through fluids like blood.

Portal of Exit

The portal of exit is the means through which a pathogen leaves a reservoir or host. The release of infectious virions from a host is known as the shedding of virus, and viruses are typically shed from the site of infection. Consequently, skin infections are spread by skin-to-skin contact; respiratory infections are shed via droplets or aerosols released through secretions that escape through the nose and mouth; and gastrointestinal viruses are shed when the host either vomits or has diarrhea, which allows the virus to be conveyed via aerosols or vehicles to a new host. If multiple types of tissues have been infected, then shedding can occur from multiple sites.[17]

Portal of Entry

Once a virus has been shed, it must then find a new and susceptible host. To infect this host, it must first pass through a portal of entry, oftentimes by exploiting a vulnerability in the host's epithelium—the protective layer of cells that line an organism's outer surface (its skin) and internal surfaces, including the respiratory tract, gastrointestinal (GI) tract, and genital tract. Natural defenses exist to prevent infection. The skin is made of a shield of dead cells that viruses cannot penetrate. The internal surfaces of the body—the GI tract, genital tract, and respiratory tract—are coated with a layer of mucus that traps pathogens and prevents them from reaching the epithelium below.

Viral transmission may also occur following the direct penetration of the skin due to an animal or insect bite, transplantation of a virally infected organ, or via placenta between mother and fetus.

Skin

The skin is composed of two layers of tissue: the epidermis and the dermis. The outer layer, the epidermis, is constantly being replaced by a new supply of cells from the inner layer, the dermis. As skin cells rise from the dermis layer, they become saturated with keratin filaments that are produced within the cell. Keratins are found in all vertebrates and form not just the outer layer of our skin but also our nails and hair. In other animals, keratins form horns, claws, and hooves for other animals.

As the cell keratinizes, it dies via programmed cell death (known as apoptosis) before reaching the epidermis, and then forms the outermost layer of the epidermis, which is known as the stratum corneum. This process, known as cornification, creates a physical barrier of dead cells (corneocytes) that pathogens cannot penetrate. As this layer of cells is no longer alive, viruses cannot use the intercellular mechanisms to replicate. However, viruses can gain entry to lower strata of the epidermis and dermis through abrasions or cuts, or they can be transported from the skin to a more permeable portal of entry, such as one's eyes, nose, or mouth.

Respiratory Tract

The respiratory tract includes the mouth, nose, throat, and lungs. Like other internal surfaces in the body, the respiratory epithelium is protected by a layer of mucus that traps pathogens, dust, and debris. Small structures known as cilia, which look like tiny hairs, then move in a sweeping motion to carry the debris-laden mucus away. Plentiful in the upper respiratory tract (nasal cavities, sinuses, pharynx, and larynx), cilia and mucus become increasingly less abundant as one moves deeper into the lower respiratory tract (trachea, bronchi, and, finally, the lungs). Pathogens that make it this deep into the respiratory tract and into the lungs are intercepted primarily by immune cells known as alveolar macrophages. Like sentries, they roam around the lungs looking for substances and pathogens that should not be there and eliminate them. They make up 95% of the white blood cells (leukocytes) that occupy airspace in the lungs.[18]

GI Tract

Much of the epithelia of the GI tract is also coated in a layer of mucus, including the mouth, esophagus, and stomach. Mucus in the latter protects the organ's lining from both pathogens and the acids produced to aid with digestion. The contents of the stomach then enter the small intestine for additional digestion and the absorption of nutrients through fingerlike projections known as villi, which are coated in membrane protrusions known as microvilli. These structures look like the teeth of a comb.

Villi and microvilli significantly increase the surface area of the intestinal epithelia to allow for more nutrient absorption, but they are also a potential liability because of increased exposure to potential viral or bacterial infections. To offer extra protection beyond mucus, the intestines possess a sophisticated defense network that relies on a healthy biota teeming with microbial life and an innate immune response system housed in the intestinal epithelia.[19] The large intestine and colon lack villi and microvilli but are home to a similar defense network of microorganisms and immune system cells.

Genital Tract

Viruses that are transmitted through the genital tract come almost solely from sexual activity. In addition to the mucosal lining of the male genital tract and the female genital tract, each system is home to a microenvironment that is regulated by microorganisms, sex hormones, and innate immune system defenses.[20]

Phases of Infection

From the time the pathogen invades the host, it rapidly multiplies and simultaneously the body's immune system mounts a defense to eliminate the infection (see Figure 2.3). In some cases, the body's immune system may clear the infection quickly enough so that the individual never experiences symptoms. The time period from the point of exposure to the onset of disease symptoms is known as the incubation period. Following this is the prodromal period, which is when early, nonspecific signs and symptoms emerge and before the major symptoms begin to affect the host. Some examples include flulike symptoms such as fatigue, muscle aches, fever, or congestion. Afterward is the illness period, which is when symptoms that are more specific to the disease present themselves. Usually, at this point, the immune system is highly active and mounts a defensive response to

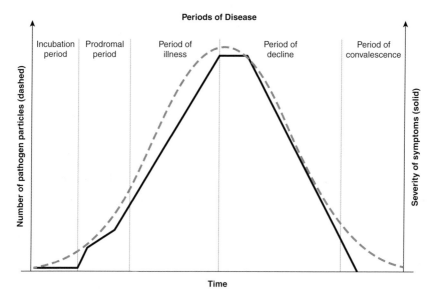

Figure 2.3 The severity of symptoms of an illness often correlates with the number of pathogens in the body.

decrease the viral load. Subsequently, the infection subsides and the host begins to feel better. This is known as the convalescent period. The length of each period is dependent on the virus.

There are two distinct immune systems that our body relies on to eliminate infections: the innate immune system and the adaptive immune system. The former is a vast network of nonspecific defense mechanisms present at birth that prevent infections from taking root. It may weaken with age, but it does not undergo significant changes. The innate immune system includes physical barriers, such as the skin and mucosa, as well as cells that work in concert to identify antigens (a substance the immune system does not recognize as part of the body) and eliminate any threats to the body before they can do any harm. The white blood cells (leukocytes) and alveolar macrophages described above are just one example of this vast, complex system.

The innate immune system is also activated when tissues are damaged due to an infection or physical trauma. Upon damage to a cell, the injured cell releases proteins known as cytokines that effectively alert the rest of the body of the trauma or infection and help mount and regulate an inflammatory response. If the site of the inflammation is near the surface of the skin, inflammation will often lead to visible redness and swelling as blood vessels dilate to bring more blood to the inflamed tissue. The increased flow of blood to the site of the inflammation makes it feel hot to the touch. While the pain associated with inflammation is undoubtedly unpleasant, it also suggests that there is an increased presence of blood at the site of the infection or trauma and that the innate immune system is eliminating the threat, clearing the site, and repairing any damaged cells. A viral infection may produce local inflammation, as well as more global physiological changes that produce the flu-like symptoms characterized by the prodromal period. In fact, this is a good thing since it means that our immune system is curtailing the spread of the viral infection.

However, should the infection persist, the adaptive immune system will be activated. This immune response may occur within a few days in younger and healthier people but may not be activated for over a week or longer in older individuals. Contrary to the innate immune system, the adaptive immune system learns to recognize specific antigens, and then creates proteins that can neutralize these threats. These proteins are known as antibodies, and they may continue to circulate in the blood after the infection has subsided. More importantly, the "blueprints" to create more antibodies are stored in memory cells, and should an infection caused by the same pathogen occur again, these antibodies can be called upon to quickly offer immune protection, though they may not always be activated quickly enough to prevent the spread of an infection or to keep individuals from experiencing symptoms of illness.

Unfortunately, viral antigens are not immutable. Viruses mutate through antigenic drift (small changes to antigens) and antigenic shift (larger changes to antigens). If the mutation is significant enough, the adaptive immune system will not recognize the antigen and will not be able to mount a rapid response to the infection, and the process of developing antibodies will have to start all over again.

As a prime example, the influenza A virus undergoes constant and rapid antigenic drift. Even within a single flu season, the initial wave of the virus may have a distinct genetic fingerprint from the virus in circulation months later. However, individuals who were infected with the early iteration of the virus are almost always protected from later iterations because the viral antigens between the two iterations are very similar and existing antibodies will recognize both. However, over the long-term, the minor changes caused by antigenic drift begin to accumulate, eventually leading to a virus that is distinct enough so that a person becomes susceptible to flu infection again because their antibodies are incapable of recognizing the new iteration of the virus.[21]

Infective Dose

If you inhale a single virion of SARS-CoV-2 or influenza A, there is a very small chance that you will become infected. To clarify: It is possible, but it is just not probable. The virion may not find a susceptible cell to infect, or the virus may be eradicated by the body's innate immune system before an infection can take root. As the number of virions introduced into the body increases, however, it also increases the risk that the innate immune system will be overwhelmed and that a sustained infection will result. In some cases, it may only take a few hundred or a few thousand individual virions to produce a sustained infection.

The lowest number of viruses needed to produce a sustained infection is known as the minimum infectious dose. Viruses with low minimum infectious doses are far more contagious than viruses with high minimum infectious doses, though a virus' minimum infectious dose is not constant across all modes of transmission.

Viral Load

Viral load is the amount of virus in an infected individual's blood. Once a cell is infected, a virus can reprogram it to start making thousands of new viruses in 12 to 24 hours. During a widespread infection, viral load can grow exponentially, and in just a few days, there may be millions or even billions of individual viruses in the blood. Viral load is frequently, but not always, correlated with symptom severity.

Cytokine Storm

There are two types of cytokines: proinflammatory and anti-inflammatory, which are regulating inflammatory responses and ensuring that inflammation occurs when it is needed and recedes once the threat has passed. In rare cases, the inflammatory response can go into overdrive, resulting in damage to healthy tissue. This exaggerated immune response may occur with or without the presence of a pathogen.

In the case of COVID-19, cytokine storm has been potentially implicated in the pathogenesis of acute respiratory distress syndrome, which can often lead to pulmonary dysfunction and death. This presents dilemmas in treatment since blocking cytokine signaling could mitigate the cytokine storm and suppress the immunoresponse to the virus, thereby inhibiting clearance of the SARS-CoV-2 and increase the risk of secondary infections.[22]

SARS-CoV-2 Transmission

SARS-CoV-2 is capable of infecting numerous types of mammals besides humans (see Figure 2.4). Natural infection has been reported in bats, pangolins, cats, dogs, minks, tigers, and lions, while experimental studies

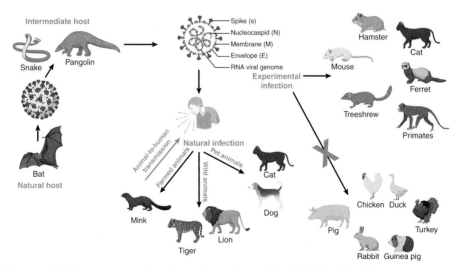

Figure 2.4 Numerous animals can be infected by SARS-CoV-2. (Illustration courtesy of Mahdy MAA, Younis W, Ewaida Z. An overview of SARS-CoV-2 and animal infection. *Front Vet Sci.* 2020;7:596391. doi:10.3389/fvets.2020.596391. Figure was created with BioRender.com)

have documented susceptibility in nonhuman primates, mice, hamsters, ferrets, and tree shrews.[23] Rabbits, guinea pigs, pigs, chickens, ducks, turkeys, geese, and Japanese quail do not appear to be susceptible to the virus.[23]

As discussed in the previous chapter, the details concerning the origin of the virus remain murky, and a purely zoonotic origin has not been confirmed. That said, bats are typically the natural hosts of coronaviruses that fall under the genera *Alphacoronavirus* and *Betacoronavirus*, and SARS-CoV-2 has been classified as a member of the *Betacoronavirus* genus. Whether via zoonotic transmission through an intermediary like a pangolin, a simple spillover event, or recombination (whether in the wild or in a laboratory), the virus responsible for the COVID-19 pandemic most likely can be traced back to a population of bats from a remote part of China or Southeast Asia.[24] In the event that it did escape from a laboratory, which remains highly speculative, there is zero evidence to support the idea that it was "weaponized" in some sinister way. Furthermore, while both a laboratory accident and natural spillover are possible, the most probable scenario remains zoonosis following an interface between a human and a wild animal.

Though SARS-CoV-2 can spread between animals and humans, the COVID-19 pandemic has been fueled by human-to-human spread, and an infective dose may be as low as just a few hundred virions.[25] Evidence of human-to-human spread is conclusive and has been noncontroversial since January 2020 though questions about the mode of transmission persist.[26]

From the beginning of the outbreak, it was presumed that droplet spread and person-to-person contact were the primary means of SARS-CoV-2 transmission. Consequently, social distancing guidelines were implemented to prevent these two types of transmission. As noted above, large droplets (measured in millimeters instead of microns) rarely travel for more than 2 m, and approximately 95% of virions carried by respiratory droplets travel 1.4 m or less even in the most conducive conditions.[10]

Airborne and fomite transmission were also believed to be possible.

Fomite Transmission

In February 2020, the WHO issued a statement claiming that it was possible for the virus to spread through contaminated surfaces (fomites). When a study was published in March 2020 showing that the virus could persist on plastic and stainless steel for days and cardboard for up 24 hours, this only caused more fear about the danger of contaminated surfaces and led more people to begin frantically disinfecting their households.[15] For a time, many families even left nonperishable grocery items outside their homes for days to prevent infection.[27] By May 2020, the WHO was recommending regular cleaning and disinfecting of surfaces, especially those that were frequently touched. Evidence clearly showed that traces of coronavirus RNA remained on surfaces, oftentimes for weeks, after an infected person had been in the vicinity. One of the most notable examples occurred when researchers boarded the *Diamond Princess*, the infamous ship that was momentarily home to more than half the world's known COVID-19 cases outside of China in early February 2020 and found viral RNA on surfaces in cabins 17 days after all passengers had been vacated.[28,29] Other studies within hospitals and outpatient settings found viral RNA on places like doorknobs, faucet handles, and other places that people regularly touch.[30]

While there is no doubt that researchers have found viral RNA on a wide variety of surfaces, this does indicate the presence of infective virions. In one study, a total of 46% of the samples taken from Assuta Ashdod University Hospital in Israel had been contaminated by viral RNA. However, the authors could not isolate viable SARS-CoV-2 virions.[30] "The viral RNA is the equivalent of the corpse of the virus," Emmanuel Goldman, a microbiologist at Rutgers New Jersey Medical School in Newark, told *Nature*'s Dyani Lewis in an article published in January 2021. "It's not infectious."[29]

This is not to say that fomite transmission is impossible. Under the right circumstances, it can happen, but the evidence that we have today suggests the risk of transmission by this route is relatively low in real-life conditions.[31] In October 2020, the WHO updated its guidance on the matter, saying that fomite transmission is "not thought to be a common way that COVID-19 spreads."[29]

While there is certainly nothing wrong with regularly cleaning spaces that become crowded or see steady daily usage, it does require a lot of resources, and reserving resources is something that becomes necessary in the midst of a pandemic. As evidence of the infrequency of fomite transmission has mounted, many have become critical of dedicating significant labor hours to preventing what appears to be a rare mode of transmission. Despite these criticisms of "hygiene theater," the practice continues to be a regular occurrence in a variety of public spaces, particularly in crowded facilities, places with significant pedestrian traffic, and on public transportation.

Airborne Transmission

The WHO maintains that SARS-CoV-2 is spread primarily via person-to-person contact or large droplets and has acknowledged that there is evidence suggesting airborne transmission. However, it is not clear if it is the primary means through which the virus is spread or if it is a secondary means.

The evidence in favor of airborne transmission is strong. Given that the threshold between an aerosol and a droplet is 5 μm and that the estimate of the minimum size of a respiratory particle containing virions is 4.7 μm, this would mean that airborne spread is possible.[32] Additionally, multiple studies have ruled out any other form of transmission besides airborne spread at multiple superspreading events (one of the earliest and most infamous of which occurred during a rehearsal of the Skagit Valley Chorale on March 10, 2020, at which one index case infected an estimated 32-52 [53%-87%] of the 60 individuals in attendance[9]), and there is evidence suggesting the existence of a fecal-oral route of transmission via particles aerosolized after toilet flushes.[33] In addition, there is evidence of airborne transmission following medical procedures,[7] as well as long-range transmission, which has been documented in quarantine hotels. Of note, there has been no direct evidence to refute the hypothesis of airborne transmission.[34]

The central argument against airborne transmission as a common route of transmission is that secondary attack rates (SARs) (the number of new cases among contacts divided by the total number of contacts) within households are far lower than they would be if SARS-CoV-2 were spread primarily by aerosols. Known airborne viruses are believed to have extremely high SARs. In the case of measles, for example, the SAR is above 90% within a household setting. A systematic review and meta-analysis of 54 relevant studies with 77,758 participants published in 2020 by Madewell and colleagues focusing on the SAR of SARS-CoV-2 within households during times of quarantine (when household units would be least mobile and exposure rates would hypothetically be at their highest) estimated that the overall SAR to be only 16.6%.[35] This is significantly higher than SARS-CoV (7.5%) and MERS-CoV (4.7%), but far lower than measles. The study also found that rates were more than twice as high among spouses (37.8%) than other family members (17.8%), suggesting that proximity plays a significant role in transmission.[35] The study seems to indicate that airborne transmission is possible but that it is not the primary means of transmission. Variants appear to have higher SARs. In a 2021 study, Madewell and colleagues noted that the SAR of SARS-CoV-2 was higher between October 2020 and June 2021 than the period under review for their first study (from the beginning of the outbreak through October 2020). They estimated that the updated household SAR is 18.9% and that the SAR of the Alpha variant is 24.5%.[36] The SAR of the Delta variant is estimated to be 20% in some settings (eg, gymnastics facility) and as high as 53% in household settings.[37] This increase in transmissibility is believed to be due to the increased viral loads of individuals infected with the Delta variant, as described in a preprint study by Li and colleagues.[38]

In sum, evidence suggests that the virus spreads via person-to-person contact and through a range of particle sizes that includes those that fall under definitions of "large droplet" and "aerosol."[39]

Viral Shedding

Viral shedding is believed to start early with SARS-CoV-2, oftentimes before symptoms have become discernible. Before the Delta variant became common, shedding was estimated to begin 0.8 days prior to the emergence of symptoms. For individuals infected with the Delta variant, shedding is believed to begin around 1.8 days before symptom onset and 4 days after infection.[40] Viral load appears to peak either shortly before or shortly after symptom onset.[25] As a higher viral load is likely associated with more viral shedding, this suggests transmission is more likely to occur in these early stages of the disease. Furthermore, since several preliminary studies (none peer-reviewed) indicate that vaccinated individuals and unvaccinated individuals carry similar viral loads, this suggests comparable contagiousness.[41]

As noted in the previous chapter, asymptomatic individuals are believed to account for as many as 59% of all transmissions, a figure which includes individuals in the presymptomatic stage of the disease. Transmission during this stage has been estimated to be in the range of 35% to 44%.[42,43] This figure is believed to be even higher in areas where the Delta variant is the predominate strain, with at least one study finding that 74% of Delta variant infections take place during the presymptomatic phase.[40] Since high viral loads can occur in asymptomatic infections, it is safe to say that high viral load is not necessarily correlated with more severe symptoms.[25] This conclusion has been buttressed by observations that the Delta variant produces a viral load in infected individuals that is many times higher than the original strain of SARS-CoV-2 but is not associated with an equally comparable increase in disease severity (ie, the Delta variant may be more deadly than the original strain, but it is not many times more deadly).[41]

After viral load peaks either in the presymptomatic phase or within a few days of symptom onset, it then steadily declines as the antibody response is ramped up (see Figure 2.5). Viral cultures created from PCR positive upper respiratory tract samples have been found to typically yield positive results for up to 9 days following symptom onset.[44] Prolonged shedding appears to occur in more severe cases. RNA has been detected in the upper respiratory tract for a mean of 17 days (maximum 83 days) following symptom onset using quantitative reverse transcription polymerase chain reaction technology, but, as noted above, the presence of viral RNA is not necessarily indicative of the presence of infective virions or infectiousness.[44]

As noted above, infections have been reported that would seem to indicate the possibility of a fecal-oral route, suggesting that fecal shedding of the virus is possible. In support of this hypothesis, nearly half of patients confirmed to have COVID-19 have detectible levels of viral RNA in stool samples, and virions have

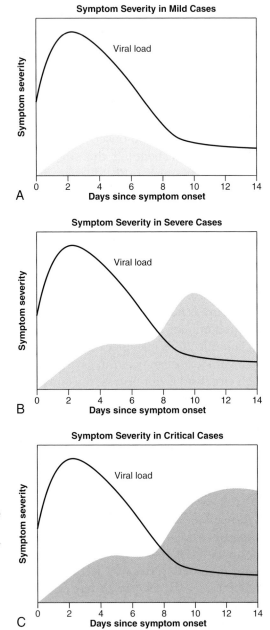

Figure 2.5 Viral load and time since symptom onset for mild (A), severe (B), and critical (C) cases. Note that emerging evidence suggests that patients infected with the Delta variant may become symptomatic within an average of just 4 days.[38] (Illustration courtesy of Cevik M, Kuppalli K, Kindrachuk J, Peiris M. Virology, transmission, and pathogenesis of SARS-CoV-2. *BMJ.* 2020;371:m3862. doi:10.1136/bmj.m3862)

demonstrated the ability to survive in simulated environments that parallel the human GI tract. In addition, several studies have isolated viable SARS-CoV-2 viruses from feces.[45] Additionally, ACE2 receptors and type II transmembrane serine protease are highly expressed in intestinal epithelial cells, meaning they are susceptible to SARS-CoV-2 infection.[17]

Though it seems rather certain that infection of the GI tract does occur, it is not clear how common or severe these infections are, or how long they persist. Furthermore, questions about the extent of fecal viral shedding remain unresolved.

Masks

One of the most controversial social issues to emerge from the pandemic was the case for and against wearing cloth masks to prevent the spread of the coronavirus. There were limited data on their efficacy at the beginning of the pandemic and guidelines issued by the CDC did frequently and drastically change, giving the impression that the rules were somewhat arbitrary and capricious.

In time, though, data did reveal that cloth masks, and especially medical-grade masks, can reduce the chances of transmitting or catching the virus.[46] There is even some evidence to suggest that wearing a mask can reduce the severity of an infection because it reduces the level of virions to which one is exposed at the time of infection. The central premise of this argument is that initial exposure to only a few hundred virions, while enough to constitute an infective inoculum, causes a less severe infection than exposure to several thousand virions. As N95 respirators are designed to protect the wearer by filtering out 95% of airborne particles measuring 0.3 µm and larger, and the minimum size of a respiratory particle that contains SARS-CoV-2 virions is 4.7 µm,[32] this would mean that wearing an N95 mask (correctly) significantly reduces the number of virions that can access portals of entry to the respiratory tract, thereby reducing the risk of severe infection.[47]

Predictably, cloth masks and disposable masks offer less protection than N95 respirators but can still inhibit community spread and may be used by the general public when proper medical masks are not available. Cloth masks should be made of three layers and should be washed daily.[48] Wet masks are less effective at filtering particles than dry masks.[48]

Prior to the approval of the Pfizer-BioNTech vaccine for emergency use authorization on December 11, 2020, the WHO website recommended medical masks for:

- Health workers in clinical settings.
- Anyone aged 60 years or above.
- Immunocompromised individuals or anyone with an underlying health condition associated with severe COVID-19:
  - Cancer
  - Cardiovascular disease
  - Chronic respiratory disease

- Diabetes mellitus
- Obesity
- Individuals with flulike symptoms (muscle aches, dry cough, fatigue, etc).
- Individuals who have received positive COVID-19 test results or are awaiting test results.
- People caring for individuals who are suspected of having COVID-19 or who have tested positive for COVID-19.[49]

As vaccination efforts progressed, the CDC became less strict in their guidance for appropriate masking. On April 27, 2021, the agency relaxed the rules on wearing masks in outdoor settings and said that vaccinated Americans can safely go without a mask unless in crowded outdoor venues like stadiums.[50] Just over 2 weeks later, on May 13, the CDC further relaxed masking guidelines for fully vaccinated individuals, saying that masks were no longer necessary in indoor settings except on public transit, in clinical settings, or in a handful of other places unless required by state or local ordinance.[51]

Unfortunately, these policies appear to have underestimated the transmissibility of the Delta variant, as well as its ability to quickly reproduce and spread even among vaccinated individuals. The unwillingness of large parts of the general public to get vaccinated has also led to surges in the virus. Consequently, on July 27, 2021, the CDC began recommending that even people who are fully vaccinated wear masks indoors if they are in an area of substantial or high transmission.[52] This includes all children over the age of 2.

Conclusion

SARS-CoV-2 appears to be primarily spread by person-to-person contact and through respiratory particles that range in size from aerosol (<5 µm) to large droplet (>5 µm). Social distancing guidelines were put in place to prevent the spread of the virus via person-to-person contact and larger respiratory particles. Masks also were recommended to reduce the chances of transmitting or catching the virus after breathing in respiratory particles discharged from infected individuals.

Viral load does not appear to be correlated with more severe COVID-19 symptoms. Higher viral load is, however, associated with increased viral shedding. As viral load is highest just before or at the onset of the prodromal period, individuals may be at their most contagious before they have developed symptoms—if they develop symptoms at all—and 59% of all transmissions are believed to have come from individuals without symptoms.

REFERENCES

1. Olival KJ, Hosseini PR, Zambrana-Torrelio C, Ross N, Bogich TL, Daszak P. Host and viral traits predict zoonotic spillover from mammals. *Nature*. 2017;546:646-650. doi:10.1038/nature22975
2. Zimmer C. Welcome to the virosphere. *New York Times*. Published March 24, 2020. Accessed May 28, 2021. https://www.nytimes.com/2020/03/24/science/viruses-coranavirus-biology.html
3. Asjo B, Kruse H. Zoonoses in the emergence of human viral diseases. *Perspect Med Virol*. 2006;16:15-41. doi:10.1016/S0168-7069(06)16003-6
4. Wolfe ND, Daszak P, Kilpatrick AM, Burke DS. Bushmeat hunting, deforestation, and prediction of zoonotic disease. *Emerg Infect Dis*. 2005;11(12):1822-1827. doi:10.3201/eid1112.040789
5. Vlasova AN, Diaz A, Damtie D, et al. Novel canine coronavirus isolated from a hospitalized pneumonia patient, East Malaysia. *Clin Infect Dis*. 2021:ciab456. doi:10.1093/cid/ciab456
6. Lednicky JA, Tagliamonte MS, White SK, et al. Emergence of porcine delta-coronavirus pathogenic infections among children in Haiti through independent zoonoses and convergent evolution. Preprint. Posted online March 19, 2021. medRxiv 21253391. doi:10.1101/2021.03.19.21253391
7. Jayaweera M, Perera H, Gunawardana B, Manatunge J. Transmission of COVID-19 virus by droplets and aerosols: a critical review on the unresolved dichotomy. *Environ Res*. 2020;188:109819. doi:10.1016/j.envres.2020.109819
8. Gwaltney JM Jr, Moskalski PB, Hendley JO. Hand-to-hand transmission of rhinovirus colds. *Ann Intern Med*. 1978;88(4):463-467. doi:10.7326/0003-4819-88-4-463
9. Miller SL, Nazaroff WW, Jimenez JL, et al. Transmission of SARS-CoV-2 by inhalation of respiratory aerosol in the Skagit Valley Chorale superspreading event. *Indoor Air*. 2021;31(2):314-323. doi:10.1111/ina.12751. Epub 2020 Oct 13
10. Zhao L, Qi Y, Luzzatto-Fegiz P, Cui Y, Zhu Y. COVID-19: effects of environmental conditions on the propagation of respiratory droplets. *Nano Lett*. 2020;20(10):7744-7750. doi:10.1021/acs.nanolett.0c03331
11. Nishiura H, Oshitani H, Kobayashi T, et al. Closed environments facilitate secondary transmission of coronavirus disease 2019 (COVID-19). Preprint 2020. Posted online April 16, 2020. medRxiv. doi:10.1101/2020.02.28.20029272
12. Ratnesar-Shumate S, Williams G, Green B, et al. Simulated sunlight rapidly inactivates SARS-CoV-2 on surfaces. *J Infect Dis*. 2020;222(2):214-222. doi:10.1093/infdis/jiaa274
13. Hirose R, Ikegaya H, Naito Y, et al. Survival of severe acute respiratory syndrome coronavirus 2 (SARS-CoV-2) and influenza virus on human skin: importance of hand hygiene in coronavirus disease 2019 (COVID-19). *Clin Infect Dis*. 2020:ciaa1517. doi:10.1093/cid/ciaa1517
14. Boone SA, Gerba CP. Significance of fomites in the spread of respiratory and enteric viral disease. *Appl Environ Microbiol*. 2007;73(6):1687-1696. doi:10.1128/AEM.02051-06
15. van Doremalen N, Bushmaker T, Morris DH, et al. Aerosol and surface stability of SARS-CoV-2 as compared with SARS-CoV-1. *N Engl J Med*. 2020;382(16):1564-1567. doi:10.1056/NEJMc2004973
16. World Health Organization (WHO). *Modes of Transmission of Virus Causing COVID-19: Implications for IPC Precaution Recommendations*. March 27, 2020. Accessed May 13, 2021. https://www.who.int/news-room/commentaries/detail/modes-of-transmission-of-virus-causing-covid-19-implications-for-ipc-precaution-recommendations
17. Jiao L, Li H, Xu J, et al. The gastrointestinal tract is an alternative route for SARS-CoV-2 infection in a nonhuman primate model. *Gastroenterology*. 2021;160(5):1647-1661. doi:10.1053/j.gastro.2020.12.001
18. Martin TR, Frevent CW. Innate immunity in the lungs. *Proc Am Thorac Soc*. 2005;2(5):403-411. doi:10.1513/pats.200508-090JS
19. Shi N, Li N, Duan X, Niu H. Interaction between the gut microbiome and mucosal immune system. *Mil Med Res*. 2017;4:14. doi:10.1186/s40779-017-0122-9

20. Nguyen P, Kafka J, Ferreira V, et al. Innate and adaptive immune responses in male and female reproductive tracts in homeostasis and following HIV infection. *Cell Mol Immunol.* 2014;11(5):410-427. doi:10.1038/cmi.2014.41

21. Centers for Disease Control and Prevention. *How the Flu Virus Can Change: "Drift" and "shift."* CDC website. Updated October 15, 2019. Accessed May 31, 2021. https://www.cdc.gov/flu/about/viruses/change.htm

22. Fajgenbaum DC, June CH. Cytokine storm. *N Engl J Med.* 2020;383(23):2255-2273. doi:10.1056/NEJMra2026131

23. Mahdy MAA, Younis W, Ewaida Z. An overview of SARS-CoV-2 and animal infection. *Front Vet Sci.* 2020;7:596391. doi:10.3389/fvets.2020.596391

24. Zhou H, Ji J, Chen X, et al. Identification of novel bat coronaviruses sheds light on the evolutionary origins of SARS-CoV-2 and related viruses. Preprint. Posted online August 3, 2021. bioRxiv 434390. doi:10.1101/2021.03.08.434390

25. Karimzadeh S, Bhopal R, Huy NT. Review of infective dose, routes of transmission and outcome of COVID-19 caused by the SARS-CoV-2: comparison with other respiratory viruses. *Epidemiol Infect.* 2021;149:e96. doi:10.1017/S0950268821000790

26. Kuo L. *China Confirms Human-to-Human Transmission of Coronavirus.* The Guardian. January 20, 2020. Accessed May 14, 2021. https://www.theguardian.com/world/2020/jan/20/coronavirus-spreads-to-beijing-as-china-confirms-new-cases

27. Lofton J. *Michigan Doctor Says Leave Groceries Outside for 3 Days if Possible, Shows How to Disinfect.* MLive website. Published March 25, 2020. Updated March 28, 2020. Accessed May 6, 2021. https://www.mlive.com/coronavirus/2020/03/michigan-doctor-says-leave-groceries-outside-for-3-days-if-possible-shows-how-to-disinfect.html

28. Baraniuk C. What the Diamond Princess taught the world about COVID-19. *BMJ.* 2020;369:m1632. doi:10.1136/bmj.m1632

29. Lewis D. COVID-19 rarely infects through surfaces. So why are we still deep cleaning? *Nature.* 2021;590(7844):26-28. doi:10.1038/d41586-021-00251-4

30. Ben-Shmuel A, Brosh-Nissimov T, Glinert I, et al. Detection and infectivity potential of severe acute respiratory syndrome coronavirus 2 (SARS-CoV-2) environmental contamination in isolation units and quarantine facilities. *Clin Microbiol Infect.* 2020;26(12):1658-1662. doi:10.1016/j.cmi.2020.09.004

31. Mondelli MU, Colaneri M, Seminari EM, Baldanti F, Bruno R. Low risk of SARS-CoV-2 transmission by fomites in real-life conditions. *Lancet Infect Dis.* 2021;21(5):E112. doi:10.1016/S1473-3099(20)30678-2

32. Lee BU. Minimum sizes of respiratory particles carrying SARS-CoV-2 and the possibility of aerosol generation. *Int J Environ Res Public Health.* 2020;17(19):6960. doi:10.3390/ijerph17196960

33. Kang M, Wei J, Yuan J, et al. Probable evidence of fecal aerosol transmission of SARS-CoV-2 in a high-rise building. *Ann Intern Med.* 2020;173(12)974-980. doi:10.7326/M20-0928

34. Greenhalgh T, Jimenez JL, Prather KA, Tufekci Z, Fisman D, Schooley R. Ten scientific reasons in support of airborne transmission of SARS-CoV-2. *Lancet.* 2021;397(10285):1603-1605. doi:10.1016/S0140-6736(21)00869-2

35. Madewell ZJ, Yang Y, Longini IM Jr, Halloran ME, Dean NE. Household transmission of SARS-CoV-2: a systematic review and meta-analysis. *JAMA Netw Open.* 2020;3(12):e2031756. doi:10.1001/jamanetworkopen.2003.31756

36. Madewell ZJ, Yang Y, Longini IM Jr, Halloran ME, Dean NE. Factors associated with household transmission of SARS-CoV-2: an updated systematic review and meta-analysis. *JAMA Netw Open.* 2021;4(8):e2122240. 10.1001/jamanetworkopen.2021.22240

37. Dougherty K, Mannell M, Naqvi O, Matson D, Stone J. SARS-CoV-2 B.1.617.2 (Delta) variant COVID-19 outbreak associated with a gymnastics facility – Oklahoma, April-May 2021. *MMWR Morb Mortal Wkly Rep.* 2021;70(28):1004-1007. doi:10.1101/2021.04.23.21255515

38. Li B, Deng A, Li K, et al. Viral infection and transmission in a large, well-traced outbreak caused by the SARS-CoV-2 Delta variant. Preprint. Posted online July 23, 2021. medRxiv. Accessed August 19, 2021. doi:10.1101/2021.07.07.21260122

39. Tang JW, Bahnfleth WP, Bluyssen PM, et al. Dismantling myths on the airborne transmission of severe acute respiratory syndrome coronavirus-2 (SARS-CoV-2). *J Hosp Infect*. 2021;110:89-96. doi:10.1016/j.jhin.2020.12.022

40. Mallapaty S. Delta's rise is fueled by rampant spread from people who feel fine. *Nature*. Published August 19, 2021. Accessed August 20, 2021. https://www.nature.com/articles/d41586-021-02259-2

41. Mishra S. Why is Delta more infectious and deadly? New research holds answers. *National Geographic*. Published August 6, 2021. Accessed August 19, 2021. https://www.nationalgeographic.com/science/article/why-is-delta-more-infectious-and-deadly-new-research-holds-answers?loggedin=true

42. Johansson MA, Quandelacy TM, Kada S, et al. SARS-CoV-2 transmission from people without COVID-19 symptoms. *JAMA Netw Open*. 2021;4(1):e2035057. doi:10.1001/jamanetworkopen.2020.35057

43. He X, Lau EH, Wu P, et al. Temporal dynamics in viral shedding and transmissibility of COVID-19. *Nat Med*. 2020;26(5):672-675. doi:10.1038/s41591-020-0869-5

44. Wölfel R, Corman VM, Guggemos W, et al. Virological assessment of hospitalized patients with COVID-2019. *Nature*. 2020;581(7809):465-469. doi:10.1038/s41586-020-2196-x

45. Guo M, Tao W, Flavell RA, Zhu S. Potential intestinal infection and faecal-oral transmission of SARS-CoV-2. *Nat Rev Gastroenterol Hepatol*. 2021;18(4):269-283. doi:10.1038/s41575-021-00416-6

46. Chang Y, Ma N, Witt C, et al. Face masks effectively limit the probability of SARS-CoV-2 transmission. *Science*. 2021;372:1439-1443. doi:10.1126/science.abg6296

47. Gandhi M, Beyrer C, Goosby E. Masks do more than protect others during COVID-19: reducing the inoculum of SARS-CoV-2 to protect the wearer. *J Gen Intern Med*. 2020;35(10):3063-3066. doi:10.1007/s11606-020-06067-8

48. Chughtai AA, Seale H, Macintyre R. Effectiveness of cloth masks for protection against severe acute respiratory syndrome coronavirus 2. *Emerg Infect Dis*. 2020;26(10):1-5. doi:10.3201/eid2610.200948

49. World Health Organization. *Coronavirus Disease (COVID-19): Masks*. World Health Organization. Updated December 1, 2020. Accessed May 31, 2021. https://www.who.int/news-room/q-a-detail/coronavirus-disease-covid-19-masks#:~:text=Fabric%20masks%20should%20be%20made,polyester%20or%20polyester%20blend

50. Stolberg SG, Rabin RC. C.D.C. eases outdoor mask guidance for vaccinated Americans. *New York Times*. Updated May 13, 2021. Accessed May 31, 2021. https://www.nytimes.com/2021/04/27/us/politics/coronavirus-masks-outdoors.html

51. Gupta S, Saey TH, Garcia de Jesús E. The CDC's changes to mask guidelines raised questions. Here are 6 answers. *Science News*. Published May 24, 2021. Accessed May 31, 2021. https://www.sciencenews.org/article/cdc-mask-guideline-question-answer-coronavirus-covid-pandemic

52. Centers for Disease Control and Prevention. *Your Guide to Masks*. CDC website. Updated August 13, 2021. Accessed August 19, 2021. https://www.cdc.gov/coronavirus/2019-ncov/prevent-getting-sick/about-face-coverings.html

3

Pathology—What We Knew and What We Know

The pathology of COVID-19 has been the most perplexing aspect of the pandemic. In early 2020, severe acute respiratory syndrome coronavirus 2 (SARS-CoV-2) infection was thought to be localized in the respiratory system and, to a lesser extent, the gastrointestinal (GI) tract. Reported symptoms of coronavirus disease of 2019 (COVID-19) included GI problems (diarrhea, nausea, vomiting, etc) and, oftentimes, severe respiratory problems, particularly pneumonia. Mild cases often include flulike symptoms and others that affect the GI tract. More severe cases of the disease are found to follow a biphasic pattern that begins with an early viral response and an inflammatory secondary phase that can often prove fatal due to aberrant immunoresponse and subsequent complications involving cytokine storm, coagulopathy, acute respiratory distress syndrome (ARDS), multiple organ dysfunction syndrome (MODS), sepsis, and death. In this chapter, I will explore the typical course COVID-19, the symptoms associated with the disease and some of its risk factors and long-term effects.

Pathogenesis

As noted in the previous chapter (*Chapter 2: Transmission of SARS-CoV-2*), SARS-CoV-2 is transmitted through respiratory particles and the virus is believed to first infect the epithelium of the respiratory tract. Larger particles laden with the virus (droplets) infect the upper respiratory tract, while smaller particles laden with the virus (aerosols) can infect the lower respiratory tract. Moreover, the virus can also infect the epithelium of the intestines.[1]

COVID-19 develops following SARS-CoV-2 infection. The median incubation period for COVID-19 is estimated to be 5.1 days and 97.5% of individuals who develop symptoms do so within 11.5 days of infection.[2] For individuals infected with the Delta variant, the median incubation period is estimated to be only 4 days, as the virus is believed to replicate far more rapidly than ancestral strains.[3] The Chinese Center for Disease Control and Prevention examined 44,500 confirmed infections and found that 81% of individuals experienced mild or asymptomatic cases, 14% of individuals developed severe disease, 5% of patients became critical, and 2.3% of all cases resulted in a fatality.[4] All fatalities in this study occurred in critical cases.

Since that study's publication, fatality rates have dropped considerably as health care workers have learned how to better treat COVID-19. A retrospective study that relied on a national surveillance database in England and included approximately 21,000 critical care patients with COVID-19 found that survival rates in intensive care units improved from 58% in late March 2020 to 80% by June 2020.[5] As of this writing, the fatality rate is believed to be in the vicinity of 0.9% to 1.0%.[6]

As discussed in Chapter 1 (particularly *Viruses*), SARS-CoV-2 attaches to angiotensin-converting enzyme 2 (ACE2) receptors with its spike protein once it has been primed and cleaved by transmembrane protease serine (TMPRSS) and/or furin, which is a ubiquitous membrane protein.[7] Both ACE2 receptors and TMPRSS are coexpressed in the epithelia of the respiratory tract and alveolar cells, GI tract, and many other locations throughout the body, including major organs like the heart and kidneys.[8] Infection of the GI tract can lead to symptoms of GI pain, nausea, diarrhea, and vomiting, while infection in the respiratory tract give rise to symptoms such as congestion, sore throat, and cough. ACE2 receptors are also expressed in the olfactory neuroepithelium, the infection of which may result in abnormalities in sense of smell and taste without nasal inflammation.[9] There is also evidence to suggest that SARS-CoV-2 can bind to neuropilin-1 (NRP1) receptors, which are also expressed in olfactory neuroepithelium and olfactory neurons, as well as in lung tissue, and may increase SARS-CoV-2 infectivity.[10] Several variants, particularly the Delta variant, have mutated in such a way that allows them to more easily invade host cells and bind to ACE2 receptors.[11]

Disease Spectrum of COVID-19

In mild infections (approximately 81% of all cases), patients experience either no symptoms or symptoms comparable to mild cases of the flu. In the vast majority of mild cases, particularly in younger individuals, symptoms can be managed and treated without the need for hospitalization. Symptoms include taste and smell disturbances, malaise, myalgia, headache, dry cough, and fever. Symptoms may also include enteric symptoms like diarrhea, abdominal pain, nausea, and vomiting. Most patients recover within one to 2 weeks, though some may develop post-acute sequelae of SARS-CoV-2 (PASC), which is more popularly known as long COVID (see *Chapter 4: Neuropsychiatric Symptoms and Postacute Sequelae of SARS-CoV-2—The Long Haulers*).

In approximately 19% of cases, the infection spreads deeper into the lower respiratory tract, affecting bilateral lobes of the lung and causing pneumonia, which typically occurs over the course of about 10 days.[12] More importantly, the histopathologic findings have determined the predominant lung pathology to be diffuse alveolar damage (DAD) characterized by hyaline membrane formation.[13] These phenomena are known as ground-glass opacities, since the infected areas of the lungs may look hazy or shadowy when seen on a computed tomography (CT) scan (see Figure 3.1).

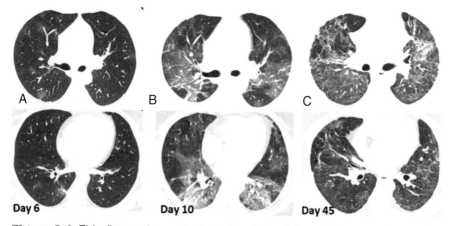

Figure 3.1 This figure shows the initial and two follow-up computed tomographic (CT) images of a 31-year-old male patient. The two lines represent two distinct cross sections. In A (Day 6 of infection), scattered ground glass opacities (GGO) can be observed in the subpleural area. In B (Day 10), the GGO have begun to consolidate bilaterally. In C (Day 45), remission is evident, but fibrous stripes and interstitial thickening persist. (Courtesy of Zhang Q, Xiong Y, Wu T, Zhu W. Very fast-progressive pulmonary opacities and high inflammatory factors levels are associated with decease of young Coronavirus Disease 2019 patients. *Medicine*. 2021;100(7):e24668.)

As the infection spreads and the pneumonia becomes more severe, the resultant lung parenchymal damage and pulmonary fibrosis, patients may experience decreased oxygen saturation and low blood oxygen levels (hypoxia). In rare cases, some patients' oxygen levels may fall dangerously low even if they do not feel particularly ill (a condition is known as silent hypoxia), though most patients experience shortness of breath (dyspnea) when in a hypoxic state. Silent hypoxia has been described as especially dangerous for patients because their condition may deteriorate significantly before seeking medical care and lead to poor prognosis.[14] Patients who are experiencing hypoxia and pneumonia may need supplemental oxygen or even require ventilator support. It is worth noting that hypoxia is associated with blood clot risk and is one of several factors contributing to the increased risk of ischemic stroke in COVID-19 patients, even in those who are otherwise healthy.[15] An overactive cytokine response is yet another factor that can contribute to coagulopathy and other complications. It has also been theorized that a persistent enteric infection may worsen viremia and further exacerbate cytokine response.[16]

In 5% of cases, aberrant host immune response results in a surge of proinflammatory cytokines, thereby leading to severe complications, particularly pulmonary edema and ARDS, which may result in respiratory failure and death.[17] Patients with severe and critical COVID-19 symptoms have tested positive for elevated levels of myriad cytokines (see Table 3.1), and elevated cytokine levels can also sometimes cause mucus hypersecretion, thereby leading to the formation of mucus plugs. As the name suggests, these plug up airways and make it difficult for patients to breathe.[8]

Damage caused by the inflammatory response is not restricted to the lungs. In severe cases, the acute inflammatory response ultimately affects other organs and can lead to MODS, sepsis, and death.[19] A combination of hypoxia, cytokine storm, and infection of heart tissue (ACE2 is highly expressed in cardiomyocytes) may lead to myocardial injury, which appears to be associated with a worse prognosis, especially in those with preexisting heart conditions.[19] Cardiac injury via myocyte necrosis, predominantly in the left ventricle, has also been reported.[20]

Acute kidney injury (AKI) (also known as acute renal failure [ARF]) occurs in up to half of those hospitalized with COVID-19 and is even more common among those who are admitted to intensive care units.[21] COVID-19 patients with kidney injury are reportedly five times more likely to suffer in-hospital mortality when compared with patients without AKI.[19] While renal failure has not been publicized as a major feature of SARS-CoV-2, the risk of severe kidney damage is well documented in other coronaviruses, particularly Middle Eastern respiratory syndrome (MERS).[22] Of note,

TABLE 3.1 Proinflammatory Cytokines Observed in Severe COVID-19 Patients[18]

Interleukin (IL) 1-β

IL-1RA

IL-6

IL-7

IL-8

IL-9

IL-10

Interferon-γ (IFNγ)

Interferon-inducible protein 10 (IP10)

Basic fibroblast growth factor 2 (b FGF2)

Granulocyte colony-stimulating factor (GCSF)

Granulocyte macrophage colony-stimulating factor (GMCSF)

Macrophage inflammatory proteins 1α (MIP1α)

MIP1ß

Monocyte chemoattractant protein-1 (MCP1)

Platelet-derived growth factor ß (PDGFß)

Tumor necrosis factor-α (TNF-α)

Vascular endothelial growth factor-A (VEGFA)

ACE2 receptors are expressed in kidney tissue and may suffer direct damage from infection, though computed tomography have also found renal abnormalities suggestive of inflammation and edema, but so far the exact mechanism remains unclear.[23] As a result of the kidney failure, some patients may require routine dialysis even after the initial infection has passed.[19]

Severity of infection has been associated with liver damage and increased levels of liver enzymes (alanine aminotransferase [ALT] and aspartate aminotransferase [AST]). Temporary liver damage has been reported in even mild infections and patients with preexisting liver comorbidities may have a heightened risk of complications. ACE2 receptors are also expressed in liver tissue suggesting that direct infection may be responsible for damage, though it is also possible that a combination of hypoxia and inflammatory responses may play a role in COVID-19–induced liver injury.[24]

As noted above, COVID-19 can trigger abnormal coagulation leading to microthrombi in tissues and cause ischemia.[18] Elevated levels of D-dimer, a breakdown product of fibrin, have been frequently reported in severe and critical cases, while D-dimer levels remain relatively static in individuals who experience mild symptoms. Consequently, D-dimer has been proposed as a biomarker to evaluate the prognosis of patients.[25] Prolonged prothrombin time has also been reported in severe cases of COVID-19 and may serve as a biomarker, as well.[26]

D-dimer levels may remain elevated for months following initial infection. This phenomenon is believed to be more common in patients who required hospital admission and are older than 50 years, but a small study found that 4 months after initial infection 29% of patients with elevated D-dimer levels had managed symptoms without the need for hospitalization. Of note, other coagulation and inflammation markers had largely returned to normal levels in convalescent patients, which suggests that symptoms of long COVID may be associated with pulmonary microvascular immunothrombosis.[27]

Clinical Presentation

It is difficult to provide accurate estimates for the symptomology of COVID-19. Many individuals may only develop minor symptoms and assume that they are not infected with the novel coronavirus. Similarly, many people who believe that they are infected with COVID-19 may only seek medical help if their symptoms become severe enough for them to realize that they may have more than just the flu. Consequently, the rate of occurrence of individual symptoms may be skewed. Estimates about the frequency of symptoms that are common among individuals with mild infections and uncommon among those with more severe infections may be far too low. Conversely, estimates about the frequency of symptoms that are common among individuals with severe infections and uncommon among those with less severe infections may be far too high. From an epidemiological perspective this is an important point, but unfortunately, there is no remedy for this issue at the present time.

That said, the symptoms of COVID-19 that are most frequently reported include fever, dry cough, dyspnea, fatigue, sore throat, congestion, and myalgia (see Table 3.2).[17] What has been surprising

TABLE 3.2 Common Symptoms Associated With COVID-19

System	Symptom
Respiratory	Fever/chills
	Cough
	Dyspnea
	Sore throat
	Congestion/rhinorrhea
Gastrointestinal	Diarrhea
	Nausea/vomiting
	Abdominal pain
	Loss of appetite
Musculoskeletal	Fatigue
	Myalgia
	Headache
	Joint pain
Dermatological	Pseudo-chilblains ("COVID toe")
	Rash containing macules and papules
	Urticarial lesions
	Vesicular lesion
	Vaso-occlusive lesion
Otolaryngeal	Anosmia
	Taste dysfunction
	Smell dysfunction
Reproductive	Menstrual volume changes
	Menstrual cycle changes

and one of the many reasons why COVID-19 is considered to be such a diagnostic chameleon is that no single sign or symptom has been universally reported across all positive cases at presentation or even during hospitalization. A report of over 370,000 confirmed COVID-19 cases compiled by the US Centers for Disease Control and Prevention (CDC) found that only 50% of patients reported a cough and that 43% had a fever.[28] The reported percentages of other symptoms were even lower:

- Myalgia (36%)
- Headache (34%)
- Dyspnea (29%)
- Sore throat (20%)
- Diarrhea (19%)
- Nausea/vomiting (12%)
- Anosmia (loss of smell) (<10%)
- Abdominal pain (<10%)
- Rhinorrhea (<10%)

Meta-analyses from multiple countries have met with similar issues. A systematic review of 24,410 adults across nine countries found that fever was reported by 78% of patients, 57% experienced a cough, and that 31% reported fatigue.[29] Meanwhile, a global meta-analysis involving 67 studies and 8302 patients found that the most common symptoms were:

- Fever (69%)
- Cough (53%)
- Anosmia (38%)
- Fatigue (31%)
- Loss of taste (31%)
- Nasal congestion (26%)
- Dyspnea (20%)
- Headache (19%)
- Sore throat (18%)
- Vertigo (16%)
- Rhinorrhea (13%)
- Diarrhea (9%)
- Nausea/vomiting (8%)
- Hearing loss (3%)[30]

To reiterate the point made at the beginning of this section, disparities in datasets makes it extremely difficult to access accurate estimates of symptomology for COVID-19.

Another curious phenomenon, one that has been observed since the first months of the pandemic, is that different symptoms appear with greater frequency in different populations. For example, in early 2020, rates of olfactory dysfunction ranged from 5.14% to 98.33% depending on the study and were found to be much more common in North America and Europe than in East Asia.[31] It is unclear if this was due to oversight while recording patient symptoms at the earlier stages of the outbreak or if there was another reason as to why these symptoms were so infrequently reported—it could possibly be due to genetic or environmental factors. Similarly, enteric symptoms appear to have been less common during the initial outbreak than they were after the virus spread to other parts of the world. A meta-analysis involving 4243 patients from six countries found that prevalence of GI symptoms was 16.2% in studies that were based in Hubei and 18.6% for all studies from outside of the province.[32] Once again the reasons are unclear.

It is also possible that certain symptom constellations may be more common in some variants than others. For example, some medical workers have observed that patients who have been infected with the Delta variant tend to report symptoms that have more in common with a bout of severe flu—headache, sore throat, runny nose, fever—and seem to less frequently report symptoms associated with ancestral strains of the virus, such as anosmia, gustatory dysfunction, cough, etc.[33] At present, this should be considered anecdotal until a peer-reviewed study has examined disparities in symptoms between variants.

Respiratory Symptoms

COVID-19 often presents as a respiratory illness, and some of the most common symptoms are akin to symptoms of other viral infections that affect the respiratory tract. More importantly, some of these symptoms, such as fever, chills, cough, and fatigue, are not predictive of severe disease. Conversely, dyspnea has been associated with an increased risk of severe disease and mortality.[34]

Additional symptoms include sore throat, rhinorrhea, and trouble breathing.

Musculoskeletal Symptoms

It is estimated that between 15% and 40% of COVID-19 patients experience fatigue, headache, joint pain, and/or myalgia. Fatigue appears to be the most common of these symptoms and is especially prevalent among individuals with long COVID. Surprisingly, post-COVID fatigue is independent of severity of infection, and more than 50% of participants in one study reported persistent fatigue 10 weeks after symptom onset. Female gender and individuals with a preexisting diagnosis of anxiety disorder and/or depressive disorder were overrepresented in this study. Several investigations have attempted to find specific inflammatory markers associated with postinfection fatigue, but no consistent change in markers has been reported across multiple studies.[35]

Myalgia and headache are also quite common. A meta-analysis involving 59,254 patients who tested positive for COVID-19 found that the former occurred in 36% of individuals.[36] A separate study found that headache has been reported between 11% and 34% of patients hospitalized with COVID-19.[37]

Gastrointestinal Symptoms

Symptoms affecting the GI tract have been widely reported and include loss of appetite, diarrhea, nausea, vomiting, and abdominal pain. These symptoms rarely occur independently of symptoms associated with respiratory infections (fever, cough, fatigue, etc). A study that examined the symptoms of 20,133 hospital in-patients who tested positive for COVID-19 in the United Kingdom found that only 4% reported GI problems without concomitant respiratory symptoms.[38] More importantly, it has been observed that there is a reduced mortality rate among patients who present with enteric symptoms, even in conjunction with other symptoms, but the reason for this association remains unclear.[39]

Dermatological Symptoms

Approximately one in five patients who tested positive for COVID-19 were found to have developed skin manifestations at different points during the disease progression. These manifestations appear to be most common among individuals of European ancestry. In one meta-analysis from around the world involving 51 articles and a database of 1211 patients, 96.9% of patients (n = 1172) who developed skin manifestations were from Europe or the United States, while only 3.1% (n = 39) were from East Asia.[40]

The most commonly reported skin manifestations were pseudo-chilblains, rashes containing macules and papules, urticarial lesions, vesicular lesions, and vaso-occlusive lesions. Whether clinically relevant or not, it is worth noting that vaso-occlusive legions were the least common but were associated with the lowest survival rate (78.9%).[40]

"COVID toe" (which can also appear on the finger) is another symptom that has been reported and involves the appearance of pseudo-chilblains and is characterized by localized swelling and discoloration of fingers or toes. The discoloration may be reddish or purplish and may result in discomfort.[41]

"COVID nails" have been reported in many patients following convalescence. The phenomenon occurs when a shock to the system interrupts nail growth and results in horizontal grooves in one's nails. These grooves, also known as Beau lines, become visible weeks or months after symptom onset.[42]

Otolaryngeal Symptoms

Anosmia (loss of smell), as well as olfactory and gustatory dysfunction, has been widely reported in mild, moderate, and severe COVID-19 cases and may be one of the most commonly experienced symptoms associated with COVID-19. Most patients develop these symptoms after the onset of other symptoms typically associated with respiratory illness. Mean duration of anosmia has been reported to be 8.4 days.[43] As noted earlier, there is some evidence to suggest that anosmia is less common among patients infected with one of the variants.

Though the symptom typically disappears within a few days, some patients have reported that it has taken months for patients to fully regain their sense of taste and/or smell. A study involving 813 health care workers who tested positive for COVID-19 found that 580 (71.34%) reported losing their sense of taste and/or smell, and 300 of those participants (51.72%) reported that they had not regained it 5 months later. It is possible that persistent loss or dysfunction in taste and smell is a sign of long COVID.[44]

Parosmia, a condition in which one's sense of smell is distorted, has also been reported. In some cases, this can have a severe impact on quality of life as patients report that scents that they once smelled pleasant are perceived as smelling putrid or in other ways foul.[45]

Reproductive System Symptoms

Many women with COVID-19 have reported changes to their menstrual cycles during acute infection, recovery, and after being vaccinated. Unfortunately, there appears to be only one study on the subject, which examined the menstrual data of 237 women in China. The study included 177 women who had had COVID-19 and found that 25% (45) of patients presented with menstrual volume changes, 28% (50) had cycle changes, and that a prolonged cycle was reported by 19% of patients. The study's authors speculated that these changes could have been brought on by ephemeral sex hormone changes due to suppressed ovarian function but could not rule out other potential physiological sources for the changes or the fact that stress associated with COVID-19 could have played a role.[46]

Asymptomatic Cases

It is estimated that a total of 30% to 40% of cases of COVID-19 are asymptomatic.[47] The frequent occurrence of transmission while asymptomatic or presymptomatic has played an unfortunate role in the spread of the virus and made SARS-CoV-2 both dangerous and difficult to trace. Infected individuals unwittingly transmitted the virus while asymptomatic because they did not take the precautions that they would have had they known that they were capable of infecting others. It is estimated that 35% of infections can be traced back to presymptomatic individuals and that asymptomatic individuals have been responsible for 24% of total infections.[48] This figure is believed to be higher among individuals infected with the Delta variant.

Asymptomatic cases appear to be far more common in younger individuals. Though patients may not be aware of infection due to symptoms, they may still exhibit clinical abnormalities if tested.[49] A study involving 24 asymptomatic patients found that 50% had ground-glass opacities or shadowing in their CT scans, while another 20% reported other imaging abnormalities.[50] Another study involving 55 patients found that CT scans showed evidence of pneumonia in 67% of participants. Only two patients went on to develop hypoxia before making a full recovery.[51]

Clinical Abnormalities

There are numerous abnormalities that clinicians may observe after running routine tests on patients that may indicate more severe illness. As noted above in *Disease Spectrum of COVID-19*, these include elevations in liver enzymes, inflammatory markers (eg, C-reactive protein, ferritin), inflammatory cytokines, and D-dimer, as well as acute kidney injury. Additional clinical abnormalities include the following:

- Elevated creatine phosphokinase[52]
- Elevated lactate dehydrogenase[53]
- Elevated troponins and B-type natriuretic peptides[54]
- Lymphopenia[55]
- Thrombocytopenia[56]

Treatment

In most cases, individuals who have COVID-19 should be able to recover at home with plenty of bed rest, liquids, and medications to relieve minor aches, pains, and fever. Diet can also help maintain a healthy immune system, specifically if one eats functional foods that are high in vitamins (particularly vitamins A, B6, B12, C, D, E, and folate) and minerals (zinc, iron, selenium, magnesium, and copper). Additionally, some foods may even have limited antiviral properties, including fermented foods (kimchi, sauerkraut, yogurt, etc), squashes, legumes, mushrooms, fish, olive oil, garlic, black pepper, and coffee.[57] For those whose symptoms get worse (eg, difficulty breathing, low oxygen saturation, high fever, or strokelike symptoms), they may require treatment in the hospital with supplemental oxygen or, in critical cases, intubation and ventilator use may be necessary.

There have been a plethora of proposed pharmaceutical treatments for COVID-19, and, at the time of this writing, the United States has indicated that it plans to spend billions of dollars more in the development of antivirals that may prove effective at treating COVID-19.[58] Studies are ongoing, and it is unclear which, if any, of the current candidates will receive FDA approval.

Therapies that are currently available for emergency use or approved by FDA include the following:

- Remdesivir (Veklury): An antiviral that is currently the only FDA-approved therapy for COVID-19.[59]
- Dexamethasone: A corticosteroid and anti-inflammatory. Alternative corticosteroids like prednisone, methylprednisolone, and hydrocortisone may also be used.[60]
- Tocilizumab: A monoclonal antibody that targets interleukin-6 used in conjunction with dexamethasone.[60]
- Baricitinib: A Janus kinase inhibitor that may be used in conjunction with dexamethasone or remdesivir.[61]
- Anticoagulants.[62]
- Convalescent plasma.[62]
- Monoclonal antibodies: bamlanivimab, etesevimab, casirivimab, and imdevimab.[63,64]

The decision to use one or several of these treatments is solely at the discretion of the physician.

Risk Factors

Not everyone is equally at risk of being infected by SARS-CoV-2 or being stricken with a severe case of COVID-19. There are multiple factors that not only make certain individuals more likely to catch the disease, but to also have a worse outcome. Socioeconomic status and vocation have played an outsized role in the former. Approximately 55 million "essential workers" employed across crucial industries like health care, emergency services, food and agriculture, and infrastructure management have continued to work in-person throughout the pandemic.[65] Particularly among health care workers in places like New York City, the first months of the pandemic saw a surge in the number of cases as supplies of personal protective equipment (PPE) ran short and hospital staff had to get creative with supplies to try to keep themselves safe. Meanwhile, nonessential workers were given the opportunity to work remotely, which significantly reduced their risk of exposure to infected individuals, though, as will be explored in later chapters, the risk of social isolation, substance use disorders, and myriad psychiatric problems by no means made the experience enviable.

The present section will focus exclusively on risk factors for prognosis, including genetics, preexisting conditions, socioeconomic background, age, and gender. Many of these subjects will be returned to again later in the book.

Preexisting Conditions and Genetics

There are numerous preexisting conditions that make individuals more susceptible to severe COVID-19 (see Table 3.3). Patients with numerous comorbidities are at an increased risk of severe illness, especially if this is in conjunction with other risk factors like old age or male gender.[66,67]

In addition to genetic predispositions that may make patients more likely to develop the above conditions, a genome-wide association study discovered a positive correlation between individuals from the type A blood group and COVID-19–related respiratory failure.[68] Conversely, individuals with type O blood have a lower risk of severe disease and possibly even infection.[69]

Gender

A meta-analysis of more than 3 million global cases confirmed that males and females are just as likely to get COVID-19, but that males are 2.84 times more likely to be admitted to intensive care units and are 1.39 times more likely to die of COVID-19.[70] COVID-19 appears to more frequently lead to an intensive inflammatory response in men, which could potentially explain the disparity. Conjectures that are based on anecdotal evidence suggest that men are more likely to develop severe COVID-19 because of poor lifestyle choices when compared to women (eg, higher rates of tobacco use, higher rates of obesity, higher rates of alcohol use). At present, these theories remain entirely speculative.

TABLE 3.3 Comorbidities the CDC Classifies as Risk Factors for Severe COVID-19

Established and probable risk factors:

- Cancer
- Cardiovascular disease (eg, heart failure, coronary artery disease, cardiomyopathies)
- Cerebrovascular disease
- Chronic kidney disease
- COPD and other lung diseases (eg, interstitial lung disease, pulmonary fibrosis, pulmonary hypertension)
- Diabetes mellitus type 1
- Diabetes mellitus type 2
- Down syndrome
- HIV/AIDS
- Neurologic conditions (eg, dementia)
- Obesity (BMI $\geq$ 30 kg/m^2) and overweight (BMI 25-29 kg/m^2)
- Pregnancy
- Sickle cell disease
- Solid organ or blood stem cell transplantation
- Substance use disorders
- Smoking
- Use of immunosuppressive medications like corticosteroids

Possible risk factors with limited evidence:

- Cystic fibrosis
- Thalassemia

Possible risk factors with mixed evidence:

- Asthma
- Hypertension
- Immune deficiencies
- Liver disease

BMI, body mass index; CDC, Centers for Disease Control and Prevention; COPD, chronic obstructive pulmonary disease; HIV/AIDS, human immunodeficiency virus/acquired immunodeficiency syndrome.

Socioeconomic Background

Statistically speaking, one of the most salient examples of the disproportionate effects the COVID-19 pandemic has had on disadvantaged communities can be seen in the life expectancy estimates from January through June 2020, which were released by the CDC in February 2021 (see Figures 3.2 and 3.3). In this report, it was found that provisional life expectancy at birth for the total US population declined by 1.0 year when compared to data from 2019 (from 78.8 to 77.8). Within the same period of time, life expectancies for non-Hispanic Black populations decreased by 2.7 years (from 74.7 to 72.0), while Hispanic populations experienced a decrease of 1.9 years (from 81.8 to 79.9) and non-Hispanic White populations saw a decrease of 0.8 year (78.8-78.0). When gender was included as a factor, the data revealed that non-Hispanic Black and Hispanic men bore the worst of the effects, with the former experiencing a decline of 3.0 years (71.3-68.3) and the latter experiencing a decline of 2.4 years (79.0-76.6).[71]

As will be discussed in *Chapter 5: Psychosocial and Economic Impact of COVID-19—A Nation Under Siege*, socioeconomic factors contribute to poor prognoses—not race or ethnicity. In fact, it appears as though non-Hispanic Black and Hispanic individuals are at no greater risk of COVID-19–related mortality than their non-Hispanic White counterparts when controlling for comorbidities, gender, and age.[72]

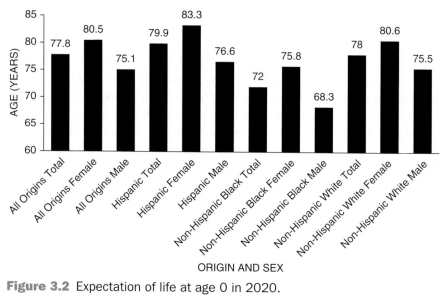

Figure 3.2 Expectation of life at age 0 in 2020.

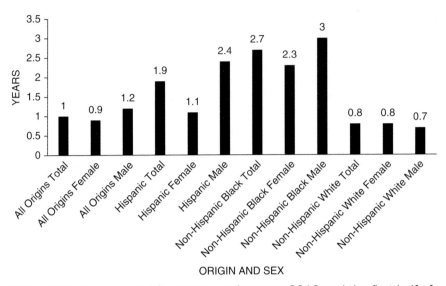

Figure 3.3 Decrease in life expectancy between 2019 and the first half of 2020.

As Black and Hispanic individuals are more likely to live in poverty than their White or Asian counterparts, and because poverty is a major social determinant of health, the consequence is that more Black and Hispanic individuals tend to experience worse health outcomes than other racial groups in the United States. These factors are difficult to properly quantify because they tend to compound one another and oftentimes occur in conjunction with or give rise to preexisting conditions like the ones mentioned above.

For example, an individual living in poverty may be forced to move into an area that has poor air quality due to its proximity to several industrial facilities. The building in which this individual resides would not receive a great deal of upkeep, leading occupants to be exposed to moderate levels of indoor allergens and mold. Finally, their lack of income means they are far more likely to consume and provide their family with a calorie-rich but nutrient-poor diet. These three factors could potentially lead to the development of asthma and/or type 2 diabetes.[73] Poverty could ultimately make them worse because individuals who live on limited resources in the United States typically do not have adequate health coverage, which means they may avoid treating the conditions until they become so severe that they require emergency care.

Socioeconomic status plays a tremendous role in determining the conditions in which people live, which then plays a vital role in determining their health. Without experiencing the first of the three conditions associated with poverty (poor outdoor air quality, poor indoor air quality, and poor diet), the individuals above would most likely not have developed either preexisting condition and consequently not have been put at a greater risk of severe COVID-19.

Old Age

Approximately 80% of the 658,754 individuals in the United States who died due to COVID-19 as of September 2021 were 65 years of age or older (see Table 3.4).[74] There is simply no question that old age is not only a major risk factor for death but is also a risk factor for more severe disease. In a modeling study from China involving over 70,000 patients, it was found that hospitalization rates increased with age in a manner akin to fatalities (see Table 3.5).[75]

TABLE 3.4 COVID-19 Deaths by Age Group, as Reported by the CDC September 11, 2021[74]

Age Range (years)	COVID-19 Deaths	As Percentage of Total Deaths (%)	As Percentage of All COVID-19 Deaths (%)
Under 1 year	105	0.331	0.016
1-4	54	0.918	0.008
5-14	145	1.547	0.022
15-24	1297	2.149	0.197
25-34	5759	4.599	0.874
35-44	14,423	7.937	2.189
45-54	37,451	11.541	5.685
55-64	87,847	11.873	13.335
65-74	147,568	13.026	22.401
75-84	176,763	13.063	26.833
85 and above	187,342	11.536	28.439
Total	658,754	11.789	100

TABLE 3.5 Estimated Proportion of all SARS-CoV-2 Infections Resulting in Hospitalization, Based on a Subset of Cases Reported in Mainland China, 2020[75]

Age Range (years)	Proportion of Infected Individuals Hospitalized (%)
0-9	0
10-19	0.041
20-29	1.04
30-39	3.43
40-49	4.25
50-59	8.16
60-69	11.8
70-79	16.6
≥80	18.4

COVID-19 in Children

In children, COVID-19 is usually experienced as a mild illness, if symptoms are experienced at all. The two most common symptoms are fever and cough.[76] Children younger than 18 years may still develop severe COVID-19, but the risk is far lower in this age group than in adults—particularly older adults. One study that examined over 277,000 students across 47 US states who tested positive for COVID-19 between March 2020 and September 2020 found that 1.2% (3240) were hospitalized, 0.1% (404) were admitted to the ICU, and 0.02% (51) died. When divided into groups aged 5 to 11 years ($n = 101,503$) and 12 to 17 years ($n = 175,782$), the data revealed that younger children were less likely than older children to be hospitalized or be admitted to the ICU—1.0% (1021) of the younger group were hospitalized, 0.14% (145) were admitted to the ICU, and 0.0197% (20) died; 1.26% (2219) of the older group were hospitalized, 0.15% (259) were admitted to the ICU, and 0.0176% (31) died.[77] According to the CDC, the total number of deaths for individuals aged 0 to 17 years was 439 as of September 11, 2021. For reference, the total number of COVID-19 deaths for all age groups as of September 2021 was 658,754.[74] For a breakdown of COVID-19 mortalities by age group, please see Table 3.4.

There is some evidence to suggest that individual variants, particularly Gamma and Delta, affect young children more than previous iterations of the virus.[78,79] It is unclear if this is proportional to the overall increase in transmissibility seen in variants. There has been some speculation about viral shedding and rates of infection being lower in younger children, too. The above study involving over 270,000 students found that the rate of infection is twice as high in children aged 12 to 17 years as it is in their peers in the 5 to 11 years age group.[77] Unfortunately, there is a fundamental flaw with this figure: It is not current policy to test all children, so the data does not include asymptomatic cases, which could mean as many 30% to 40% of cases are simply not being counted.[80]

Why children are less likely to develop severe symptoms remains a mystery. It has been speculated that ACE2 receptors are expressed differently in the lungs of younger children, and that this may be a potential reason why severe disease is relatively rare in people younger than 18 years.[38]

Long-Term Effects

The next chapter (*Chapter 4: Neuropsychiatric Symptoms and Postacute Sequelae of SARS-CoV-2—The Long Haulers*) will focus mostly on what most people typically think of when they hear the words "long-term" COVID-19, which are primarily nonspecific or neuropsychiatric symptoms that persist following the acute phase of COVID-19 (eg, brain fog, difficulty concentrating, difficulty sleeping, malaise). Independent of these symptoms, there are reports of patients who are still experiencing respiratory problems many weeks after the acute phase of the illness has passed. In some cases, the SARS-CoV-2 infection has resolved, but CT scans continue to show inflammation. Presenting at the European Respiratory Society International Congress in September 2020, researchers from Austria reported that of the 86 patients they monitored as part of an on-going study, 88% showed signs of lung inflammation 6 weeks after being discharged from the hospital, but that figure had dropped to 56% after 12 weeks.[81] Other patients' scans show clear signs of lung tissue scarring, which remains present even months after the infection and can be extremely detrimental to patients' quality of life.[82]

It is worth noting that many patients who recovered from SARS still had persistent respiratory impairment months and years after the initial infection. An observational cohort study published in 2020 that followed 71 health care providers from Peking University's People's Hospital from the time they contracted SARS (2003) to 2018 examined the recovery curve of lung injury in patients and found that lesions rapidly decreased between

2003 and 2004, and then largely plateaued from 2004 to 2018. Even after 15 years, 38% of the study's participants still had reduced diffusion capacity and 4.6% had visible lesions on their lungs.[83]

While it is far too early to draw conclusions about the long-term effects of COVID-19 and potentially fallacious to equate SARS-CoV and SARS-CoV-2, there have been numerous parallels between the two illnesses caused by the viruses. Unfortunately, this may be yet another one.

Immunity Following Infection and Reinfection

Patients develop significant serum antibodies while fighting a SARS-CoV-2 infection, and antibody levels are reportedly higher in severe infection than in mild infection.[84] Neutralizing antibodies then decline over what appears to be several months. It is unclear how long the antibody response remains effective against reinfection, but it is safe to say that immunity extends at least for several months in most individuals. Recent evidence suggests that serum antibodies decline relatively rapidly within the first few months after infection, but that a long-lived humoral response can be called upon to fight reinfection.[85] This appears to be supported by researchers from the Cleveland Clinic, who concluded in a June 2021 report that has not been peer reviewed at this time, "The cumulative incidence of SARS-CoV-2 infection remained almost zero among previously infected unvaccinated subjects, previously infected subjects who were vaccinated, and previously uninfected subjects who remained unvaccinated."[86] Consequently, the report does provide some evidence to support the claim that vaccination may not be necessary for those who have developed immunity from natural infection. However, it should be noted that this study has not been peer reviewed at this time.

Other reports have concluded that there is some risk of reinfection for individuals with natural immunity, but that case severity appears to be far milder than the initial infection.[87] Still others have found that those who have experienced natural infection but have not been vaccinated face a notably greater risk of reinfection. A case-control study based in Kentucky between May and June 2021 found that, among individuals who had already been infected with the virus, those who were unvaccinated were 2.34 times more likely to become reinfected than those who were vaccinated.[88] Meanwhile, an Israeli study that has yet to be peer reviewed and focused explicitly on immunity against the Delta variant found that those who had both been previously infected and received one dose of the vaccine were better protected against breakthrough cases than those who had been infected with the virus and remained unvaccinated. This study also found that individuals who had received two doses of the Pfizer/BioNTech vaccine were at a 13.06-fold greater risk for breakthrough infection than those who had had previously been infected with SARS-CoV-2.[89]

Suffice to say, the science is far from settled on the matter, especially since so many of the studies on vaccine efficacy in real-world scenarios, the Delta variant, and how well vaccines protect against the Delta variant have yet to be peer reviewed. These preliminary findings suggesting improved immunity against the Delta variant for vaccinated individuals who were previously infected warrant cautious optimism about the potential dangers posed by future variants. Similarly, some evidence has emerged to suggest that individuals who received a full vaccine series but were never infected with the virus have a risk of breakthrough infection of between 1 in 5000 and 1 in 10,000.[90] This is all good news, especially if SARS-CoV-2 becomes endemic and continues to circulate around the globe for years to come.

Conclusion

Most cases of COVID-19 tend to be mild and characterized by flulike and enteric symptoms. The larger threat posed by the disease concerns the patient's immunoresponse. If it is properly targeted, the viral infection is cleared and the patient experiences full convalescence. Improper cytokine response can lead to numerous potentially life-threatening complications, the most common of which appear to be ARDS and coagulopathy. It is possible that errant immunoresponse also results in lingering symptoms. Multiple factors can influence patient immunoresponse, including age, genetics, preexisting conditions, gender, and socioeconomic status.

REFERENCES

1. Devaux CA, Lagier JC, Raoult D. New insights into the physiopathology of COVID-19: SARS-CoV-2-associated gastrointestinal illness. *Front Med (Lausanne)*. 2021;8:640073. doi:10.3389/fmed.2021.640073

2. Lauer SA, Grantz KH, Bi Q, et al. The incubation period of coronavirus disease 2019 (COVID-19) from publicly reported confirmed cases: estimation and application. *Ann Intern Med*. 2020;172(9):577-582. doi:10.7326/M20-0504

3. Mallapaty S. Delta's rise is fueled by rampant spread from people who feel fine. *Nature*. Published August 19, 2021. Accessed August 20, 2021. https://www.nature.com/articles/d41586-021-02259-2

4. Wu Z, McGoogan JM. Characteristics of and important lessons from the coronavirus disease 2019 (COVID-19) outbreak in China: summary of a report of 72,314 cases from the Chinese Center for Disease Control and Prevention. *JAMA*. 2020;323(13):1239-1242. doi:10.1001/jama.2020.2648

5. Dennis JM, McGovern AP, Vollmer SJ, Mateen BA. Improving survival of critical care patients with coronavirus disease 2019 in England: a national cohort study, March to June 2020. *Crit Care Med*. 2021;49(2):209-214. doi:10.1097/CCM.0000000000004747

6. Ioannidis JPA. Infection fatality rate of COVID-19 inferred from seroprevalence data. *Bull World Health Organ.* 2021;99(1):19-33F. doi:10.2471/BLT.20.265892

7. Peacock TP, Goldhill DH, Zhou J, et al. The furin cleavage site in the SARS-CoV-2 spike protein is required for transmission in ferrets. *Nat Microbiol.* 2021;6:899-909. Accessed June 5, 2021. doi:10.1038/s41564-021-00908-w. https://www.nature.com/articles/s41564-021-00908-w

8. Cevik M, Kuppalli K, Kindrachuk J, Peiris M. Virology, transmission, and pathogenesis of SARS-CoV-2. *BMJ.* 2020;371:m3862. doi:10.1136/bmj.m3862

9. Chen M, Shen W, Rowan NR, et al. Elevated ACE-2 expression in the olfactory neuroepithelium: implications for anosmia and upper respiratory SARS-CoV-2 entry and replication. *Eur Respir J.* 2020;56(3):2001948. doi:10.1183/13993003.01948-2020

10. Mayi BS, Leibowitz JA, Woods AT, Ammon KA, Liu AE, Raja A. The role of neuropilin-1 in COVID-19. *PLoS Pathog.* 2021;17(1):e1009153. doi:10.1371/journal.ppat.1009153

11. Mishra S. Why is Delta more infectious and deadly? New research holds answers. *National Geographic.* Published August 6, 2021. Accessed August 19, 2021. https://www.nationalgeographic.com/science/article/why-is-delta-more-infectious-and-deadly-new-research-holds-answers?loggedin=true

12. Marjot T, Webb GJ, Barritt AS, et al. COVID-19 and liver disease: mechanistic and clinical perspectives. *Nat Rev Gastroenterol Hepatol.* 2021;18(5):348-364. doi:10.1038/s41575-021-00426-4

13. Martines RB, Ritter JM, Matkovic E, et al. Pathology and pathogenesis of SARS-CoV-2 associated with fatal coronavirus disease, United States. *Emerg Infect Dis.* 2020;26(9):2005-2015. doi:10.3201/eid2609.202095

14. Teo J. Early detection of silent hypoxia in COVID-19 pneumonia using smartphone pulse oximetry. *J Med Syst.* 2020;44(8):134. doi:10.1007/s10916-020-01587-6

15. Pilli VS, Datta A, Afreen S, Catalano D, Szabo G, Majumder R. Hypoxia downregulates protein S expression. *Blood.* 2018;132(4):452-455. doi:10.1182/blood-2018-04-841585

16. Stanifer ML, Kee C, Cortese M, et al. Critical role of type III interferon in controlling SARS-CoV-2 infection in human intestinal epithelial cells. *Cell Rep.* 2020;32(1):107863. doi:10.1016/j.celrep.2020.107863

17. Hosoki K, Chakraborty A, Sur S. Molecular mechanisms and epidemiology of COVID-19 from an allergist's perspective. *J Allergy Clin Immunol.* 2020;146(2):285-299. doi:10.1016/j.jaci.2020.05.033

18. Shanmugam C, Mohammed AR, Ravuri S, Luthra V, Rajagopal N, Karre S.COVID-2019 – a comprehensive pathology insight. *Pathol Res Pract.* 2020;216(10):153222. doi:10.1016/j.prp.2020.153222

19. Lopes-Pacheco M, Silva PL, Cruz FF, et al. Pathogenesis of multiple organ injury in COVID-19 and potential therapeutic strategies. *Front Physiol.* 2021;12:593223. doi:10.3389/fphys.2021.593223

20. Pellegrini D, Kawakami R, Guagliumi G, et al. Microthrombi as a major cause of cardiac injury in COVID-19. *Circulation.* 2021;143(10):1031-1042. doi:10.1161/CIRCULATIONAHA.120.051828

21. Nugent J, Aklilu A, Yamamoto Y, et al. Assessment of acute kidney injury and longitudinal kidney function after hospital discharge among patients with and without COVID-19. *JAMA Netw Open.* 2021;4(3):e211095. doi:10.1001/jamanetworkopen.2021.1095

22. Hu T, Liu Y, Zhao M, Zhuang Q, Xu L, He Q. A comparison of COVID-19, SARS, and MERS. *PeerJ.* 2020;8:e9725. doi:10.7717/peerj.9725

23. Huang Q, LI J, Lyu S, et al. COVID-19 associated kidney impairment in adult: qualitative and quantitative analyses with non-enhanced CT on admission. *Eur J Radiol.* 2020;131:109240. doi:10.1016/j.ejrad.2020.109240

24. Clark R, Waters B, Stanfill AG. Elevated liver function tests in COVID-19. *Nurse Pract.* 2021;46(1):21-26. doi:10.1097/01.NPR.0000722316.63824.f9

25. Berger JS, Kunichoff D, Adhikari S, et al. Prevalence and outcome of D-dimer elevation in hospitalized patients with COVID-19. *Arterioscler Thromb Vasc Biol.* 2020;40(10):2539-2547. doi:10.1161/ATVBAHA.120.314872

26. Levi M, Thachil J, Iba T, Levy JH. Coagulation abnormalities and thrombosis in patients with COVID-19. *Lancet Haematol.* 2020;7(6):E438-E440. doi:10.1016/S2352-3026(20)30145-9

27. Townsend L, Fogarty H, Dyer A, et al. Prolonged elevation of D-dimer levels in convalescent COVID-19 patients is independent of the acute phase response. *J Thromb Haemost.* 2021;19(4):1064-1070. doi:10.1111/jth.15267

28. Stokes EK, Zambrano LD, Anderson KN, et al. Coronavirus disease 2019 case surveillance – United States, January 22-May 30, 2020. *MMWR Morb Mortal Wkly Rep.* 2020;69(24):759-765. doi:10.15585/mmwr.mm6924e2

29. Grant MC, Geoghegan L, Arbyn M, et al. The prevalence of symptoms in 24,410 adults infected by the novel coronavirus (SARS-CoV-2; COVID-19): a systematic review and meta-analysis of 148 studies from 9 countries. *PLoS One.* 2020;15(6):e0234765. doi:10.1371/journal.pone.0234765

30. Mair M, Singhavi H, Pai A, et al. A meta-analysis of 67 studies with presenting symptoms and laboratory tests of COVID-19 patients. *Laryngoscope.* 2021;131(6):1254-1265. doi:10.1002/lary.29207

31. Tong JY, Wong A, Zhu D, Fastenberg JH, Tham T. The prevalence of olfactory and gustatory dysfunction in COVID-19 patients: a systematic review and meta-analysis. *Otolaryngol Head Neck Surg.* 2020;163(1):3-11. doi:10.1177/0194599820826473

32. Cheung KS, Hung IFN, Chan PPY, et al. Gastrointestinal manifestations of SARS-CoV-2 infection and virus load in fecal samples from a Hong Kong cohort: systematic review and meta-analysis. *Gastroenterology.* 2020;159(1):81-95. doi:10.1053/j.gastro.2020.03.065

33. Fiore K. Are COVID symptoms different with Delta? *Medpage Today.* Published August 11, 2021. Accessed August 31, 2021. https://www.medpagetoday.com/special-reports/exclusives/93997

34. Shi L, Wang Y, Wang Y, Duan G, Yang H. Dyspnea rather than fever is a risk factor for predicting mortality in patients with COVID-19. *J Infect.* 2020;81(4):647-679. doi:10.1016/j.jinf.2020.05.013

35. Townsend L, Dyer AH, Jones K, et al. Persistent fatigue following SARS-CoV-2 infection is common and independent of severity of initial infection. *PLoS One.* 2020;15(11):e0240784. doi:10.1371/journal.pone.0240784

36. Widyadharma IPE, Sari NNSP, Pradnyaswari KE, et al. Pain as clinical manifestations of COVID-19 infection and its management in the pandemic era: a literature review. *Egypt J Neurol Psychiatr Neurosurg.* 2020;56(1):121. doi:10.1186/s41983-020-00258-0

37. Bolay H, Gül A, Baykan B. COVID-19 is a real headache! *Headache.* 2020;60(7):1415-1421. doi:10.1111/head.13856

38. Docherty AB, Harrison EW, Green CA, et al. Features of 20,133 UK patients in hospital with COVID-19 using the ISARIC WHO clinical characterization protocol: prospective observational cohort study. *BMJ.* 2020;369:m1985. doi:10.1136/bmj.m1985

39. Livanos AE, Jha D, Cossarini F, et al. Intestinal host response to SARS-CoV-2 infection and COVID-19 outcomes in patients with gastrointestinal symptoms. *Gastroenterology.* 2021;160(7):2435-2450.e34. doi:10.1053/j.gastro.2021.02.056

40. Tan SW, Tam YC, Oh CC. Skin manifestations of COVID-19: a worldwide review. *JAAD Int.* 2021;2:119-133. doi:10.1016/j.jdin.2020.12.003

41. Rabin RC. What is 'COVID toe'? Maybe a strange sign of coronavirus infection. *New York Times.* Updated September 11, 2021. Accessed June 6, 2021. https://www.nytimes.com/2020/05/01/health/coronavirus-covid-toe.html

42. Chiu A. Are 'COVID nails' a sign that you had the virus? Experts weigh in. *Washington Post.* Published May 12, 2021. Accessed June 6, 2021. https://www.washingtonpost.com/lifestyle/wellness/covid-nails-symptoms-beaus-lines/2021/05/11/c449243e-b1b4-11eb-9059-d8176b9e3798_story.html

43. Lechien JR, Chiesa-Estomba CM, Hans S, Barillari MR, Jouffe L, Saussez S. Loss of smell and taste in 2013 European patients with mild to moderate COVID. *Ann Intern Med.* 2020;173(8):672-675. doi:10.7326/M20-2428

44. Drillinger M. *Post-COVID-19, It Can Take Over 5 Months for Sense of Smell to Return.* Healthline. Published February 24, 2021. Accessed June 6, 2021. https://www.healthline.com/health-news/post-covid-19-it-can-take-over-5-months-for-sense-of-smell-to-return
45. Brewer K. Parosmia: 'Since I had COVID, food makes me want to vomit.' *BBC News.* Published January 28, 2021. Accessed June 7, 2021. https://www.bbc.com/news/stories-55824567
46. Li K, Chen G, Hou H, et al. Analysis of sex hormones and menstruation in COVID-19 women of child-bearing age. *Reprod Biomed Online.* 2021;42(1):260-267. doi:10.1016/j.rbmo.2020.09.020
47. Oran DP, Topol EJ. Prevalence of asymptomatic SARS-CoV-2 infection. *Ann Intern Med.* 2020;173(5):362-367. doi:10.7326/M20-3012
48. Johansson MA, Quandelacy TM, Kada S, et al. SARS-CoV-2 transmission from people without COVID-19 symptoms. *JAMA Netw Open.* 2021;4(1):e2035057. doi:10.1001/jamanetworkopen.2020.35057
49. Kasper MR, Geibe JR, Sears CL, et al. An outbreak of COVID-19 on an aircraft carrier. *N Engl J Med.* 2020;383(25):2417-2426. doi:10.1056/NEJMoa2019375
50. Hu Z, Song C, Xu C, et al. Clinical characteristics of 24 asymptomatic infections with COVID-19 screened among close contacts in Nanjing, China. *Sci China Life Sci.* 2020;63(5):706-711. doi:10.1007/s11427-020-1661-4
51. Wang Y, Liu Y, Liu L, et al. Clinical outcomes in 55 patients with severe acute respiratory syndrome coronavirus 2 who were asymptomatic at hospital admission in Shenzhen, China. *J Infect Dis.* 2020;221(11):1770-1774. doi:10.1093/infdis/jiaa119
52. Orsucci D, Trezzi M, Anichini R, et al. Increased creatine kinase may predict a worse COVID-19 outcome. *J Clin Med.* 2021;10(8):1734. doi:10.3390/jcm10081734
53. Henry BM, Aggarwal G, Wong J, et al. Lactate dehydrogenase levels predict coronavirus disease 2019 (COVID-19) severity and mortality: a pooled analysis. *Am J Emerg Med.* 2020;38(9):1722-1726. doi:10.1016/j.ajem.2020.05.073
54. Manocha KK, Kirzner J, Ying X, et al. Troponin and other biomarker levels and outcomes among patients hospitalized with COVID-19: derivation and validation of the HA2T2 COVID-19 mortality risk score. *J Am Heart Assoc.* 2021;10(6):e018477. doi:10.1161/JAHA.120.018477
55. Huang I, Pranata R. Lymphopenia in severe coronavirus disease-2019 (COVID-19): systematic review and meta-analysis. *J Intensive Care.* 2020;8:36. doi:10.1186/s40560-020-00453-4
56. Mei H, Luo L, Hu Y. Thrombocytopenia and thrombosis in hospitalized patients with COVID-19. *J Hematol Oncol.* 2020;13(1):161. doi:10.1186/s13045-020-01003-z
57. Alkhatib A. Antiviral functional foods and exercise lifestyle prevention of coronavirus. *Nutrients.* 2020;12(9):2633. doi:10.3390/nu12092633
58. Zimmer C. A pill to treat COVID-19? The U.S. is betting on it. *New York Times.* Published June 17, 2021. Accessed June 17, 2021. https://www.nytimes.com/2021/06/17/health/covid-pill-antiviral.html?action=click&module=Well&pgtype=Homepage&section=Health
59. U.S. Food and Drug Administration. *FDA Approves First Treatment for COVID-19.* FDA website. Published October 22, 2020. Accessed June 17, 2021. https://www.fda.gov/news-events/press-announcements/fda-approves-first-treatment-covid-19
60. Basen R, D'Ambrosio A. *COVID-19 Treatments: What's in, What's Out.* Medpage Today. Updated June 3, 2021. Accessed June 17, 2021. https://www.medpagetoday.com/special-reports/exclusives/91680
61. Kalil AC, Patterson TF, Mehta AK, et al. Baricitinib plus remdesivir for hospitalized adults with COVID-19. *N Engl J Med.* 2021;384:795-807. doi:10.1056/NEJMoa2031994
62. U.S. Food and Drug Administration. *FDA Combatting COVID-19 with Therapeutics.* FDA website. Published December 2, 2020. Accessed June 17, 2021. https://www.fda.gov/media/136832/download
63. Taylor PC, Adams AC, Hullford MM, de la Torre I, Winthrop K, Gottlieb RL. Neutralizing monoclonal antibodies for treatment of COVID-19. *Nat Rev Immunol.* 2021;44(1):7-17. doi:10.1016/j.bj.2020.11.011

64. Walker M. Antibody cocktail cut death rate in certain severe COVID patients. *Medpage Today*. Published June 16, 2021. Accessed June 17, 2021. https://www.medpagetoday.com/infectiousdisease/covid19/93140

65. McNicholas C, Poydock M. *Who Are Essential Workers? A Comprehensive Look at Their Wages, Demographics, and Unionization Rates*. Economic Policy Institute. Published May 19, 2020. Accessed June 8, 2021. https://www.epi.org/blog/who-are-essential-workers-a-comprehensive-look-at-their-wages-demographics-and-unionization-rates/

66. Centers for Disease Control and Prevention. *Underlying Medical Conditions Associated with High Risk for Severe COVID-19: Information for Healthcare Providers*. CDC website. Updated May 13, 2021. Accessed June 8, 2021. https://www.cdc.gov/coronavirus/2019-ncov/hcp/clinical-care/underlyingconditions.html

67. Centers for Disease Control and Prevention. *Science Brief: Evidence Used to Update the List of Underlying Medical Conditions that Increase a Person's Risk of Severe Illness from COVID-19*. CDC website. Updated May 12, 2021. Accessed June 8, 2021. https://www.cdc.gov/coronavirus/2019-ncov/science/science-briefs/underlying-evidence-table.html?CDC_AA_refVal=https%3A%2F%2Fwww.cdc.gov%2Fcoronavirus%2F2019-ncov%2Fhcp%2Fclinical-care%2Funderlying-evidence-table.html

68. The Severe COVID-19 GWAS Group. Genomewide association study of severe COVID-19 with respiratory failure. *N Engl J Med*. 2020;383:1522-1534. doi:10.1056/NEJMoa2020283

69. Ray JG, Schull MJ, Vermeulen MJ, Park AL. Association between ABO and Rh blood groups and SARS-CoV-2 infection or severe COVID-19 illness: a population-based cohort study. *Ann Intern Med*. 2021;174(3):308-315. doi:10.7326/M20-4511

70. Peckham H, de Gruijter NM, Raine C, et al. Male sex identified by global COVID-19 meta-analysis as a risk factor for death and ITU admission. *Nat Commun*. 2020;11(1):6317. doi:10.1038/s41467-020-19741-6

71. Arias E, Tejada-Vera B, Ahmad F. *Provisional Life Expectancy Estimates for January through June, 2020. Vital Statistics Rapid Release; No 10*. National Center for Health Statistics; 2021. Accessed February 18, 2021. doi:10.15620/cdc:100392. https://www.cdc.gov/nchs/data/vsrr/VSRR10-508.pdf

72. Kabarriti R, Brodin NP, Maron MI, et al. Association of race and ethnicity with comorbidities and survival among patients with COVID-19 at an urban medical center in New York. *JAMA Netw Open*. 2020;3(9):e2019795. doi:10.1001/jamanetworkopen.2020.19795

73. Mendy A, Wu X, Keller JL, et al. Long-term exposure to fine particulate matter and hospitalization in COVID-19 patients. *Respir Med*. 2021;178:106313. doi:10.1016/j.rmed.2021.106313

74. Centers for Disease Control and Prevention. *Provisional COVID-19 deaths by sex and age*. Updated September 11, 2021. Accessed September 15, 2021. https://data.cdc.gov/NCHS/Provisional-COVID-19-Deaths-by-Sex-and-Age/9bhg-hcku/data

75. Verity R, Okell LC, Dorigatti I, et al. Estimates of the severity of coronavirus disease 2019: a model-based analysis. *Lancet Infect Dis*. 2020;20(6):669-677. doi:10.1016/S1473-3099(20)30243-7

76. Viner RM, Ward JL, Hudson LD, et al. Systematic review of reviews of symptoms and signs of COVID-19 in children and adolescents. *Arch Dis Child*. 2020;archdischild-2020-320972. doi:10.1136/archdischild-2020-320972

77. Leeb RT, Price S, Sliwa S, et al. COVID-19 trends among school-aged children—United States, March 1-September 19, 2020. *MMWR Morb Mortal Wkly Rep*. 2020;69(39):1410-1415. doi:10.15585/mmwr.mm6939e2

78. Hoetz PJ, Ko AI. Why are so many children in Brazil dying from COVID-19? *New York Times*. Published June 4, 2021. Accessed June 6, 2021. https://www.nytimes.com/2021/06/04/opinion/Brazil-covid-children.html

79. Havers FP, Whitaker M, Self JL, et al. Hospitalization of adolescents aged 12-17 years with laboratory-confirmed COVID-19 – COVID.net, 14 states, March 1, 2020-April 24, 2021. *MMWR Morb Mortal Wkly Rep*. 2021;70(23):851-857. doi:10.15585/mmwr.mm7023e1

80. Lewis D. Why schools probably aren't COVID hotspots. *Nature*. 2020;587(7832):17. doi:10.1038/d41586-020-02973-3

81. European Lung Foundation. COVID-19 patients suffer long-term lung and heart damage but it can improve with time. *Science Daily*. Published September 6, 2020. Accessed June 12, 2021. https://www.sciencedaily.com/releases/2020/09/200906202950.htm

82. Marshall M. The lasting misery of coronavirus long-haulers. *Nature*. 2020;585:339-341. doi:10.1038/d41586-020-02598-6

83. Zhang P, Li J, Huixan L, et al. Long-term bone and lung consequences associated with hospital-acquired severe acute respiratory syndrome: a 15-year follow-up from a prospective cohort study. *Bone Res*. 2020;8:8. doi:10.1038/s41413-020-0084-5

84. Lynch KL, Whitman JD, Lacanienta NP, et al. Magnitude and kinetics of anti-severe acute respiratory syndrome coronavirus 2 antibody responses and their relationship to disease severity. *Clin Infect Dis*. 2021;72(2):301-308. doi:10.1093/cid/ciaa979

85. Turner JS, Kim W, Kalaidina E, et al. SARS-CoV-2 infection induces long-lived bone marrow plasma cells in humans. *Nature*. 2021;595:421-425. doi:10.1038/s41586-021-03647-4

86. Shreshta NK, Burke PC, Nowacki AS, Terpeluk P, Gordon SM. Necessity of COVID-19 vaccination in previously infected individuals. medRxiv. doi:10.1101/2021.06.01.21258176

87. Qureshi AI, Baskett WI, Huang W, Lobanova I, Naqvi SH, Shyu CR. Re-infection with SARS-CoV-2 in patients undergoing serial laboratory testing. *Clin Infect Dis*. 2021;ciab345. doi:10.1093/cid/ciab345

88. Cavanaugh AM, Spicer KB, Thoroughman D, Glick C, Winter K. Reduced risk of reinfection with SARS-CoV-2 after COVID-19 vaccination – Kentucky, May-June 2021. *MMWR Morb Mortal Wkly Rep*. 2021;70:1081-1083. doi:10.15585/mmwr.mm7032e1

89. Gazit S, Schlezinger R, Perez G, et al. Comparing SARS-CoV-2 natural immunity to vaccine-induced immunity: reinfections versus breakthrough infections. MedRxiv. doi:10.1101/2021.08.24.21262415

90. Leonhardt D. One in 5,000. *New York Times*. Published September 7, 2021. Accessed September 12, 2021. https://www.nytimes.com/2021/09/07/briefing/risk-breakthrough-infections-delta.html

4

Neuropsychiatric Symptoms and Postacute Sequelae of SARS-CoV-2—The Long Haulers

The previous chapter focused on the pathology and symptomology of COVID-19 but purposely neglected to mention many of the neuropsychiatric symptoms associated with the disease. This chapter will examine these symptoms, as well as how neuroinflammation, chronic systemic inflammation, and psychosocial factors may all converge and define the constellation of neuropsychiatric symptoms frequently reported by patients ranging from those with mild acute cases to those who have experienced persistent problems believed to be related to their initial bout with the disease. This chapter will also include a description of multisystem inflammation syndrome in children (MIS-C) and a discussion of some of the theories that have been proposed to explain the mechanisms of long COVID (or postacute sequelae of SARS-CoV-2 [PASC]), a poorly understood syndrome with a diverse symptomology that may actually be an umbrella term for multiple conditions with heterogeneous etiologies.

COVID-19 and the Central Nervous System

Initial reports about COVID-19 focused primarily on the disease's severe respiratory symptoms. This should come as no surprise since the reports out of Wuhan in December 2019 characterized COVID-19 as an atypical pneumonia, and some of the first media stories to be associated with the outbreak included an 11-second video clip of a computed tomography (CT) scan showing ground-glass opacities in the lungs of a patient and an image of a report showing a false positive for SARS both taken by Dr Ai Fen, Head of Emergency Medicine at Wuhan Central Hospital.[1] Even today, most people tend to associate COVID-19 with respiratory complications, particularly acute respiratory distress syndrome (ARDS).

As research into the pathogenesis of COVID-19 has progressed, evidence has emerged to suggest that it is in fact a multisystem disease that can cause systematic inflammation, blood clotting, organ failure, and sepsis via multiple routes.[2] Apart from these system-wide effects, there are also numerous neurological effects of SARS-CoV-2 infection, though the etiology and the route of infection remain unclear. Moreover, it has yet to be elucidated if SARS-CoV-2 directly invades the central nervous system (CNS) or if neurological complications are due to secondary or systemic effects like hypoxemia, immune dysfunction, or coagulopathy.[2]

Direct evidence of CNS infection was well documented during the SARS-CoV and MERS-CoV outbreaks, indicating that coronaviruses are capable of infecting the CNS; moreover, viral RNA was detected in brain tissue during autopsies of individuals who had tested positive for both viruses.[3] SARS-CoV-2 also appears capable of infecting neural tissue and has been detected in the cortical neurons during autopsy,[4] as well as in cerebrospinal fluid.[5] The route the virus takes to infect the brain remains a mystery, but SARS-CoV-2 may infect the CNS by traveling along nerves from other parts of the body. It is also possible that it may cross the blood-brain barrier after the membrane has been weakened due to the frenzied and systemic inflammatory response, the so-called "cytokine storm" described before (see *Chapter 3: Pathology—What We Knew and What We Know*).

While direct infection of neural tissue appears possible, it has only infrequently been observed in real-world scenarios. Autopsies of 41 consecutive patients with SARS-CoV-2 infections found low to very low levels of viral RNA in the majority of brains, suggesting that neural infection is not core pathology of COVID-19.[6] This would suggest that neuropsychiatric symptoms arise due to a combination of abnormal inflammatory response, hypoxia, and ischemia. Conversely, a study that has yet to be peer reviewed examined the brain scans of 394 COVID-19 patients before and after becoming ill and found deleterious effects to the olfactory and gustatory cortical systems that especially impacted gray matter thickness and volume in the left parahippocampal gyrus, the left superior (dorsal) insula, and the left lateral orbitofrontal cortex. The disease's impact was also observed in the left cingulate cortex, the left supramarginal gyrus, and the right temporal pole. The 15 patients from the group who were hospitalized due to COVID-19 also showed damage to the right hippocampus and amygdala.[7]

One of the most commonly described neurological symptoms is encephalopathy, which is more common in severe cases of COVID-19.[8] Encephalopathy is associated with increased morbidity and mortality, independent of the severity of any COVID-19-related respiratory disease.[9] One case series reported encephalopathy to be present in approximately two-thirds of patients with COVID-19-related ARDS,[10] while another case series found that 31.8% of hospitalized patients had comorbid encephalopathy.[9] Most importantly, a study of 817 older patients in a hospital setting who were diagnosed with COVID-19 infection reported that 226 (28%) had delirium at presentation and 37% of those patients did not present with symptoms typically characterized with COVID-19 (fever, cough, dyspnea, etc). Within the subgroup, 16% presented with delirium as the primary symptom.[11] Risk factors for encephalopathy include male sex, old age, cancer, history of neurologic disorder, cerebrovascular disease, heart failure, kidney disease, diabetes, dyslipidemia, hypertension, and smoking.[9]

Instances of ischemic stroke and hemorrhagic stroke have been reported and may be influenced by a myriad of factors, including coagulopathy, systemic inflammation, and preexisting risk factors typically associated with strokes (hypertension, dyslipidemia, obesity, smoking, etc).[12] Despite relatively infrequent occurrence, the phenomenon was given ample attention in the press, especially because reports of COVID-19-related stroke emerged at the height of the first wave of the pandemic in late April 2020 and because those who were affected were often young, otherwise healthy, and ostensibly were experiencing mild cases of COVID-19.[13] Despite the small panic that this set off that spring, further studies have found that frequency of stroke is correlated with severity of illness and that patients with mild illness have a <1% risk of having a stroke, while the risk for patients admitted to intensive care units may be as high as 6%.[14]

Seizures have been reported far less frequently than stroke or encephalopathy, but they still do occur. Moreover, subclinical or electrographic seizures appear to be quite common, especially in critically ill patients.[15] Meanwhile, meningoencephalitis and acute encephalitis have been reported in connection with COVID-19, and the former appears to be rarer than the latter.[2] In both instances, patients may present with headache and altered consciousness, especially confusion, with or without respiratory symptoms.[16,17]

Microglia and Neuroinflammation

CNS is not just composed of neurons; glial cells play a supportive role by helping clear debris, providing structural and synaptic support for neurons, insulating neurons from one another, maintaining the integrity of the blood-brain barrier, and regulating blood flow. Specialized cells known as microglia serve as the resident innate immune system cells of the CNS and are responsible for responding to pathogens through an inflammatory response known as microgliosis.[18]

Should a pathogen manage to invade the CNS by breaking through the blood-brain barrier or the blood-cerebrospinal fluid barrier, hitching a ride along an infected peripheral nerve, or another means, microgliosis may also be triggered. In ideal scenarios, microglia respond to these insults in a well-orchestrated process that eliminates injury to the neural tissue with as little damage as possible by releasing a balance of proinflammatory and anti-inflammatory cytokines. However, in other instances, microgliosis may occur without the presence of a pathogen when the insult to the neural tissue may be due to hypoxic brain injury or is activated by systemic cytokines that manage to cross the blood-brain barrier. In other words, even if SARS-CoV-2 is incapable of invading the CNS, it can still indirectly cause neuroinflammation (see Figure 4.1).[18]

As Gonçalves de Andrade and colleagues very astutely summed up in a paper published in February 2021, "In the context of a cytokine storm or after exposure to chronic psychosocial stress, microglia can become altered in their function and then increase the release of inflammatory mediators, generating pathogenic effects associated with neurological and psychiatric conditions."[18]

Neurological Symptoms

As described in *Chapter 3: Pathology—What We Knew and What We Know*, it is extremely common for patients with COVID-19 to present with nonspecific features of systemic illness that can also manifest as neurological symptoms. A meta-analysis of 215 studies published between January 2020 and July 2020 involving 105,638 patients found that the most common neurological or neuropsychiatric symptoms included anosmia, weakness, fatigue, dysgeusia, myalgia, sleep disorder, depression, and headache (for a full listing, see Ref. 19). One of the study's limitations is that it overrepresented patients with severe COVID-19, as most of the participants from the 215 studies were recruited from a hospital setting. Consequently, some of the prevalence rates of

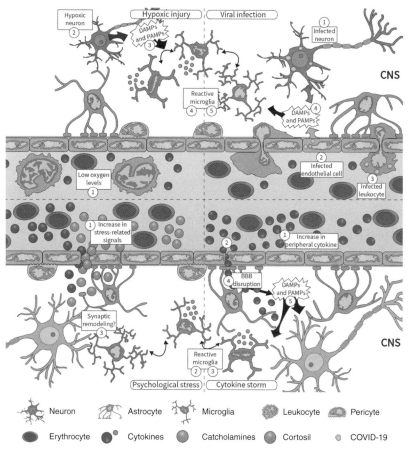

Figure 4.1 Illustration of the ways in which microglia respond to different kinds of insults to the central nervous system (CNS), including hypoxic injury, viral infection, psychological stress, and cytokine storm. As demonstrated in the upper left panel, hypoxia occurs in many cases of COVID-19. When the CNS is deprived of oxygen, oxygen-starved neurons release damage-associated molecular patterns (DAMPs) and pathogen-associated molecular patterns (PAMPs) that then trigger microgliosis and the release of proinflammatory cytokines. The upper right panel illustrates the effects of viral infection should SARS-CoV-2 breach the blood-brain barrier (BBB) via infected peripheral neurons, microvascular brain endothelial cells, or leukocytes. Infected neural tissue may then release DAMPs and PAMPs, triggering microgliosis and the release of proinflammatory cytokines. In the lower left panel, systemic increases in stress-related signals like cortisol, catecholamines, and cytokines may induce microgliosis and dysfunctional synaptic remodeling. In the lower right panel, excessive circulating cytokines may induce a proinflammatory response in the CNS or disrupt BBB function, thereby increasing levels of DAMPs, PAMPs, and cytokines in the CNS while also leading to increases in cytokine production due to microgliosis. (Illustration courtesy of Gonçalves de Andrade E, Šimončičová E, Carrier M, Vecchiarelli HA, Robert ME, Tremblay ME. Microglia fighting for neurological and mental health: on the central nervous system frontline of COVID-19 pandemic. *Front Cell Neurosci.* 2017;15:647378.)

individual symptoms may be skewed, but the study still provides an accurate look at the diversity of neurological and psychiatric symptoms associated with COVID-19.

As noted above, encephalopathy appears to be somewhat common in older patients who may present with delirium and agitation but may also experience tiredness and lapses in memory.[8] Similarly, COVID-19-related ischemic strokes or transient ischemic attacks may result in neuronal damage, and symptoms will depend upon the brain region affected by the ischemic event.

Anosmia

Many of the neurological and neuropsychiatric symptoms[19] are common during the prodrome of numerous diseases and are not unique to COVID-19. However, the anosmia described by COVID-19 patients has been the focus of intense discussion and research because patients do not report experiencing concurrent nasal obstructions. As anyone who has suffered through a run-of-the-mill rhinovirus infection knows, one's sense of smell and taste are disrupted because of congestion and blockage. Of note, most COVID-19 patients report no such blockages but still experience significant olfactory dysfunction.

Initially, researchers wondered if this would mean that the virus was capable of infecting the olfactory bulb. More than just a part of the brain that processes sensory information pertaining to scent, the olfactory bulb is one of the physiological antechambers leading to the CNS (in this metaphor, the figurative door would be the olfactory neuroepithelium and the walkway would be the nasal cavity). Consequently, an infection of the olfactory bulb would allow the virus to access the CNS and could potentially lead to infection of the neural tissue.

Criticism of the theory of CNS infection via the olfactory system has focused on the fact that olfactory receptor neurons do not express ACE2 receptors—the primary receptors to which the SARS-CoV-2 virus binds and uses to invade cells. However, ACE2 expression has been observed in the olfactory neuroepithelium (the door from the above metaphor), which could inhibit cell functionality, disrupt olfactory pathways, and lead to partial or total loss of smell.[20] Furthermore, SARS-CoV-2 has demonstrated binding affinity with another receptor protein, neuropilin-1 (NRP-1).[21] As NRP-1 is highly expressed in olfactory neuroepithelia and the olfactory bulb, it is possible that anosmia results from NRP-1-facilitated infiltration of olfactory neurons.[22] Additionally, and far more concerning, is the fact that SARS-CoV-2 may also be able to infect the CNS through the olfactory system. More research is needed to confirm if this is indeed the mechanism behind

COVID-19-related anosmia and if CNS invasion, even if uncommon, can be mediated by infection of olfactory neurons and NRP-1 receptors.

Guillain-Barré Syndrome

Guillain-Barré syndrome (GBS) is a rare autoimmune disorder in which the immune system targets the body's peripheral nervous system. Patients suffering from GBS can experience a diverse set of symptoms depending on the severity of the disease that range from feelings of weakness all the way to paralysis, and in extreme cases, individuals with GBS may require mechanical ventilation. However, in most cases, GBS is a temporary condition though some patients may experience prolonged sensations of weakness after recovery.[23]

Several clinicians have reported concurrent cases of GBS with COVID-19, suggesting that the hyperactive inflammatory response characterized by COVID-19 may trigger GBS. Preliminary evidence suggests that this complication is more common in elderly men but still quite rare (1 or 2 cases per 100,000 adults) and even rarer in children (0.4-1.4 cases per 100,000).[24] Additionally, approximately 100 of the 12.5 million Americans who have received the Johnson & Johnson vaccine have reportedly developed GBS. So far, one fatality has been reported as of September 2021.[25] Similarly, a study that examined the risk of relapse of GBS after receiving Comirnaty, the Pfizer/BioNTech vaccine, showed that only 1 individual out of the 702 patients previously diagnosed with GBS required brief medical care for relapse of previous syndrome and quickly recovered.[26]

The Neuroinflammation-Chronic Disease Nexus and COVID-19

As troubling as the word "neuroinflammation" may be, it is unfortunately a relatively common phenomenon. Furthermore, neuroinflammation has been linked with diseases that arise when the body is in a chronic proinflammatory state due to lifestyle choices that include poor diet, lack of exercise, smoking, and excessive alcohol consumption. These choices often manifest as pathologic obesity, hypertension, dyslipidemia, insulin resistance, diabetes, or thrombophilia and increase individuals' risk of cardiovascular disease or stroke. Research has also found an association between these chronic inflammatory conditions, poor lifestyle choices, and poor gut microbiome health, and research into the association between the microbiome and COVID-19 has found that there is correlation between poor biome health, increased cytokine levels, and worse outcomes with slower recovery from COVID-19.[27,28]

Inflammation does not just lead to physiological problems or immune system impairment. As Gonçalves de Andrade and colleagues noted above, chronic inflammation and neuroinflammation have been linked with sleep disturbances, anxiety, depression, and other psychiatric disorders.[18] Furthermore, there seems to be a degree of bidirectionality.[29] Neuroinflammation can manifest as physiological distress and psychological distress—be it depression, anxiety, or trauma- and stressor-related disorders like posttraumatic stress disorder—which can lead to neuroinflammation. These implications provide a partial theory as to why patients with conditions like hypertension, diabetes, and Alzheimer disease (of which neuroinflammation appears to be a core pathology[30]) have been more susceptible to severe cases of COVID-19 than children and individuals without these preexisting conditions. The underlying mechanism seems to be that being in a proinflammatory state primes the cytokine response and increases the risk of cytokine storm in COVID-19, significantly worsening prognosis. (Why this occurs with COVID-19 and not with other viral infections remains an open question.) It also provides an explanation as to why so many individuals who tested positive for COVID-19 reported symptoms of new-onset anxiety and depression, as described below.[31] It may even help to explain some of the symptoms associated with long COVID.

In many ways, this phenomenon seems to parallel a frequent observation that has been made when discussing COVID-19 and the social problems that unfolded throughout 2020 and 2021, which is that the pandemic did not create novel problems in the United States; it exacerbated existing ones. This is a subject that will be explored more thoroughly in *Chapter 5: Psychosocial and Economic Impact of COVID-19—A Nation Under Siege*.

Psychiatric Symptoms and Psychosocial Aspects of COVID-19

The most notable psychiatric symptoms observed after COVID-19 infection include traumatic distress, depression, anxiety, sleep problems, and altered consciousness. Surveys conducted by the National Center for Health Services have found that an average of 38% of adults have reported symptoms of anxiety or depressive disorders in surveys conducted between the spring of 2020 and the spring of 2021. That's a threefold jump when compared to the first 6 months of 2019, when the number of adults experiencing these symptoms held steady at approximately 11%.[32]

As noted above, these symptoms are often associated with high levels of systemic proinflammatory cytokines and neuroinflammation.[8] However, psychiatric symptoms may also emerge in the context of psychosocial stresses associated with the pandemic. By no means, complete or exhaustive but a cursory list of stresses includes home confinement, fear of exposure to the virus, fear of exposing loved ones and family members to the virus if infected, and inconsistent messaging about precautions and directives from authority figures and the press. There is no doubt that these stresses exacerbated symptoms in patients with preexisting anxiety and mood disorders, as well as led to new onset symptoms, though it is difficult to determine to what degree individuals' symptoms were influenced by environmental stressors, neuroinflammation, or a combination of two.

As a consequence of stay-at-home orders and social distancing recommendations, individuals became more sedentary by simply remaining at home whenever possible. While this may have prevented transmission of the SARS-CoV-2 virus, it also led to people exercising less, feeling frustrated as a result of being cooped up, and oftentimes resorting to unhealthy coping mechanisms—i.e., excessive use of substances, overeating, overworking—which can all lead to a proinflammatory state. According to a February 2021 poll conducted by the American Psychological Association, 23% of adults reported drinking more to cope with the stress of COVID-19.[33] This should come as no surprise since alcohol sales reportedly skyrocketed during much of the pandemic.[34] Additionally, 61% of respondents in the same survey stated that they experienced undesired changes in weight with an average gain of 29 lb.[33] An even larger number of those polled, 67%, said that they had experienced sleep disturbances since the beginning of the pandemic.[33]

This confluence of cause and effect is in many ways a positive feedback loop, which is a self-affirming process. In a positive feedback loop, the product of a reaction amplifies the reaction, which further amplifies the product. In other words, A produces more of B, which leads to more A, which leads to more B, which leads to more A, and so on.

A very clear example occurs during a stampede. If a single cow is alarmed because they perceive a threat, they may respond by taking flight. This solitary cow's response causes multiple cows to panic and take flight, which causes more cows to panic. The panic rapidly spreads through the entire herd, resulting in a stampede.

A similar phenomenon occurred when the Colonial Pipeline was shut down due to a cyberattack in May 2021. The pipeline supplies approximately half of the gasoline supplied to the East Coast and runs 5500 miles from Texas to New Jersey. Though there were no gas shortages when the pipeline was shut down, individuals began to take precautions against a potential gas shortage by stockpiling gas. When others saw their neighbors taking these precautions, they started taking precautions, as well. Eventually, gas stations began running out of gas. Once the news spread that gas stations were running out of gas, this caused panic buying, resulting in long gas lines and further outages.[35] The same phenomenon can occur with virtually any commodity or staple. As many of us learned at the beginning of the pandemic, this includes toilet paper.[36]

There are clear parallels between this dynamic and the interplay between inflammation, neuroinflammation, increased anxiety and depressive symptoms, and unhealthy behaviors. This is illustrated in Figure 4.2, where one can see the feedback loop that involves four components: chronic inflammatory states, neuroinflammation, increased anxiety and depressive symptoms, and unhealthy behaviors/coping mechanisms. These

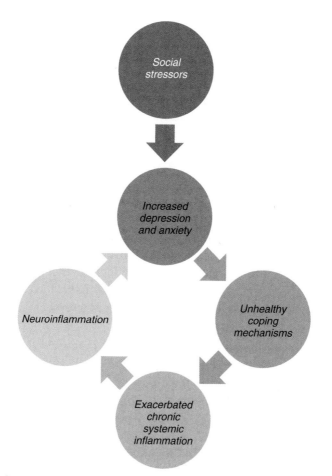

Figure 4.2 Social stressors can lead to anxiety and mood disorders leading to unhealthy coping mechanisms, which not only cause immune system dysfunction and neuroinflammation but also reinforce feelings of depression and anxiety.

four components tend to reinforce one another, resulting in deteriorating health as the body works overtime to try and maintain a healthy homeostasis. To begin with, a person experiencing feelings of anxiety and/or depression may feel distressed, which may lead to unhealthy coping mechanisms; that further exacerbates the underlying chronic inflammatory state, leading to neuroinflammation, thereby worsening feelings of anxiety and/or depression.

By no means is this a predetermined model, as individuals can break the loop by adopting healthier behaviors or coping mechanisms to deal with stress. However, it is difficult even in the best of circumstances. Given the amount of stress that the pandemic placed on individuals and the fact that many support networks were unavailable to those who were struggling with mental health problems, substance use disorders, or eating disorders, it should come as no surprise that anecdotal evidence suggests that backsliding was widespread among those with established conditions and that countless others may have developed addictions or compulsive unhealthy behaviors.

It is far too early to tell if individuals will be able to rectify these behaviors as we adapt to the new normal and begin to gingerly resume routines that feel similar to life prior to the pandemic. Considering the impact of stress on our individual psyches as well as on the society as a whole, the toll the pandemic took on the economy, and the fact that we may be dealing with SARS-CoV-2 variants for years to come, it may be best to temper our optimism.

Long COVID PASC

In late spring of 2020, many patients who recovered from their initial SARS-CoV-2 infection and survived COVID-19 began to report lingering respiratory problems, musculoskeletal symptoms like headache and myalgia, and a foggy feeling that made it difficult to concentrate. Others said that they were sporadically plagued by bouts of fatigue that made it hard to even get out of bed.

The syndrome has become known as either long COVID or PASC, and those who struggle with these symptoms are often referred to as COVID long haulers.

At first glance, this was not particularly surprising. COVID-19 causes numerous complications that do not resolve immediately. Furthermore, evidence of lung tissue scarring has persisted for years following some individuals' struggle with SARS-CoV and has had significant impact on the quality of their life.[37] Since SARS-CoV-2 also causes significant damage to the lungs, as well as the kidneys, heart, and immune system, persisting symptoms associated with the initial infection were to be expected in those who recovered from severe infections.[38]

However, not everyone who experiences these lingering symptoms had a severe case of COVID-19. Many were never hospitalized and yet are reporting new, nonspecific, and bizarre symptoms well after recovering from initial infection. A survey of 3762 people from around the world described 205 symptoms from 10 different organ systems.[39] Meanwhile, a study tracking nearly 2 million people who had COVID-19 found that 23.2% sought medical treatment for at least one new condition 1 month or more following infection. Of those who reported these lingering symptoms, 55% were asymptomatic while infected with the virus, approximately 40% who had symptoms recovered at home, and only 5% were hospitalized.[40]

Symptoms of PASC

The symptoms of PASC or long COVID may persist for weeks or months following a case of COVID-19. Exactly how long symptoms tend to last or if they eventually fade away is still unknown. Long COVID can affect anyone who has had COVID-19, even if they only experienced mild symptoms of acute illness, and it is still too early to determine prevalence. Reports suggest that women are affected slightly more than men and that individuals between 35 and 49 years of age most frequently develop symptoms of long COVID.[41] Estimates of prevalence 4 weeks after the acute onset of COVID-19 symptoms range from 32.6% to 87.4%, while at least one estimate of prevalence after 12 weeks shows a drop to 13.7%.[41] Huang and colleagues painted a far less rosy picture in a paper published in August 2021, where they reported that 49% of patients still had at least one sequela symptom at 12-month follow-up (down from 68% at 6-month follow-up). The cohort study, which involved 1276 COVID-19 survivors, also found that the number of patients still experiencing fatigue and muscle weakness declined between the 6-month and 12-month follow-ups (from 52% to 20%), but that the proportion of patients reporting symptoms of anxiety/depression and dyspnea increased between the 6-month and 12-month follow-ups from 26% to 30% and from 23% to 26%, respectively.[42] Keep in mind that these are preliminary findings and that a clearer picture of the long-term effects of COVID will become apparent as more data become available and as the definition of the condition is better refined.

Some of the most commonly reported symptoms among long haulers include the following:[43]

- Headache
- Chronic fatigue or tiredness

- Difficulty concentrating (brain fog)
- Anosmia
- Dysgeusia
- Dizziness on standing
- Heart palpitations
- Chest pain
- Dyspnea
- Cough
- Joint or muscle pain
- Depression
- Anxiety
- Fever

Symptoms reportedly become worse after physical or mental exertion for many individuals and patients often say that they can become significantly winded after even mild physical activity. A paper that has not been peer reviewed at this time reports that the most common symptoms 6 months after the initial infection appear to be fatigue, postexertional malaise, and cognitive dysfunction.[39]

PASC Etiology and Skepticism

As reports of this condition began to emerge, many clinicians initially thought that the problem was purely psychiatric and related to the stresses of being diagnosed with a potentially deadly disease in addition to the stresses of living through a pandemic. Simultaneously, less sympathetic individuals derided it as being a condition manufactured by the media. One op-ed in the *Wall Street Journal* published in 2021 even characterized it as "largely an invention of vocal patient activist groups," particularly Body Politic, "a feminist wellness collective merging the personal and the political." The author had the wherewithal to not use the phrase "mass hysteria" when mocking those with the condition, which is perhaps the sole merit of the piece.[44]

It is true that suggestion can be very powerful, but the story of medicine, and psychiatry in particular, is riddled with stories of people who were effectively told they were "faking it" or malingering only to be vindicated either later in life or by posterity. This is especially true in cases where signs and discernible etiologies are lacking, and diagnostic criteria are often guided more by symptomology. A prime example of this kind of controversy can be observed by examining the history of PTSD (*see* Box 4.1).

BOX 4.1   How Nostalgia Became PTSD

What we know as posttraumatic stress disorder (PTSD) today was initially referred to as "nostalgia." First coined by the French physician Johannes Hofer in 1688, he described a malady that seemed to affect Swiss mercenaries more often than any other group.

Over the next 200 years, nostalgia was recognized as a condition that affected people throughout Europe, though it continued to be most widely reported among soldiers. During the American Civil War, cases of nostalgia were reportedly occurring at a rate of 2.34 per 1000 during the first year of the war and 3.3 during its second year among White Union soldiers.[45]

The Civil War would be the last major conflict where the term would be used to describe patients with symptomologies that align with our diagnostic criteria for PTSD. As the process of industrialization accelerated in the second half of the 19th century, industrial accidents and railroad crashes became more common, and more physicians became acquainted with patients suffering from symptoms that would today warrant a diagnosis of PTSD. What members of the medical community came to realize is that there was an etiological source to the phenomena, which they called "shock" or trauma, and this led to the popularization of the term "traumatic neurosis" following a traumatic event.

During the First World War, cases of "fright neurosis" and "war neurosis" grew exponentially, while the term "shell shock" was introduced and gained wide traction in the media.[46] In a war primer published in 1915, neurologist Wilfred Harris observed that symptoms reported by patients who had been injured due to the concussive force of an exploding shell while in the trenches were often indistinguishable from those who had escaped bodily harm. Some of the symptoms he noted were "profuse perspiration," sleep disturbances, lack of concentration, shaky hands, tachycardia, dreams about the traumatic event, and "excessive nervousness connected with the actual incidents of the original injury."[47]

"War neurosis" and "shell shock" would remain in use, as would the broader term "traumatic neurosis," during and following World War II, but the diagnostic category fell by the wayside, and there was no mention of any stress- or trauma-related disorders in DSM II, which was published in 1968. Veterans' rights groups argued that the omission was more political than science-based and demanded that the condition be recognized. During the 1970s, they were joined by other social movements in the United States, particularly, feminist groups, who argued that people who had survived sexual assault and sexual violence experienced symptoms akin to those reported by soldiers long after their traumatic experiences.

> **BOX 4.1   How Nostalgia Became PTSD   (Continued)**
>
> The publication of DSM III in 1980 saw the creation of diagnostic criteria for PTSD, and any patient who had persistent symptoms of reexperiencing the event, avoidance, negative mood, and hyperarousal following any form of trauma, whether combat-related or arising from childhood abuse or sexual assault, could be diagnosed with the disorder. Since that time, our understanding of PTSD and trauma has evolved and the most recent edition of DSM (DSM-5) now includes a section on trauma- and stress-related disorders, of which PTSD is but one. Since that time, advances in neuroimaging technology over the past 20 years have revealed that there are clear neural correlates in the bilateral motor regions, dorsolateral prefrontal cortices, medial prefrontal cortex, hippocampi, and the amygdala.[48-50]

At the time of this writing, it is unclear what causes long COVID. This is cold comfort for those who are experiencing symptoms at present and simply do not know when or if their condition will improve. What does seem likely is that "long COVID" is an umbrella term for several conditions with different etiologies. Causes may be tied to tissue damage suffered during the initial acute infection (as discussed in *Chapter 3: Pathology—What We Knew and What We Know*), lingering viral fragments, or an autoimmune disorder that manifests following initial viral infection and continues despite the absence of a pathogen.

In the two latter cases, the mechanisms causing long COVID may not be particularly different from "mystery diseases" like posttreatment Lyme disease syndrome, fibromyalgia, and myalgic encephalomyelitis/chronic fatigue syndrome.[51,52] The lingering fragments theory postulates that a small number of pathogens may manage to avoid complete destruction by the immune system and survive in anatomical sanctuaries. Even if the pathogens remain somehow sheltered from the host's immune system, the presence of viral antigens continues to be detected, prompting a persistent immunoresponse and chronic inflammation.[53] The autoimmune theory suggests that a sustained neuroinflammatory response following initial infection may be the root cause of such symptoms.[54] At this time, these just remain theories.

Reports that some patients experience symptom improvement following vaccination became widespread in spring 2021, but data suggest the response was more mixed than these stories made it seem. A survey of 900 long haulers taken after the participants had received vaccinations found that 56.7% reported symptom improvement. Unfortunately, 6.7%

said either all symptoms deteriorated further or that some symptoms deteriorated while others remained the same.[55] Furthermore, research into the vaccine's efficacy in preventing long COVID is ongoing, and it is not clear if vaccinated individuals have the same risk of developing long COVID should they experience a breakthrough infection.

Multisystem Inflammation Syndrome in Children

For the most part, young children have fared far better than older individuals during the pandemic. To make a very broad generalization, younger and/or healthier individuals typically experience mild symptoms, while older individuals who oftentimes have comorbid inflammatory disorders seem to have more severe symptoms and face a far greater risk of mortality.

One of the exceptions has been MIS-C (also known as pediatric inflammatory multisystem syndrome), which seems to erupt 4 to 6 weeks after children experience a mild case of COVID-19. Similar to Kawasaki disease, MIS-C is a condition where multiple organs become inflamed and may include the kidneys, heart, lungs, spleen, eyes, gastrointestinal (GI) tract, skin, and brain. Symptoms include fever, vomiting, diarrhea, nausea, abdominal pain, neck pain, rash, bloodshot eyes, and drowsiness.[56] Patients typically present with GI symptoms but can go on to develop myocarditis, cardiac dysfunction, and coronary artery dilation. These three complications occurred in approximately 30% of patients.[57]

While it is rare (occurring in 2.1 per 100,000 persons younger than 21 years in the United States), an estimated 60% of individuals who develop MIS-C are admitted to intensive care units.[57] As of September 14, 2021, a total of 4661 cases have been reported in the United States and 41 (0.9%) have proven fatal.[58] Very young children aged 0 to 4 typically had fewer complications and fewer admissions to intensive care, while patients in the age group of 18 to 20 years with recent infection of COVID-19 were more likely to experience myocarditis, ARDS, or pneumonia.[57] The median age of patients with MIS-C in the United States is 9 years while half of all reported cases have been children between the ages of 5 and 13 years and 60% of reported patients have been males.[59]

Like COVID-19, MIS-C disproportionately impacted Black and Hispanic children—30% and 32% of cases, respectively.[59,60] Social determinants in health, particularly poverty, housing, and employment dynamics, and insurance status have placed both Hispanic and Black individuals at greater risk of COVID-19 infection and greater risk of severe complications, including MIS-C.[57]

Conclusion

COVID-19 is far more than a respiratory disease. COVID-19 links the neurological, neuropsychiatric, psychological, psychosocial, and immunological conditions and is associated with a broad range of either clear neurological or mixed neuropsychiatric symptoms. These symptoms may be mediated by neuroinflammation and can be influenced by individual patients' responses to the psychosocial effects of the pandemic, physiological effects of the virus, as well as their underlying mental and physical health. Systemic inflammation plays a major role in the pathologies of COVID-19, long COVID, and MIS-C, and learning how to better control and mitigate chronic inflammation as well as neuroinflammation will be key to understanding the connections between these three diseases, as well as treating them without any prolonged sequela.

REFERENCES

1. Lawrence SV. *COVID-19 and China: A Chronology of Events (December 2019-January 2020)*. Congressional Research Service. Updated May 13, 2020. Accessed May 21, 2021. https://crsreports.congress.gov/product/pdf/r/r46354
2. Norouzi M, Miar P, Norouzi S, Nikpour P. Nervous system involvement in COVID-19: a review of the current knowledge. *Mol Neurobiol.* 2021;58(7):3561-3574. doi:10.1007/s12035-021-02347-4
3. Xu J, Zhong S, Liu J, et al. Detection of severe acute respiratory syndrome coronavirus in the brain: potential role of the chemokine mig in pathogenesis. *Clin Infect Dis.* 2005;41(8):1089-1096. doi:10.1086/444461
4. Song E, Zhang C, Israelow B, et al. Neuroinvasion of SARS-CoV-2 in human and mouse brain. *J Exp Med.* 2021;218(3):e20202135. doi:10.1084/jem.20202135
5. Yavarpour-Bali H, Ghasemi-Kasman M. Update on neurological manifestations of COVID-19. *Life Sci.* 2020;257:118063. doi:10.1016/j.lfs.2020.118063
6. Thakur KT, Miller EH, Glendinning MD, et al. COVID-19 neuropathology at Columbia University Irving Medical Center/New York Presbyterian Hospital. *Brain.* 2021;144(9):2696-2708. doi:10.1093/brain/awab148
7. Douaud G, Lee S, Alfaro-Almagro F, et al. Brain imaging before and after COVID-19 in UK Biobank. Published June 20, 2021. MedRxiv. doi:10.1101/2021.06.11.21258690
8. Fotuhi M, Mian A, Meysami S, Raji CA. Neurobiology of COVID-19. *J Alzheimers Dis.* 2020;76(1):3-19. doi:10.3233/JAD-200581
9. Liotta EM, Batra A, Clark JF, et al. Frequent neurologic manifestations and encephalopathy-associated morbidity in COVID-19 patients. *Ann Clin Transl Neurol.* 2020;7(11):2221-2230. doi:10.1002/acn3.51210
10. Helms J, Kremer S, Merdji H, et al. Neurologic features in severe SARS-CoV-2 infection. *N Engl J Med.* 2020;382:2268-2270. doi:10.1056/NEJMc2008597
11. Kennedy M, Helfand BKI, Gou RY, et al. Delirium in older patients with COVID-19 presenting to the emergency department. *JAMA Netw Open.* 2020;3(11):e2029540. doi:10.1001/jamanetworkopen.2020.29540
12. McAlpine LS, Zubair AS, Maran I, et al. Ischemic stroke, inflammation, and endotheliopathy in COVID-19 patients. *Stroke.* 2021;52(6):e233-e238. doi:10.1161/STROKEAHA.120.031971
13. Hamilton J. *Doctors Link COVID-19 to Potentially Deadly Blood Clots and Strokes*. NPR. Published April 29, 2020. Accessed June 9, 2021.

https://www.npr.org/sections/health-shots/2020/04/29/847917017/
doctors-link-covid-19-to-potentially-deadly-blood-clots-and-strokes

14. Mao L, Hin H, Wang M, et al. Neurologic manifestations of hospitalized patients with coronavirus disease 2019 in Wuhan, China. *JAMA Neurol.* 2020;77(6):683-690. doi:10.1001/jamaneurol.2020.1127

15. Lin L, Al-Faraj A, Ayub N, et al. Electroencephalographic abnormalities are common in COVID-19 and are associated with outcomes. *Ann Neurol.* 2021;89(5):872-883. doi:10.1002/ana.26060

16. Hafizi F, Kherani S, Shams M. Meningoencephalitis from SARS-CoV-2 infection. *ID Cases.* 2020;21:e00919. doi:10.1016/j.idcr.2020.e00919

17. Benameur K, Agarwal A, Auld SC, et al. Encephalopathy and encephalitis associated with cerebrospinal fluid cytokine alterations and coronavirus disease, Atlanta, Georgia, USA, 2020. *Emerg Infect Dis.* 2020;26(9):2016-2021. doi:10.3201/eid2609.202122

18. Gonçalves de Andrade E, Šimončičová E, Carrier M, Vecchiarelli HA, Robert ME, Tremblay ME. Microglia fighting for neurological and mental health: on the central nervous system frontline of COVID-19 pandemic. *Front Cell Neurosci.* 2017;15:647378. doi:10.3389/fncel.2021.647378

19. Rogers JP, Watson CJ, Badenoch J, et al. Neurology and neuropsychiatry of COVID-19: a systematic review and meta-analysis of the early literature reveals frequent CNS manifestations and key emerging narratives. *J Neurol Neurosurg Psychiatry.* 2021;92(9):932-941. doi:10.1136/jnnp-2021-326405

20. Bauers S. *Penn Researcher Explains Why COVID-19 Affects Our Sense of Smell | 5 Questions.* Philadelphia Inquirer. Published May 19, 2021. Accessed June 9, 2021. https://www.inquirer.com/health/coronavirus/covid-loss-of-smell-test-penn-20210519.html

21. Kyrou I, Randeva HS, Spandidos DA, Karteris E. Not only ACE2—the quest for additional host cell mediators of SARS-CoV-2 infection: neuropilin-1 (NPR1) as a novel SARS-CoV-2 host cell mediator implicated in COVID-19. *Signal Transduct Target Ther.* 2021;6(1):21. doi:10.1038/s41392-020-00460-9

22. Mayi BS, Leibowitz JA, Woods AT, Ammon KA, Liu AE, Raja A. The role of neuropilin-1 in COVID-19. *PLoS Pathog.* 2021;17(1):e1009153. doi:10.1371/journal.ppat.1009153

23. Guillian-Barré syndrome fact sheet. *National Institute of Neurological Disorders and Stroke.* Published June 2018. Accessed June 9, 2021. https://www.ninds.nih.gov/disorders/patient-caregiver-education/fact-sheets/Guillain-barr%C3%A9-syndrome-fact-sheet

24. Rahimi K. Guillian-Barre syndrome during COVID-19 pandemic: an overview of the reports. *Neurol Sci.* 2020;41(11):3149-3156. doi:10.1007/s10072-020-04693-y

25. FDA News Release. *Coronavirus (COVID-19) Update: July 13, 2021.* U.S. Food and Drug Administration. Published July 13, 2021. Accessed August 20, 2021. https://www.fda.gov/news-events/press-announcements/coronavirus-covid-19-update-july-13-2021

26. Shapiro Ben David S, Potasman I, Rahamin-Cohen D. Rate of recurrent Guillain-Barré syndrome after mRNA COVID-19 vaccine BNT162b2. *JAMA Neurol.* 2021. doi:10.1001/jamaneurol.2021.3287

27. Zuo T, Zhang F, Lui GCY, et al. Alterations in gut microbiota of patients with COVID-19 during time of hospitalization. *Gastroenterology.* 2020;15(3):944-955. doi:10.1053/j.gastro.2020.05.048

28. Yeoh YK, Zuo T, Lui GCY, et al. Gut microbiota composition reflects disease severity and dysfunctional immune response in patients with COVID-19. *Gut.* 2021;70(4):698-706. doi:10.1136/gutjnl-2020-323020

29. Pierce GL, Kalil GZ, Ajibewa T, et al. Anxiety independently contributes to elevated inflammation in humans with obesity. *Obesity (Silver Spring).* 2017;25(2):286-289. doi:10.1002/oby.21698

30. Kinney JW, Bemiller SM, Murtishaw AS, Leisgang AM, Salazar AM, Lamb BT. Inflammation as a central mechanism in Alzheimer's disease. *Alzheimers Dement (N Y).* 2018;4:575-590. doi:10.1016/j.trci.2018.06.014

31. Hurissi E, Abu-jabir E, Mohammed A, et al. Assessment of new-onset depression and anxiety associated with COVID-19. *Middle East Curr Psychiatry.* 2021;28(1):33. doi:10.1186/s43045-021-00112-w

32. Panchal N, Kamal R, Cox C, Garfield R. *The Implications of COVID-19 for Mental Health and Substance Use.* KFF website. Published February 10, 2021. Accessed April 5, 2021. https://www.kff.org/coronavirus-covid-19/issue-brief/the-implications-of-covid-19-for-mental-health-and-substance-use/

33. American Psychological Association. *Stress in America: One Year Later, a New Wave of Pandemic Health Concerns.* Accessed June 6, 2021. https://www.apa.org/news/press/releases/stress/2021/sia-pandemic-report.pdf

34. Mann B. *Hangover from Alcohol Boom Could Last Long after Pandemic Ends.* NPR. Published September 11, 2020. Accessed April 5, 2021. https://www.npr.org/2020/09/11/908773533/hangover-from-alcohol-boom-could-last-long-after-pandemic-ends#:~:text=According%20to%20Nielsen's%20market%20data,27%25%20increase%20over%20last%20year

35. Englund W, Nakashima E. Panic buying strikes Southeastern United States as shuttered pipeline resumes operations. *Washington Post.* Published May 12, 2021. Accessed June 12, 2021. https://www.washingtonpost.com/business/2021/05/12/gas-shortage-colonial-pipeline-live-updates/

36. Shih WC. Global supply chains in a post-pandemic world: companies need to make their networks more resilient. Here's how. *Harv Bus Rev.* Published September-October 2020. Accessed June 12, 2021. https://hbr.org/2020/09/global-supply-chains-in-a-post-pandemic-world

37. Zhang P, Li J, Huixan L, et al. Long-term bone and lung consequences associated with hospital-acquired severe acute respiratory syndrome: a 15-year follow-up from a prospective cohort study. *Bone Res.* 2020;8:8. doi:10.1038/s41413-020-0084-5

38. Marshall M. The lasting misery of coronavirus long-haulers. *Nature.* 2020;585:339-341. doi:10.1038/d41586-020-02598-6

39. Davis HE, Assaf GS, McCorkell LM, et al. Characterizing long COVID in an international cohort: 7 months of symptoms and their impact. 2021. MedRxiv. doi:10.1101/2020.12.24.20248802

40. FAIR Health. *A Detailed Study of Patients with Long-Haul COVID: An Analysis of Private Healthcare Claims.* Published June 15, 2021. Accessed June 20, 2021. https://s3.amazonaws.com/media2.fairhealth.org/whitepaper/asset/A%20Detailed%20Study%20of%20Patients%20with%20Long-Haul%20COVID--An%20Analysis%20of%20Private%20Healthcare%20Claims--A%20FAIR%20Health%20White%20Paper.pdf

41. Marshall M. The four most urgent questions about long COVID. *Nature.* 2021;594(7862):168-170. doi:10.1038/d41586-021-01511-z

42. Huang L, Yao Q, Gu X, et al. 1-year outcomes in hospital survivors with COVID-19: a longitudinal cohort study. *Lancet.* 2021;398(10302):747-758. doi:10.1016/S0140-6736(21)01755-4

43. Centers for Disease Control and Prevention. *Post-COVID Conditions.* Updated April 8, 2021. Accessed June 12, 2021. https://www.cdc.gov/coronavirus/2019-ncov/long-term-effects.html

44. Devine J. The dubious origins of long COVID. *Wall St J.* Published March 22, 2021. Accessed June 4, 2021. https://www.wsj.com/articles/the-dubious-origins-of-long-covid-11616452583

45. Ellis PS. The origins of the war neuroses (Part I). *J Roy Nav Med Serv.* 1984;70:168-177. Accessed on June 22, 2020. https://archive.org/details/JRNMSVOL70Images/page/n185/mode/2up

46. Ellis PS. The origins of the war neuroses (Part II). *J Roy Nav Med Serv.* 1985;71:32-44. Accessed on June 4, 2021. https://archive.org/details/JRNMSVOL71Images/page/n43/mode/2up

47. Harris W. *Nerve Injuries and Shock.* Oxford University Press; 1915. Accessed June 4, 2021. https://archive.org/stream/nerveinjuriessho00harruoft?ref=ol#page/100/mode/2up

48. Bremner JD. Neuroimaging in posttraumatic stress disorder and other stress-related disorders. *Neuroimaging Clin N Am.* 2007;17(4):523-538. ix. doi:10.1016/j.nic.2007.07.003

49. Badura-Brack AS, Heinrichs-Graham E, McDermott TJ, et al. Resting-state neurophysiological abnormalities in posttraumatic stress disorder: a magnetoencephalography study. *Front Neurosci.* 2017;11:205. doi:10.3389/fnhum.2017.00205

50. Xiong K, Zhang Y, Qiu M, et al. Negative emotion regulation in patients with posttraumatic stress disorder. *PLoS One.* 2013;8(12):e81957. doi:10.1371/journal.pone.0081957

51. Bäckryd E, Tanum L, Lind AL, Larsson A, Gordh T. Evidence of both system inflammation and neuroinflammation in fibromyalgia patients, as assessed by a multiplex protein panel applied to the cerebrospinal fluid and to plasma. *J Pain Res.* 2017;10:515-525. doi:10.2147/JPR.S128508

52. VanElzakker MB, Brumfield SA, Lara Mejia PS. Neuroinflammation and cytokines in myalgic encephalomyelitis/chronic fatigue syndrome (ME/CFS): a critical review of research methods. *Front Neurol.* 2019;9:1033. doi:10.3389/fneur.2018.01033. eCollection 2018.

53. Cox D. What COVID-19's long tail is revealing about disease. *BBC.* Published June 9, 2021. Accessed June 13, 2021. https://www.bbc.com/future/article/20210609-how-long-will-long-covid-last

54. Coughlin JM, Yang T, Rebman AW, et al. Image glial activation in patients with post-treatment Lyme disease symptoms: a pilot study using [11C]DPA-713 PET. *J Neuroinflammation.* 2018;15(1):346. doi:10.1186/s12974-018-1381-4

55. Sherwood O, Strain WD, Rossman J. *The Impact of COVID Vaccinations on Symptoms of Long COVID. An International Survey of 900 People with Lived Experience.* LongCovidSOS. Published May 2021. Accessed June 12, 2021. https://3ca26cd7-266e-4609-b25f-6f3d1497c4cf.filesusr.com/ugd/8bd4fe_a338597f76bf4279a851a7a4cb0e0a74.pdf

56. *Multisystem Inflammatory Syndrome (MIS-C).* Centers for Disease Control and Prevention. Updated February 25, 2021. Accessed June 10, 2021. https://www.cdc.gov/mis-c/

57. Belay ED, Abrams J, Oster ME. Trends in geographic and temporal distribution of US children with multisystem inflammatory syndrome during the COVID-19 pandemic. *JAMA Pediatr.* 2021;175:837-845. doi:10.1001/jamapediatrics.2021.0630

58. Centers for Disease Control and Prevention. *Health Department – Reported Cases of Multisystem Inflammatory Syndrome in Children (MIS-C) in the United States.* Updated August 27, 2021. Accessed September 14, 2021. https://www.cdc.gov/mis-c/cases/index.html

59. Centers for Disease Control and Prevention. *Health Department – Reported Cases of Multisystem Inflammatory Syndrome in Children (MIS-C) in the United States.* Updated June 2, 2021. Accessed June 13, 2021. https://www.cdc.gov/mis-c/cases/index.html

60. Frey WH. *Less than Half of US Children under 15 Are white, Census Shows.* Brookings Institute. Updated July 17, 2019. Accessed June 13, 2019. https://www.brookings.edu/research/less-than-half-of-us-children-under-15-are-white-census-shows/

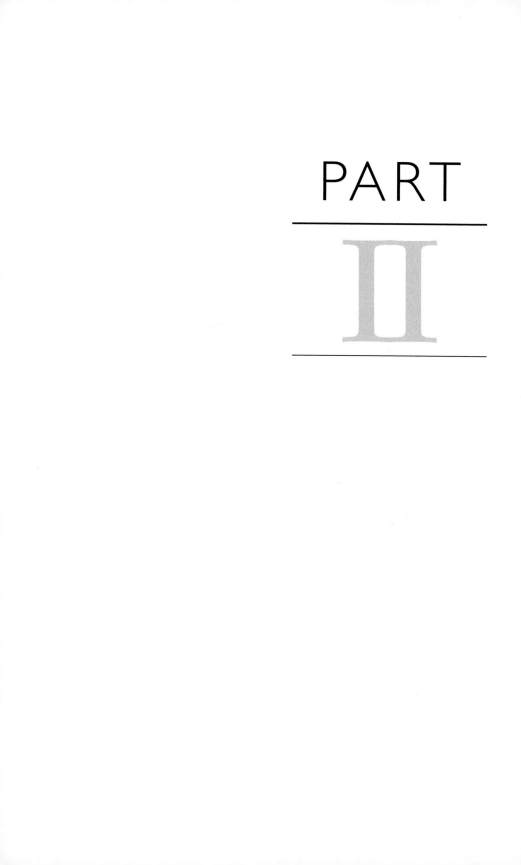

PART

II

Understanding the full impact of the pandemic will likely be the subject of debates for years, largely because there are so many different and often subjective metrics that we can use to measure its effects. While an understanding of a virus' R_0 value or a rolling count of the number of cases or deaths can begin to sketch out how bad a particular strain of a virus is from an epidemiologist's perspective, it does not fully illustrate what it is like to have the disease. It does not fully explain why patients are reporting symptoms associated with major depressive disorders, anxiety disorders, adjustment disorder, and posttraumatic stress disorder following recovery. Moreover, it does not explain what it is like to live under the threat of catching the virus when virtually nothing is known about it or worrying about what happens should a loved one become ill. Empathy simply does not play a role in this kind of calculus.

Similarly, data about lost jobs, ruined businesses, and boarded up storefronts can start to give some impression of how deep the economic impact of the pandemic has been, but there is once again an empathy gap. The data do not take into account the psychological effect of losing a job, losing a business, or even walking through the town or city that one has known for years and seeing its avenues of commerce barren. No amount of data mining will ever be able to provide a panoramic view of the pain and destruction caused by the pandemic.

Another reason why we cannot understand the full scale of the event is because it is still happening and will likely continue for years to come; even the defining features of the pandemic's acute phase—overburdened hospitals, strictly enforced social distancing measures, shelter-in-place orders, and widespread mask wearing—is largely becoming a thing of the past, at least in the parts of the United States where vaccination rates have been high.

If we continue to define the time before the pandemic as normal, we will never emerge from the COVID Era. We must recognize that many of the features that we currently identify as being unique to 2020 and 2021 will be absorbed either consciously or subconsciously by a significant portion of the population well after the majority of Americans have processed the traumas of the pandemic and moved on. Some people will likely continue to wear masks when they become sick with even minor illnesses. Some people will continue to regularly use hand sanitizer after touching unfamiliar surfaces. Some people may find it exceptionally difficult just to leave their homes.

Some may argue that these are manifestations of a common feature of psychological trauma. As Bessel van der Kolk has observed in beautiful works like *The Body Keeps the Score*, trauma anchors people to a moment in time and prevents them from fully moving forward.[1] The trauma then comes to define them, and it can ultimately devour them. However, it may also be the case that these behaviors, especially the wearing of a mask when ill, become cultural norms in the United States. Again, *if we continue to define normal as the return to life before the pandemic, there is a good chance that we will never return to a sense of normal again.* We need to absorb the experiences of the past 2 years, learn from them, and create a new normal if we are to be healthy and functioning adults, especially if the SARS-CoV-2 virus becomes endemic.

So much of our day-to-day lives have been affected by COVID-19. It is difficult to even understand it as a singular phenomenon since the pandemic introduced new stressors, exacerbated existing ones, and produced a wide range of secondary and tertiary effects that all occurred simultaneously. For example, at the same time that some individuals were struggling with anxieties caused by the sudden appearance of an unfamiliar virus, they were also losing their jobs, access to their houses of worship, and oftentimes physical contact with their family and friends.

Research into trauma- and stress-related disorders, most notably posttraumatic stress disorder, has found that a majority of people experience a traumatic event in their life.[2] Those from disadvantaged communities appear to be at an even greater risk, with incidence rates of traumatic events as high as 90% in areas that struggle with high rates of poverty, unemployment, and various environmental burdens.[3] Despite the unfortunately high frequency of traumatic events, the majority of people do not develop a trauma- or stress-related disorder.[4]

Why not?

Through my years of research, I have found that people who have strong social support networks or a sense of purpose are more resilient and better able to cope with stressors and trauma than those who do not.[5] I say this not only as a clinician practicing in New York City but in response to my experience as part of a team researching resilience in remote villages and towns in the Northwestern Frontier Province of Pakistan following the October 8, 2005, earthquake that caused an estimated quarter million casualties and left approximately 3.5 million homeless.[6] It is believed to be the deadliest earthquake to have ever occurred in the area. Even in this extremely devastating scenario, those who were the most resilient in the aftermath of the event were those who had strong social bonds. That these social bonds were ripped away precisely when they were needed most almost certainly made it more difficult for individuals to endure traumatic experiences. We are still waiting for data to see how social isolation impacted rates of resilience.

Of course, not all of the stress caused by COVID was nearly so cataclysmic. For hundreds of millions of people throughout the world, the pandemic has been instead a source of constant, low-level stress that has added up over time. Our world really began to revolve around the virus, and this was the case even for those who were not directly harmed by it. For those who are predisposed to anxiety disorders or depressive disorders, being forced to shut themselves away while watching the world fall apart around them had a debilitating effect. For individuals with severe and persistent mental illnesses like schizophrenia or bipolar disorder, the combination of these stressors and disruptions in mental health services has been catastrophic.

Even for those who were not struggling with a mental illness or never got infected or never lost anyone close to them or managed to keep their job and stay in a relatively healthy living situation, it is not as though they have necessarily escaped unscathed. True, they fared far better than others, but the stresses of being cooped up in a house by oneself or with a few other adults or with very young children were also very difficult for people in all age groups and from all kinds of backgrounds. Add to this the uncertainty of how or when one resumes normal activities in the face of new developments like the Delta variant and it becomes clear why signs of increased stress and anxiety have been ubiquitous.

With very rare exception, the stresses of the COVID-19 pandemic have been felt by everyone to some degree, and the *status quo* that had been accepted by billions of people as the natural or normal state of affairs evaporated, virtually overnight. This provided fodder for a certain kind of existential questioning as people considered what kind of world should replace the old one. Thoughts about happiness and the meaning of life that had may have been common among people when they were in young adulthood but had been suppressed because of the need to earn a living suddenly came roaring back. Meanwhile, fervent calls for social change erupted across the globe and especially in the United States in a way that had not been seen since the dawn of the Arab Spring in countries like Egypt, Libya, Tunisia, Yemen, and Syria or in the West since the student uprisings of 1968.

When George Floyd was murdered by former police officer Derek Chauvin in Minneapolis on May 25, 2020, it served as a flashpoint that ultimately led to a summer of protests against police brutality and racism. Had people not been locked inside for several months and searching for meaning, and had Chauvin's excessive cruelty not been vividly documented, it is impossible to say if the protests would have erupted with the same fervor and the same level of participation. What is clear is that there was a sense that transformation, whether welcomed or feared, that permeated the summer and fall of 2020 in the United States as activists poured into the streets, the 2020 presidential elections kicked into high gear, the pandemic continued to rage, and the economic and social fallout of the first wave of the pandemic continued to reverberate across the globe. 2021 offered little to no reprieve from this sense of crisis as it started with the mayhem at the Capitol, the rise of the Delta variant, a sputtering economy, and seemingly weekly political crises at home and abroad.

Suffice to say, COVID-19 has radically altered our culture; it has fundamentally changed how we live our lives; and it will have dramatic effects on the way we think, behave, socialize, and receive medical care whether it becomes an endemic disease or not. It will certainly impact how governments approach issues of public health, particularly mental health. Consequently, it will no doubt rank among September 11, the fall of the Berlin Wall, and the dropping of the first atomic bomb with respect to historical significance because such a violent paradigm shift has created an uncrossable rift between the before and the after. This may seem a bit hyperbolic at first, but life in the COVID-19 Era has come to resemble life during a time of war in the sense that the destruction and anguish that have been caused by the virus are not tied to a singular event, but rather an extended tragedy. In addition, one has had to become inured to survive, even if it is simultaneously impossible to ignore because not a day has gone by for almost 2 years without various cultures around the world obsessing over the latest developments surrounding the virus, and counting the number of sick, and the number of dead.

The next seven chapters will try to assess how all these converging forces affected us and hopefully begin to shine a light on some of the work we will ultimately have to undertake to reclaim a new sense of normalcy in the wake of this calamity.

REFERENCES

1. van der Kolk BA. *The Body Keeps the Score: Brain, Mind, and Body in the Healing of Trauma.* Penguin Books; 2014.
2. Benjet C, Bromet E, Karam EG, et al. The epidemiology of traumatic event exposure worldwide: results from the World Mental Health Survey Consortium. *Psychol Med.* 2016;46(2):327-343. doi:10.1017/S0033291715001981
3. Gillikin C, Habib L, Evces M, Bradley B, Ressler KJ, Sanders J. Trauma exposure and PTSD symptoms associate with violence in inner city civilians. *J Psychiatr Res.* 2016;83:1-7. doi:10.1016/j.jpsychires.2016.07.027
4. Korte KJ, Jiang T, Koenen KC, Gradus J. Trauma and PTSD: epidemiology, comorbidity, and clinical presentation in adults. In: Forbes D, Bisson JI, Monson CM, Berliner L, eds. *Effective Treatments for PTSD: Practical Guidelines From the International Society for Traumatic Stress Studies.* The Guilford Press; 2020:13-29.
5. Feder A, Ahmad S, Lee EJ, et al. Coping and PTSD symptoms in Pakistani earthquake survivors: purpose in life, religious coping and social support. *J Affect Disord.* 2013;147(1-3):156-163. doi:10.1016/j.jad.2012.10.027
6. Ahmad S, Feder A, Lee EJ, et al. Earthquake impact in a remote South Asian population: psychosocial factors and posttraumatic symptoms. *J Trauma Stress.* 2010;23(3):408-412. doi:10.1002/jts.20535

5

Psychosocial and Economic Impact of COVID-19— A Nation Under Siege

SARS-CoV-2 has radically transformed our society not only because of widespread infections among people all over the globe but also due to its profound social and economic impact. Together, these two factors exacerbated the levels of stress experienced not only by individuals who were infected by SARS-CoV-2 but also those whose lives were irrevocably changed by the direct and indirect effects of the pandemic. This chapter examines some of the specific psychological, economic, environmental, and psychosocial effects of the pandemic, as well as the way in which individuals' stress responses can adversely affect their mental health and wellbeing. While SARS-CoV-2 is a viral disease with a specific pathology that has already been discussed, the COVID-19 pandemic has proven to be a psychosocial disease with truly devastating social, economic, and psychological consequences.

Understanding COVID-19 as a Psychosocial Disease

There is a popular belief in some circles that human nature is defined almost entirely by experience. In the most basic terms, those who advocate this view believe that the human mind is largely a blank slate (or tabula rasa) when an individual is in infancy and over time it is filled in by experience. Of a similar vein, there is a belief that humans are almost endlessly adaptable and that we are capable of thriving in an almost infinite number of social conditions so long as the physical environment into which we have been placed is not too hostile. In other words, so long as we have the most basic needs for survival (water, food, air, etc), we will be able to endure and possibly even thrive.

Endure? Yes. Thrive? Hardly.

As psychoanalyst Erich Fromm wrote over 60 years ago, "The statement that man can live under almost any condition is only half true; it must be supplemented by the other statement, that if he lives under conditions which are contrary to his nature and to the basic requirements for human growth and sanity, he cannot help reacting."[1] As humans, we have our physical, social, and psychological limits, and they are all interconnected. We are not infinitely malleable. We can adapt and endure a great deal, but, eventually, we reach a breaking point. As a result, there are conditions to which we cannot adapt.

For hundreds of thousands of years, we have persevered and thrived in tribes and in clans. Survival was only possible if we worked together to overcome environmental dangers and to ward off attacks from other animals (and other humans). In time, this process of collaboration gave way to language and highly sophisticated cultures and further ingrained the need for social interaction into our psychological DNA. Human beings are social animals, and this requires us to interact with other humans. Consequently, when we are placed in isolation, we deteriorate psychologically and physically and these two have a reciprocal effect—meaning psychological deterioration accelerates physical deterioration and vice versa (more on that below). After all, if we were not social creatures, solitary confinement would not be considered a form of torture.

One of the core elements of human nature is the need for physical interactions with other humans—and not just over the phone or through Zoom. The sense of smell and touch is an essential part of being human. The pandemic and social distancing robbed us of being able to be physically close to others and took away these essential elements of our existence. We need to feel other people's presence, to share space with them, and to touch and even smell them. Virtual meetings may have been an acceptable solution in the short-term and may allow us to fulfill certain professional duties, but it became apparent relatively quickly that these ersatz interactions are flat and alienating ordeals that cannot substitute authentic social interactions. They simply do not satisfy our need for social engagement, and many of us have learned during the pandemic that this lack of real human interaction can lead to a deterioration of mental health, even if we may not develop a diagnosable mental illness.

Social interaction and social engagement provide us with two vital sources of comfort. On the one hand, it gives us a sense of belonging, that we are part of a group, and makes us feel accepted and validated. On the other, it makes us feel safe and gives us a sense of security, which is another basic requirement for human beings to thrive. This is not to say that we need to be coddled or babied or meticulously kept out of harm's way. We absolutely do need to be challenged in order to learn and to grow. However, when these challenges are constant and one feels as though they need to remain hypervigilant and fear for their life, it takes a toll on one's mental health. This was the reality for many essential workers during the first phase of the pandemic who had no security blanket, no protection via natural immunity or vaccination, and oftentimes limited supplies. They were forced to confront the persistent threat of infection and the possibility that they might even spread the virus to others, including their loved ones at a time when very little was known about the acute or long-term effects of the virus.

The human race did not evolve to be placed under this kind of solitary and persistent stress—be it due to social isolation or due to months-long fear of a pathogen without respite. We evolved specifically to avoid these kinds of issues by forming strong social networks and working together, thereby giving us the opportunity of repose. The pandemic led to the disintegration of our social fabric, which under normal circumstances provides us with a sense of tranquility and inner calm. As a result of quarantine, being cut off from our social supports which function as emotional and psychological sustenance, as well as a barrage of psychosocial stressors amidst a backdrop of extreme political polarization, violent rhetoric, mass protests, and a cavalcade of terrifying economic and geopolitical news, it seemed as though the social order that we had come to recognize as the bedrock of our day-to-day existence began to crack and crumble.

This environment has been noxious and conducive only to cultivating psychological distress, which is why many people without preexisting conditions or genetic predispositions or a history of mental illness have reported struggles with their mental health. Throughout the pandemic, nearly everyone has exhibited some of the symptoms of affective, anxiety, or substance abuse disorders. Having these conditions does not mean that one is mentally ill, an addict, or in any way weak. Rather, it suggests that one could not thrive in conditions that are contrary to the needs of humans. If anything, it is a proof of their humanity, a reminder to practice humility, and a reason that each one of us should wear our empathy on our sleeve.

What is reassuring is that the vast majority of those who were forced into long periods of social isolation or perpetual fear during the pandemic will ultimately recover. As I have said elsewhere, humans are exceptionally resilient.

Despite this, many people will not be so lucky, and it is therefore important to understand why we need to examine COVID-19 not merely through the lens of a disease that produces specific physical symptoms but also as a social phenomenon that produced not only direct psychosocial effects but also indirect effects that exacerbated many of the preexisting health problems that are common throughout the United States. Without a doubt, the greatest tragedy during this pandemic has been the deaths of millions of people around the globe, including hundreds of thousands of Americans. However, despite that horrendous number of deaths, one cannot minimize the everlasting physical and psychological scars among the sick who survived but had to be hospitalized and continue to struggle with the onslaught of lingering symptoms associated with long COVID. In addition to those who became sick, there are millions who will experience some degree of secondary and tertiary tragedies that could play out for years to come. An unfathomable number of people across the United States and the world were inundated by stress—struggling with their living situations, employment status, or the fact that they or their loved ones could become sick—and the fear and stress of contracting COVID-19 or lack of economic or social supports have been the root cause of depleting their psychological reserve and resilience.

Additionally, the biological and psychosocial aspects of COVID-19 have been intertwined such that the pathology of COVID-19 and numerous social aspects of the pandemic led to pernicious effects on an individual's health and in particular mental health. As described in *Chapter 3: Pathology—What We Knew and What We Know*, even mild cases of COVID-19 can lead to an errant immune response and systemic inflammation. Furthermore, as explored in *Chapter 4: Neuropsychiatric Symptoms and Postacute Sequelae of SARS-CoV-2— The Long Haulers*, systemic inflammation can lead to neuroinflammation which may contribute to or exacerbate symptoms of anxiety and depression. Needless to say, when social stressors are added to this mix, it further amplifies these symptoms and may worsen one's mental health.

Hard evidence is now starting to emerge about the colossal impact of the COVID-19 pandemic on individuals' mental health, and we are finding that those who were the most vulnerable before the pandemic and were already struggling with multiple stressors—particularly those tied to socioeconomic difficulties (food insecurity, housing instability, precarity of transportation, interpersonal violence, etc)—appear to have suffered the most.[2] As was observed multiple times in the early stages of the pandemic, most of these problems were not new; they were merely exacerbated by COVID-19.

Considering the abovementioned facts, a psychosocial approach to these issues should not be in any way controversial. Social stressors seem to have played a direct and significant role in the pathology of COVID-19 and have also impacted the mental health of millions of people who were never infected by the novel coronavirus. To fully understand and describe every social component that potentially contributed to COVID-related anxiety or depression would require a vast chronicle of the COVID Era, which is something that is beyond the scope of this book. However, there are crucial social components to the story of COVID-19 that need to be touched upon before moving on to discuss the larger issue of stress and some of the specific manifestations of that stress.

Economic and Social Effects of COVID-19

What follows is by no means an exhaustive list of the economic and social effects of COVID-19. These are, rather, the tips of the iceberg that either caused increased stresses or were the results of stresses on individuals who were suddenly deprived of their familiar support networks and often incapable of moving freely, working, socializing, or taking part in activities that had given their life meaning.

COVID-19 either set off or contributed to multiple domino effects that all seemed to collide in a spectacular fashion in early 2020. The result was widespread chaos, collapses in supply chains and local economies, shortages of staples, and unprecedented layoffs in virtually every sector of the economy from which we are still recovering. Within the United States, an estimated 22 million jobs disappeared in the 4 weeks after a national emergency was declared on March 13, 2020. A record 6.9 million people filed for unemployment the week ending March 28, 2020, alone.[3] One cannot underestimate the colossal impact of this economic loss that halted the lives of millions and caused mayhem, confusion, anxiety about the future, and in many cases, a deep sense of fear and depression.

Domestic Abuse

By April 2020, 95% of the U.S. population lived in an area where people were under instructions to remain at home, which meant that most individuals who lost their job were not going to be able to find a new one quickly.[4] This, combined with the widespread job losses and other stressors described above, appears to have forced many individuals into living situations that would have been untenable in less dire circumstances. Despite the abominable domestic situation, many of these individuals, who were often women with children, opted to remain in place, and endure the abuse, as they understood that leaving their homes could mean living on the streets, potential exposure to the virus, as well as the many dangers associated with homelessness. In fact, domestic abuse was even characterized in *Time Magazine* as "a pandemic within the COVID-19 pandemic."[5]

Studies that have analyzed the types of injuries reported in emergency room visits since the beginning of the pandemic have found evidence to suggest that incidence of intimate partner violence and child abuse increased as more victims were forced to choose between the abuse and the street.[6] A systematic review and meta-analysis of officially reported domestic violence in multiple countries showed similar results.[7]

Unfortunately, an accurate picture of just how pervasive domestic abuse has been during the pandemic has not emerged at this time. Preliminary studies and anecdotal stories indicate that rates of incidence have increased and that this will be an enduring source of trauma for countless individuals who may go on to develop either trauma- and stressor-related disorders or dissociative disorders. The latter may be particularly common among victims of child abuse who faced serious maltreatment by a relative or friend of the family who was given shelter during the pandemic.[8]

Depopulation of Urban Centers

The past 30 years has seen a growing number of young professionals and "creative" office workers from around the world move to a handful of what urban studies theorist Richard Florida termed "superstar cities" in his 2017 work, *The New Urban Crisis*.[9] This has led to increased gentrification of neighborhoods in cities that were originally home to lower middle-class and working-class communities, while a simultaneous dearth of affordable housing projects has made it increasingly difficult for the affected communities to remain in their home cities. Simply put, these working class and lower middle-class individuals who work in sectors of the economy like retail, hospitality, manufacturing, construction, and education are being pushed out, and professionals, who typically work in offices, are moving in.

When the pandemic began, many professionals were told that they would be allowed to work remotely for the foreseeable future and, consequently, many fled their homes in urban areas. Those who had cottages or houses in the country took up residence there. Others began a mad scramble to purchase homes in suburban and exurban areas.[10] Some even moved into so-called "Zoom towns" in more rural areas.[11]

Meanwhile, many younger people moved back home with their parents. As of September 2020, for the first time since the Great Depression, a majority of young adults between the ages of 18 and 29 years were living with at least one of their parents.[12] While young professionals in this situation were able to work remotely, nonprofessionals often struggled to find work and exert their financial independence.

The effects of this mass exodus were immediate. The urban centers that had attracted people for generations looked deserted overnight. Within just a few weeks, the cacophony of some of the most illustrious global cities fell to a murmur. The volume of foot traffic that had justified stratospheric rents in central business districts areas plummeted as more office workers were told to do their jobs remotely and stay-at-home orders were issued. Millions of construction, manufacturing, hospitality, and retail workers subsequently lost their jobs, meaning they were not only unemployed but also forced to remain at home and were unable to look for a job. While many retail and hospitality workers continue to face significant headwinds finding comparable jobs that pay more than minimum wage, the cornucopia of bars, restaurants, and retail stores in major business districts simply cannot return to normal business without the spending power of a professional class who have moved to suburban areas and no longer need to venture downtown areas.

Should the virus become endemic, which does seem highly probable, this will likely have long-lasting impacts on urban centers, as people amend their lifestyle to account for the increased risks posed by the virus. At this point in time, it is far too early to tell what these impacts will look like.

Substance Use

With the sudden economic downturn and millions of individuals becoming unemployed, the natural outcome was boredom, familial friction, increased domestic violence, and increased substance use, particularly alcohol. Studies have found that no amount of alcohol use is healthy, but the negative health effects of limited and occasional alcohol use are relatively minor so long as the individual drinking is not pregnant, has no significant medical comorbidities, is not taking certain medications, or is not planning to operate heavy machinery or drive a car. If done in excess, alcohol can lead to a host of health problems that affect the liver, heart, GI tract, and brain. Overuse of alcohol can also wreak havoc on one's familial, social, and work lives.

Anecdotal evidence suggests that people started drinking more to cope with the stresses of the pandemic and surveys have found that consumption of alcohol increased manyfold when compared to prepandemic levels. At least, one survey conducted by the American Psychological Association found that 23% of adults reported drinking more.[13] Meanwhile, retail alcohol sales have skyrocketed as people have consumed more alcohol at home, but this begs the question: Are people drinking more at home, or are they consuming more alcohol than they once did?

What this question sidesteps is the cultural importance of alcohol in many societies, including the United States. As Kate Julian observed in a very well-written article published in *The Atlantic's* July/August 2021 issue, humans have consumed alcohol socially for millennia and getting inebriated with one's friends and family has social benefits because it strengthens social bonds.[14] Alcohol becomes problematic when drinking begins to occur without friends and family or in excessive amounts, which is precisely what happened during the COVID-19 pandemic.

Meanwhile, individuals with histories of substance use disorders were confronted with disruptions in treatment access and social programs designed to assist the most in need. Networks like Alcoholics Anonymous and Narcotics Anonymous are built around the sharing of personal stories and participating in group work. The pandemic made these kinds of in-person meetings impossible, while also causing the temporary suspension of outreach programs and the closure of facilities to help homeless and mentally ill patients, many of whom, unfortunately, have comorbid substance use disorders. As we have learned to adapt to live with the virus, many of these programs have since come back online.

However, these interruptions in service, in conjunction with the more universal stresses associated with the pandemic, almost certainly fueled a wave of relapses, especially in the first months of the pandemic.[15] Instances of opioid overdoses also spiked in the early months of the pandemic and have not fully returned to pre-COVID levels. Data suggest that the opioid crisis, which was already costing as many as 60,000 lives per year, kept burning unnoticed through 2020 like a mine fire.[16] Approximately 93,000 overdose deaths were reported nationwide in 2020.[17] The exact number of accidental overdoses compared to suicide by poisoning is unclear.[18]

Collective Panic

Yet another unfortunately salient example of how the psychological, social, and economic triad can converge is when collective panic takes place. As mentioned earlier in the case of the stampede and how panic buying during perceived gas shortages creates a positive feedback loop, the pandemic initially caused panic buying in grocery stores (especially with toilet paper) and was one of the defining cultural moments of early 2020. It was shocking to see throughout the United States, the land of abundance, empty shelves in stores everywhere one looked.

Even before the first stay-at-home order was issued, the spread of the virus spurred panicky runs to grocery stores and frantic online buying. As China was still in the midst of their tight lockdown, and since many of our supply chains are reliant on Chinese manufacturing, shortages began to be reported just as retail supply chains were being strained to the limit.[19] The spike in demand combined with interruptions in production and distribution resulted in empty shelves in grocery stores, which only encouraged more frenzied hoarding behavior throughout the spring of 2020 as people stockpiled things like flour, yeast, and, of course, toilet paper.

Meanwhile, farmers who had contracts with restaurants and schools that had suddenly shuttered were unable to quickly accommodate this shift in demand.[20] Over the course of decades, they had developed and manufactured products that specifically met the demands of these outlets, and as a result of the pandemic, they could not suddenly alter the production, distribution, and supply chain, which put tremendous strain on their bottom line. Even local food banks were unprepared for the surge in supply and could not accommodate all the fresh produce and dairy.[21]

The end result was a cruel juxtaposition: Empty store shelves in the city and farmers overwhelmed with millions of pounds of rotting fruits and vegetables they could not sell. Outbreaks of COVID-19 at meatpacking plants also forced processors to scale back or in some cases temporarily close to avoid seeing their workforces decimated by the disease.[22]

It was not just grocery items. Health care workers faced severe shortages of personal protection equipment as supply chains failed and hospitals ended up competing with one another and with the public for items like N95 masks. Supplies of many drugs, particularly analgesics, sedatives, and paralytics, also became strained.[23] These drugs are necessary for patients who need to undergo invasive mechanical ventilation, which is routinely used to treat acute respiratory distress syndrome,[24] one of the more common and dangerous complications associated with COVID-19.[25] These shortages proved to be particularly stressful for medical personnel who were on the frontlines of the fight against COVID-19 and no doubt contributed to the higher levels of posttraumatic stress disorder (PTSD) reported among the health care staff.[26]

Crime

Reported crime appears to have dropped during the first days of the pandemic as states shut down and people remained inside. Crime rates then remained low for several weeks.[27] After a brief respite, however, these rates began to rise once again. In the United States, a very pronounced surge in gun violence began in the spring of 2020 and has continued well into 2021.[28] Precisely, what is causing it is unclear, but it is yet another social factor that can contribute to stress, especially among individuals in large urban areas, where homicide rates have been particularly high.[29] As the summer of 2021 comes to a close, it appears as though the uptick in murders is slowing and that other violent crimes have fallen when compared to their 2020 levels, though it is far too early to properly place this into a larger context about trends in crime.[30]

Stress

Stress is a ubiquitous word in modern society and a normal part of everyday life. Anyone reading this is familiar with the feeling, and we typically associate it with the feeling of being overburdened or when circumstances do not go our way. Physically, it can feel like a valve has been shut off somewhere in our bodies and that there is a pressure building up within us. This is reflected in our idioms about stress, and we complain about feeling "under pressure," or "about to burst," or "about to snap," or "at the breaking point."

Somewhat more formally, stress can be defined as any type of change that causes physical, emotional, or psychological strain.

In some cases, stress can be a good thing. For example, exercise is a form of stress. It puts strain on muscles, but this strain is relatively short-lived and controlled. Similarly, fear is oftentimes a good thing. As unpleasant as it may be, it is key to our emotional lives and our very survival. In fact, one could think of our fear response as really no different than a threat response. That feeling of stress or dread or terror or aggression is precipitated by perceived threats, and they start a cascade of neurochemical signals to ready our bodies to be more capable of responding to threats.[31] This physiological reaction is known as the acute stress response or, more famously, the fight or flight response.

The Science of the Stress Response

Central to this response are two small, almond-shaped regions on the left and the right sides of the brain known collectively as the amygdala (see Figure 5.1). In addition to playing a role in triggering the body's stress response, the amygdala also plays a major role in fear, memory, and aggression. Like a properly functioning smoke detector, the amygdala jumps into action when stimuli that are recognized as potentially threatening are observed. The smoke detector is programmed to respond to smoke; when there is smoke, there is fire. Similarly, the amygdala only sends out distress signals when specific stimuli are observed that could potentially mean threat.

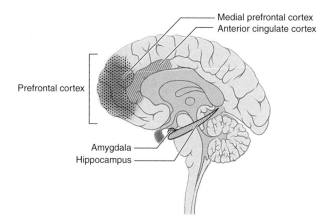

Figure 5.1 Parts of the brain central to fear response: the amygdala, hippocampus, prefrontal cortex, medial prefrontal cortex, and anterior cingulate cortex. (Illustration courtesy of Patrick J. Lynch, medical illustrator and C. Carl Jaffe, MD, cardiologist.)

What is amazing is just how integral the amygdala is to our fear response. To illustrate this point, consider the case of a Kentucky woman known only as S.M. whose amygdala was destroyed by a rare genetic condition known as Urbach-Wiethe disease. Dubbed *"the woman without fear"* by various media outlets, she simply does not experience any kind of fight or flight response whether she is watching a scary movie, wandering through a reportedly haunted facility, holding a tarantula, or even being robbed at gunpoint—something that evidently happens frequently because she has a hard time recognizing when she is in a threatening situation.[32] She recognizes that she should feel fear on an intellectual level but actual sensation of fear simply does not occur to her.

The takeaway from this should be that, while not living in fear may sound like a liberating experience, it can actually be quite dangerous. It is a bit like unplugging an overreactive smoke detector in your kitchen because it tends to go off whenever you broil something in the oven. While it may mean that you can cook without being deafened by the wail of the alarm, it also means that you might sleep through an actual fire and only wake up once the flames have gotten out of control.

The amygdala also plays a role in our learning the difference between innocuous stimuli and potentially dangerous stimuli and does so by working in concert with the hippocampus, which is the part of the brain responsible for recording and recalling episodic memories. Most memories are not merely collections of sense perceptions—sights, sounds, physical sensations, or, as French novelist Marcel Proust so famously observed, smell and taste. Memories tend to include emotional information, too, and we remember the way we felt at specific moments because the amygdala and the hippocampus act in concert to encode memories with emotion. This conditions us to repeatedly participate in activities that are tied to positive emotions. It also gives rise to what is known as fear conditioning: Our tendency to avoid activities that are tied to negative emotions.[33] This can be reversed through what is known as fear extinction, which is when we participate in these types of activities we once feared without concomitant negative emotions. Research has shown a correlation between impaired fear extinction circuitry and trauma-related disorders, particularly PTSD.[34]

To illustrate how this system works, consider an individual who manages to escape a dangerous situation. They may become conditioned to avoid not only the situation itself but also activities or stimuli associated with that situation. Such a fear is not based on instinct but rather on memory. As an extreme example, if one almost drowns in the ocean at a young age, this may create a fear not only of the ocean but also of any body of water. While this interplay between emotion and memory may lead to various phobias that can be disruptive to one's normal life, the connection is integral to survival. Without it, we would not be able to remember potential threats or dangerous activities. In the last year, living with the fear of COVID-19 has led to a prolonged stress response, which has numerous biological and psychological consequences. The following discussion about the role of various brain regions, neurotransmitters, and hormonal regulation is integral to understanding the stress response system so as to better learn and how to manage associated symptoms.

This alarm system is not ruled by emotion and memory alone. The medial prefrontal cortex, a region in the brain that is crucial for executive functioning and includes the cingulate gyrus, subcallosal gyrus, and orbitofrontal cortex, attenuates the fear response mediated by the amygdala.[35] The medial prefrontal cortex is quite literally the voice of reason that tells the amygdala to stay calm. You can think of the amygdala as your overly dramatic friend and the medial prefrontal cortex as the one in the group who can talk them down and keep them from overreacting and getting the rest of the group in trouble.

These three regions of the brain tie emotion, reason, and memory together to ensure that we make prudent decisions and only respond to legitimate threats.

When the amygdala does recognize a legitimate threat, it sends distress signals out to what is known as the hypothalamus-pituitary-adrenal (HPA) axis. The signal first activates the hypothalamus, which in turn sends chemical messages to the pituitary gland and the adrenal glands, which release epinephrine (adrenaline) into the bloodstream. This boost in adrenaline activates what is known as the sympathetic nervous system (SNS), which we will get to momentarily. Additional excretion of corticotropin-releasing hormone and arginine vasopressin from the hypothalamus induces the pituitary gland to release adrenocorticotropic hormone (ACTH). ACTH then signals to the adrenal glands to produce cortisol, which keeps the SNS engaged. For this reason, cortisol is often referred to as the "stress hormone."

Of course, the fear response does not occur solely in our brains. The hypothalamus does not only interact with the pituitary gland; it can also be thought of as the body's control center because it regulates much of the autonomic nervous system, which is responsible for controlling vital bodily functions that we do not have to think about (see Figure 5.2). Some of these functions include breathing, blood pressure, body temperature, and heart rate, to name a few. When the HPA axis is engaged by the stress response, the hypothalamus initiates a body-wide fight or flight response that involves the SNS. When the SNS is activated, we feel that familiar adrenaline rush and get primed for action as glucose is released to give us an extra burst of energy, our airways become dilated to bring more oxygen into our blood, and our heart rate increases to push more blood into skeletal muscles for added strength and endurance. The mirror image of the SNS is the parasympathetic nervous system (PNS), which is known for rest and digest. When the PNS is activated, our heart rates decrease, saliva production is increased, and blood flow is directed to the GI tract to aid in digestion.

An extremely simplified way of envisioning the roles of the SNS and PNS is to think about a car. The SNS is the gas pedal and the PNS is the brake.

Pathological Stress

Under normal conditions, the SNS and PNS are complimentary and help keep us balanced. When I say "us," I am referring to all mammals. These systems are extremely old and predate the emergence of our species, let alone Twitter and Gmail, by millions of years. They were designed to help animals navigate the stresses of the prehistoric world and to survive in an environment that is filled with other animals trying to kill and eat them. The amygdala and the HPA axis did not evolve to consider a lot of nuances or the kinds of stresses of modern life, which are a lot less dramatic but far more persistent and chronic.

This is a crucial point in understanding the distinction between normal and pathological stress. The amygdala, the HPA axis, and the greater SNS have evolved to respond to immediate and life-threatening situations that spur us into action, though in our normal lives, we do not come across these

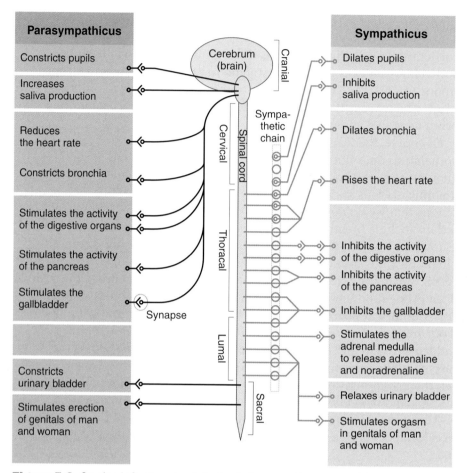

Figure 5.2 On the left, the physiological changes that occur following the activation of the parasympathetic nervous system (Parasympathicus). On the right, the physiological changes that occur following the activation of the sympathetic nervous system (Sympathicus).

situations very often. A good example of this would be the need to suddenly swerve to avoid hitting another vehicle while we are driving or having an altercation with another person. While these types of incidents do certainly happen, they are exceptionally rare. Most of the stress we experience is of a persistent and low- or mid-grade in nature. Our stresses manifest in the form of deadlines, worries about social engagements, financial insecurities, and, more recently, fear of being infected with COVID-19 or having a friend or loved one infected with the virus. This fear has of course been amplified by social media, television, newspapers, and cable news. From the spring of 2020 through at least the fall of 2021, every major media outlet in the country has run breaking news stories on the coronavirus or some novel and terrifying way it can harm us. It may be true, but the alarming and dramatic way in which it is broadcast 24/7 is not just meant to inform; it is meant to hijack our attention by manipulating our primal responses to fearful stimuli.

This perpetual drumming of bad news and anxiety-provoking headlines can leave us feeling, to use the phrase favored by the late Bruce S. McEwan's terminology, "stressed out."[36] This is pathological stress.

When we experience sustained, pathological stress, it means that our SNS remains engaged for extended periods of time, and we ultimately end up with notably higher levels of stress hormones, particularly cortisol, in our blood. This leads to a cascade of physiological changes that translates into higher heart rate, elevated blood pressure, improper digestion, disrupted sleep, tense muscles, anxiety disorders, affective disorders, and imbalances in cytokines, which, to call back to previous chapters, are vital to inter cell-cell messaging and for the proper functioning of our immune systems. Over the long term, this can lead to higher lipid levels, imbalances in blood sugar (predisposing one to diabetes), obesity, heart arrhythmias, kidney damage, and increases in inflammatory markers—precisely the kinds of preexisting conditions that can negatively impact a COVID-19 prognosis and exactly the kinds of conditions that appear to come in the wake of acute infections of SARS-CoV-2. A study involving approximately 2 million patients who were diagnosed with COVID-19 found that 23.2% had at least one new condition following recovery. Post-COVID conditions have been found to affect 50% of individuals who were hospitalized, 27.5% of individuals who were symptomatic but not hospitalized, and 19% of individuals who remained asymptomatic during infection. The five most common new conditions experienced 30 days or more following first COVID-19 diagnosis include pain, breathing difficulties, hyperlipidemia, malaise and fatigue, and hypertension. Anxiety and depression ranked sixth and fourteenth, respectively.[37]

To return to the figure seen in the previous chapter (see Figure 5.3), the central point of all this is that persistent activation of the acute stress response system that can start a vicious cycle, which leaves us feeling more stressed out, more susceptible to chronic health conditions (including anxiety and depression), and more susceptible to severe COVID-19. While it seems plausible that chronic inflammatory conditions can increase the likelihood of developing postacute sequela of SARS-CoV-2, there is not enough evidence available at this time to support that hypothesis.[38] What is clear, however, is that COVID-19 can be considered a psychosocial disease since physical stress affects our psychological well-being and vice-versa.

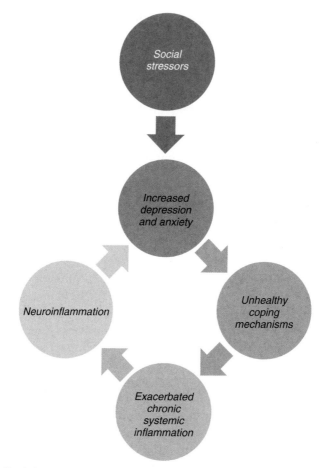

Figure 5.3 Social stressors can lead to anxiety and mood disorders leading to unhealthy coping mechanisms, which not only cause immune system dysfunction and neuroinflammation, but reinforce feelings of depression and anxiety.

Trauma Among Patients and Health Care Workers

Traumatic distress has been felt across the world and has been particularly prevalent in those who were hospitalized for COVID-19. A cross-sectional study of 381 such patients who had recovered following hospitalization found that over 30% of them met the criteria for PTSD.[39] This seems to align with a meta-analysis involving patients who were admitted to the intensive care unit (ICU) during the severe acute respiratory syndrome (SARS) and Middle East respiratory syndrome (MERS) outbreaks. Six months after being discharged, 39% met criteria for PTSD, 33% were diagnosed with clinical depression, and 30% had developed an anxiety disorder.[40]

It remains to be seen as to how many individuals from around the world who have experienced trauma directly or indirectly associated with COVID-19 will later be diagnosed with PTSD. Data suggest that in addition to those who suffered from severe COVID-19, the groups that had a higher risk of developing pandemic-related PTSD appear to be family members of patients with severe infections or who died, as well as frontline health care workers.[41]

Without a doubt, the health care workers have been exposed to traumatic stress in a unique way. In conjunction with confronting a high level of risk while on the front lines in the fight against the virus, they have also been exposed to a tremendous degree of death and human suffering. No amount of medical experience can prepare a person for such an onslaught of tragedy and death. Hospital workers have repeatedly compared the worst months of the pandemic to working in a warzone.

A meta-analysis of health care staff tasked with working to manage a novel viral outbreak, including MERS and SARS, found that distress levels persisted for up to 3 years following each of the outbreaks and that staff were almost twice as likely to experience acute or posttraumatic stress compared with controls in a typical health care environment.[42] Given the increased scope and magnitude of the current pandemic, it seems at the very least reasonable to assume that its psychosocial impact will persist for significantly longer among health care workers and that a large number of hospital staff will struggle with PTSD symptoms and remains to be seen as to how many will recover. A poll released earlier this year found that over 60% of health care workers say that their mental health has suffered because of the pandemic.[43] A poll involving 1327 poll workers conducted between February and March 2021 found that 29% of health care workers have reportedly considered leaving the profession.[44] Meanwhile, a meta-analysis of 65 studies involving over 97,000 health care workers from across 21 countries founds rates of depression, anxiety, and PTSD to be 21.7%, 22.1%, and 21.5%, respectively.[26]

Residents and workers in long-term care facilities and nursing homes have faced similar trauma, as they have been hit especially hard by the pandemic and have also suffered from loneliness and anxiety tied to feelings of uncertainty, helplessness, and exhaustion.[45] As of the end of May 2021, 655,110 COVID-19 cases had been confirmed in nursing homes across the United States, 132,608, about one in five, of those cases proved fatal (see Figure 5.4A and B). The total number of confirmed cases among nursing home staff was 583,756 (see Figure 5.5A and B). 1931, about 1 in 330, lost their lives.[46] There are currently no hard data comparing rates of anxiety and depressive symptoms at present compared to historical averages, but it would be very fitting to see significant increases in these conditions.

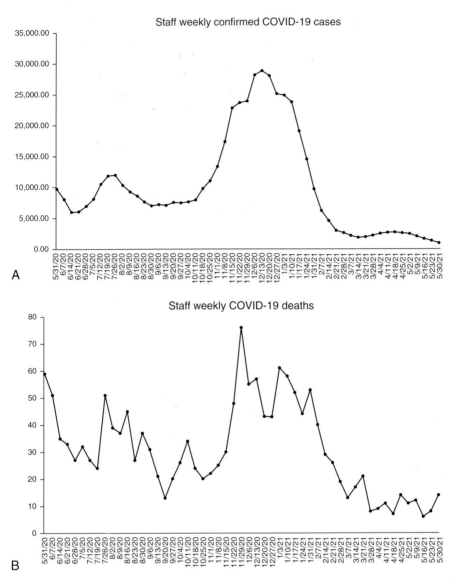

Figure 5.4 Number of nursing home staff who tested positive for COVID-19 (A) and who died of COVID-19 (B).

Environmental and Dietary Stressors

Unrelated to COVID-19, environmental phenomena can also serve as stressors or be associated with specific chronic diseases and even brain damage. Researchers in South Korea discovered a link between Parkinson disease and nitrogen dioxide (NO_2), a common air pollutant.[47] Meanwhile,

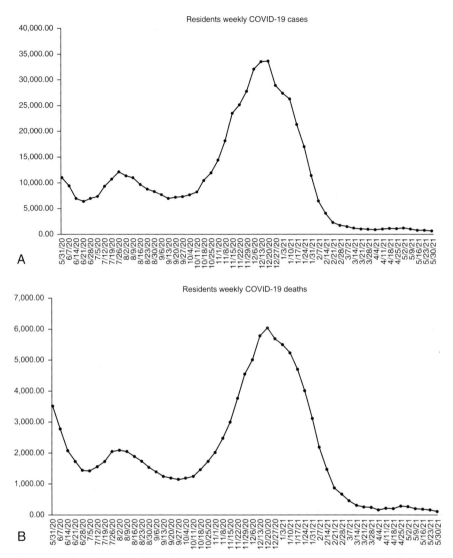

Figure 5.5 Number of nursing home residents who tested positive for COVID-19 (A) and who died of COVID-19 (B).

increased exposure to fine particulate matter (particular matter measuring 2.5 microns or less in diameter and commonly abbreviated as PM 2.5) has been associated with episodic memory decline and may increase risk of Alzheimer disease.[48] Finally, lead has been associated with brain damage and a host of other problems, which is why it is no longer in paint or gasoline, and why water crises in places like Flint, Michigan, cause so much alarm and outrage among the public.[49]

Of course, exposure to environmental toxins is not equal across all groups. Higher levels of environmental toxins affect marginalized communities more than they impact people from more affluent backgrounds. This is yet another reason why chronic conditions are more prevalent among individuals from less privileged backgrounds and why there have been growing calls for what is known as environmental justice.[50] It is grounded in the belief that no individual or group of individuals should be relegated to an area where their homes become inundated with toxic materials, thereby leading to chronic inflammatory conditions.

Complementary to this notion is the idea that all people should have access to healthy and nutrient-dense foods, as a poor diet, like environmental toxins, can play a role in the development of systemic inflammation. There are well-established associations with poor dietary choices and hypertension, insulin resistance, dyslipidemia, and chronic inflammation as evinced by elevations in proinflammatory markers such as C-reactive protein, tumor necrosis factor-α, and interleukin-6. This association also extends to psychiatric disorders like anxiety and depression.[51]

Additionally, research has found rather unsurprisingly that instances of stress eating correlate with increases in cortisol and that people tend to make very poor dietary decisions when they engage in stress eating. This again circles around the idea of the positive feedback loop: A diet that is high in saturated fats and processed sugars can lead to neural inflammation, which leads to anxiety, which leads to increased levels of cortisol, which leads to the "stress eating" of more foods that are high in saturated fats and processed sugars.[52]

What this all suggests is that individuals who are exposed to high levels of environmental stressors and who have a poor diet are more likely to be in a proinflammatory state, which could play a crucial role in the regulation of innate and adaptive immune responses and, consequently, COVID-19 prognosis. It is reasonable to assume that prognosis improves when these stressors are absent and preliminary evidence supports this hypothesis. A COVID-19 case-control study involving 2884 frontline health care workers from six countries (France, Germany, Italy, Spain, the United Kingdom, the United States) found that individuals who consumed diets that were higher in vegetables, legumes, and nuts and lower in processed meats, red meats, and poultry reported fewer instances of moderate-to-severe cases of COVID-19.[53] Meanwhile, an observational study that has yet to be peer-reviewed and used data from 592,571 participants in the United States and United Kingdom via smartphone similarly found similar results and concluded that a diet characterized by healthy plant-based foods was associated with lower risk of COVID-19 infection, as well as symptom severity.[54]

Loneliness

Recently, one of my colleagues at New York University presented at the grand rounds on the neuroscience of loneliness. To my surprise and the surprise of many of our colleagues, the lonely brain does not look all that different from the stressed brain because lonely brains exhibit the kind of heightened HPA axis activity that is the calling card of chronic stress. For those who spent the majority of the pandemic alone, this meant that they experienced both the stresses of the pandemic era— the news cycle, the political upheaval, the worry of getting infected or having a loved one get infected—in conjunction with the stresses of loneliness. Social isolation and loneliness have also been associated with cardiovascular disease and stroke, dementia and other problems with cognition, depression and anxiety, chronic health conditions, and suicidal ideation.[55]

Far more will be said about loneliness and social isolation in *Chapter 8: Extended Social Impact*. However, it is important to note here that this issue affects far more people than we probably realize. One recent example is Harvard University's Making Caring Common program, which conducted a survey in late October 2020 involving 950 people in the United States. Though they are still in the preliminary stages of analyzing the data, they found that 36% of respondents said that they experienced "serious loneliness," while 61% of individuals between the ages of 18 and 25 years reported "miserable degrees of loneliness."[56]

Many seniors have experienced extended periods of isolation to maintain social distancing protocols. In some cases, this isolation was just a more extreme version of an already solitary lifestyle, since an estimated 24% of community-dwelling Americans over the age of 65 years and older are considered socially isolated.[55] Meanwhile, 27% of adults over the age of 60 years lived by themselves prior to the pandemic—a larger percentage than anywhere else in the world.[57] Loneliness appears to be more pronounced among seniors with lower socioeconomic statuses.[58]

Spousal Bereavement in Seniors

It is not just loneliness affecting seniors; this demographic has also been hit the hardest by the pandemic. Roughly 8 out of every 10 deaths caused by COVID-19 have occurred in adults over the age of 65 years.[59] Dig a little deeper and one also finds that the disease is also more fatal for men. The total number of fatal cases among men is 362,187 compared to 296,567 women.[60] This suggests that a relatively large number of older women will have to endure the death of a spouse.

Regardless of age or cause of death, the death of a spouse is an extremely traumatic event. It can leave the bereaved feeling rudderless and helpless. While it should come as no surprise that the disruptive effects of a spouse's death can have negative effects on one's mental health, the impact appears to contribute to a significantly increased mortality rate. By some accounts, there may be as high as a 40-fold increase in the risk of a bereaved spouse developing a new illness or allowing an existing one to worsen within the first 2 months after their loss.[61] Similarly, depression-like symptoms are frequently reported and may lead the bereaved to engage in health-threatening behaviors or the neglect of health-promoting activities, particularly during the first 6 months following the death. Given the additional stressors associated with the pandemic, it seems at the very least likely that a recently widowed individual may abuse alcohol or other drugs, change their diet for the worse, fail to comply with medical regimes, or give up on maintaining their home because these responsibilities had been within the domain of the recently departed spouse.[62]

Symptoms and Behaviors Associated With Stress and Adverse Psychosocial Factors

As this chapter has shown, a wide variety of COVID-19–related stressors play a role in the development of systemic inflammation and potentially neuroinflammation. In turn, this can affect mood and cognition or lead to increased levels of anxiety and depression. Persistent stress can also lead to issues that have already been covered, including poor dietary choices and substance use disorders, as well as issues that will be addressed here: anxiety, depression, sleep problems, and suicide.

Anxiety and Depression

A survey conducted by the National Center for Health Services found that the average share of adults reporting symptoms of anxiety or depressive disorders was holding steady around 11% during the first 6 months of 2019, with 8.2% of adults describing experiencing symptoms of only an anxiety disorder, while 6.6% described symptoms of only a depressive disorder. Unfortunately, this seems to be in line with historical averages.[63,64] Since the late spring of 2020, the average has been closer to 38%, with a low of 33.9% and a peak of 42.6% following the election. In March 2021, 36.8% of participants reported experiencing these symptoms. That is more than a threefold jump from prepandemic levels.[65]

There are many reasons why we experience anxiety or depression. As discussed above, one route is through neuroinflammation and chronic systemic inflammation. Additionally, as described above, traumatic stress and excessive rumination also contribute to these conditions.[66]

Without a doubt rumination was difficult to avoid during the pandemic. After all, the year 2020 was effectively an extended fever dream that seemed to alternate between events that were absolutely terrifying, horrifying, and almost comically surreal (remember murder hornets?). It was hard not to constantly think about these things and the possibility that everything was about to collapse, especially since so many people suddenly had a lot of free time on their hands, and it seemed as if everything was actually close to collapsing. The structures, responsibilities, and obligations that had for years determined how we spent our time had vanished.

When the pandemic hit, so many of the things that were central to our social or professional lives were suddenly muted. Our priorities radically changed, and what we were left with at the dawn of the pandemic was a blank canvas. Many experienced this with a sense of dread.

For years, several of my patients have confided that their anxiety is at its worst when they first get into bed. The noise and distractions of contemporary life fade away, leaving them alone with the darkness and their thoughts. Some may relish this as a time of introspection, but these patients saw it as an opening of the book of disquiet.

In many respects, the periods of quarantine that we have had to endure have been kind of like a protracted night, and many likely experienced prolonged periods of forced introspection that led to rumination and, consequently, feelings of anxiety, as they reassessed their careers and their social lives and possibly begin to fret about some of the decisions that have led them to this point in their lives—their friends, their lovers, their habits, their choice of city, their career. Given the gravity of the pandemic, many perhaps realized that they had not taken a career path that truly inspired them or that allowed them to do monumental things.

In *The House of the Dead*, Dostoyevsky's semiautobiographical novel about his imprisonment in Siberia, the famed protoexistentialist writer mused, "The thought once occurred to me that if one wanted to crush and destroy a man entirely, to mete out to him the most terrible punishment, one at which the most fearsome murderer would tremble, shrinking from it in advance, all one would have to do would be to make him do work that was completely and utterly devoid of usefulness and meaning."[67] It is not an uplifting quote by any means, but it does speak to the need for humans to feel as though their actions are imbued with meaning, and the sense of despondency, anxiety, and even depression that can wash over someone who has found themselves incapable of seeing the purpose in following a routine that seems more cyclical than linear. This kind of rumination, in conjunction with any of the myriad stresses described throughout this chapter, no doubt led many to feel anxious, to be depressed, and to have difficulty sleeping.

Sleep Deprivation

Sleep disturbances have been very widely reported and a recent meta-analysis found that, during the pandemic, sleep problems have affected approximately one-third of the general population and slightly more (36%) health care workers reported disturbances.[68] This is troublesome on many levels. Sleep duration of 4 hours or less per night is associated with anxiety, difficulty concentrating, higher blood pressure, increased cortisol and insulin levels, hardier appetite, increased rates of obesity, and mood and behavior disturbances, particularly with respect to aggression.[69] As anyone who has pulled an all-nighter knows sleep disturbances are also strongly associated with reduced cognitive performance and executive function. Persistent lack of sleep can lead to fatigue or burnout, and for that reason, many professions are limited to the number of hours that they can work. One would not want burned-out pilot flying their plane nor would anyone want to undergo a procedure performed by a surgeon who has not slept in 24 hours.[i]

Lack of sleep is also associated with depressive disorders. In a 2008 paper, David Nutt and colleagues summed this point up rather succinctly when they wrote, "The link between the two is so fundamental that some researchers have suggested that a diagnosis of depression in absence of sleep complaints should be made with caution."[70]

For some, sleep problems mean low-sleep efficiency, which is defined as spending less than 85% of the amount of time in bed asleep. For others, this means protracted sleep-onset latency, which is amount of time it takes for one to fall asleep—which should, ideally, be between 15 and 20 minutes. For others still, it can mean a reduced amount of slow wave sleep and rapid eye movement sleep. These two stages of sleep are vital for memory consolidation and serve a restorative function for the body and brain.

Suicide

Despite how traumatic the experience of COVID-19 has been and despite the rise in rates of depression and anxiety, as well as the likely increase in

---

[i] New York State, for example, prevents residents from working more than 80 hours per week or 24 consecutive hours due to the infamous Libby Zion case. In 1984, two residents who were operating on very little sleep made several critical errors that ultimately led to Zion's death.

instances of substance abuse, there were fewer overall suicides in the United States in 2020 than there were in 2019. In fact, the number of suicides fell by 5%—from 47,511 to 44,834.[71]

This decline occurred amidst significant fluctuations in suicide rates. According to data released by the National Center for Health Statistics National Vital Statistics System, suicides fell in the early days of the pandemic before picking up later in the year. It is possible that the initial decline occurred because there was a sense of common purpose in defeating the virus and this gave individuals something for which to live. As the pandemic dragged on into the later months of 2020, however, suicide rates rose. Whether this can be linked to anxiety, depression, financial stress, existential distress, or other stressors is unlikely to ever be known. Furthermore, how the persistence of the pandemic through 2021 and beyond will affect suicide rates continues to be an open question as of this writing.

There does seem to be some evidence that there were increases in suicide among young people of color, particularly young Black men since Black communities have been particularly hard hit by the pandemic. It is possible that the many stresses articulated in this chapter were all factors leading to this increase in suicides, but it is far too early to make any conclusive statements on the matter.[18] More resources need to be dedicated to understanding what is happening so that the crisis can be resolved.

Conclusion

Psychosocial and economic factors have played an enormous role in amplifying the stresses that people experienced during the pandemic, and this has contributed to significant decline in mental wellbeing. As we begin to heal and to address the mental health crisis left in the wake of the COVID-19 pandemic, we would be remiss to not also bear in mind the role that psychosocial factors play in patients' total health and to, therefore, seek to ameliorate some of these factors to our best abilities.

REFERENCES
1. Fromm E. *The Sane Society*. Fawcett Publications, Inc; 1955:27.
2. Lindau ST, Makelarski JA, Body K, et al. Change in health-related socioeconomic risk factors and mental health during the early phase of the COVID-19 pandemic: a national survey of U.S. women. *J Womens Health (Larchmt)*. 2021;30(4):502-513. doi:10.1089/jwh.2020.8879
3. Long H. U.S. now has 22 million unemployed, wiping out a decade of job gains. *Washington Post*. Published April 16, 2020. Accessed June 16, 2021. https://www.washingtonpost.com/business/2020/04/16/unemployment-claims-coronavirus/

4. Mervosh S, Lu D, Swales V. See which states and cities have told residents to stay home. *New York Times*. Updated April 20, 2020. Accessed May 25, 2021. https://www.nytimes.com/interactive/2020/us/coronavirus-stay-at-home-order.html

5. Kluger J. Domestic violence is a pandemic within the COVID-19 pandemic. *Time*. Published February 3, 2021. Accessed April 1, 2021. https://time.com/5928539/domestic-violence-covid-19/

6. Holland KM, Jones C, Vivolo-Kantor AM, et al. Trends in US emergency department visits for mental health, overdose, and violence outcomes before and during the COVID-19 pandemic. *JAMA Psychiatry*. 2021;78(4):372-379. doi:10.1001/jamapsychiatry.2020.4402

7. Piquero AR, Jennings WG, Jemison E, Kaukinen C, Knaul FM. Domestic violence during the COVID-19 pandemic—evidence from a systematic review and meta-analysis. *J Crim Justice*. 2021;74:101806. doi:10.1016/j.crimjus.2021.101806

8. Loewenstein RJ. Dissociation debates: everything you know is wrong. *Dialogues Clin Neurosci*. 2018;20(3):229-242. doi:10.31887/DCNS.2018.20.3/rloewenstein

9. Florida R. *The New Urban Crisis: How Our Cities Are Increasing Inequality, Deepening Segregation, and Failing the Middle Class—And what We Can Do about it*. Basic Books; 2018.

10. Frey WH. *America's Largest Cities Saw the Sharpest Population Losses during the Pandemic, New Census Data Shows*. The Brookings Institution; Published June 8, 2021. Accessed June 16, 2021. https://www.brookings.edu/research/the-largest-cities-saw-the-sharpest-population-losses-during-the-pandemic-new-census-data-shows/

11. Johanson M. The 'Zoom towns' Luring Remote Workers to Rural Enclaves. *BBC*. Published June 8, 2021. Accessed June 16, 2021. https://www.bbc.com/worklife/article/20210604-the-zoom-towns-luring-remote-workers-to-rural-enclaves

12. Fry R, Passel JS, Cohn D. *A Majority of Young Adults in the U.S. Live with Their Parents for the First Time since the Great Depression*. Pew Research Center; Published September 4, 2020. Accessed June 16, 2021. https://www.pewresearch.org/fact-tank/2020/09/04/a--majority-of-young-adults-in-the-u-s-live-with-their-parents-for-the-first-time-since-the-great-depression/

13. American Psychological Association. *Stress in America: One Year Later, a New Wave of Pandemic Health Concerns*. Accessed June 6, 2021. https://www.apa.org/news/press/releases/stress/2021/sia-pandemic-report.pdf

14. Julian K. America has a drinking problem. *The Atlantic*. Published June 1, 2021. Accessed June 4, 2021. https://www.theatlantic.com/magazine/archive/2021/07/america-drinking-alone-problem/619017/

15. Alfonso FIII. *The Pandemic Is Triggering Opioid Relapses across Appalachia*. CNN; Published May 14, 2020. Accessed April 5, 2021. https://www.cnn.com/2020/05/14/health/opioids-addiction-appalachia-coronavirus-trnd/index.html

16. *Overdosing Deaths Accelerating During COVID-19*. CDC website; Published December 17, 2020. Accessed April 5, 2021. https://www.cdc.gov/media/releases/2020/p1218-overdose-deaths-covid-19.html

17. Ahmad FB, Rossen LM, Sutton P. *Provisional Drug Overdose Death Counts*. National Center for Health Statistics; Updated August 11, 2021. Accessed September 1, 2021. https://www.cdc.gov/nchs/nvss/vsrr/drug-overdose-data.htm

18. Rabin RC. U.S. suicides declined over all in 2020 but may have risen among people of color. *New York Times*. Published April 15, 2021. Accessed June 17, 2021. https://www.washingtonpost.com/health/2021/04/22/health-workers-covid-quit/

19. Shih WC. Global supply chains in a post-pandemic world: companies need to make their networks more resilient. Here's how. *Harvard Business Review*. Published September-October 2020. Accessed February 18, 2021. https://hbr.org/2020/09/global-supply-chains-in-a-post-pandemic-world

20. Mulvany L, Patton L, Hirtzer M. Farmers dump milk in latest blow to battered U.S. dairy. *Bloomberg*. Published April 2, 2020. Updated April 3, 2020. Accessed February 18, 2021. https://www.bloomberg.com/news/articles/2020-04-02/farmers-are-dumping-milk-in-latest-blow-to-battered-u-s-dairy

21. Yaffe-Bellany D, Corkery M. Dumped milk, smashed eggs, plowed vegetables: food waste of the pandemic. *New York Times*. Published April 11, 2020. Accessed February 18, 2021. https://www.nytimes.com/2020/04/11/business/coronavirus-destroying-food.html

22. Balagtas J, Cooper J. *The Impact of Coronavirus COVID-19 on U.S. Meat and Livestock Markets*. U.S. Department of Agriculture, Office of the Chief Economist; March 2021. Accessed June 17, 2021. https://www.usda.gov/sites/default/files/documents/covid-impact-livestock-markets.pdf

23. Berg S. *COVID-19 Exacerbates Drug Shortages. AMA Details Next Steps*. AMA Website. Published November 17, 2020. Accessed February 18, 2021. https://www.ama-assn.org/delivering-care/public-health/covid-19-exacerbates-drug-shortages-ama-details-next-steps

24. Lepper PM, Muellenbach RM. Mechanical ventilation in early COVID-19 ARDS. *EClinicalMedicine*. 2020;28:100616. doi:10.1016/j.eclinm.2020.100616

25. Gibson PG, Qin L, Puah SH. COVID-19 acute respiratory distress syndrome (ARDS): clinical features and differences from typical pre-COVID-19 ARDS. *Med J Aust*. 2020;213(2):54-56.e1. doi:10.5694/mja2.50674

26. Li Y, Scherer N, Felix L, Kuper H. Prevalence of depression, anxiety and post-traumatic stress disorder in health care workers during the COVID-19 pandemic: a systematic review and meta-analysis. *PLoS One*. 2021;16(3):e0246454. doi:10.1371/journal.pone.0246454. eCollection 2021.

27. Nivette AE, Zahnow R, Aguilar R, et al. A global analysis of the impact of COVID-19 stay-at-home restrictions on crime. *Nat Hum Behav*. 2021;5:868-877. Accessed June 16, 2021. doi:10.1038/s41562-021-01139-z

28. Thebault R, Fox J, Tran AB. 2020 was the deadliest gun violence year in decades. So far, 2021 is worse. *Washington Post*. Published June 14, 2021. Accessed June 15, 2021. https://www.washingtonpost.com/nation/2021/06/14/2021-gun-violence/?itid=hp-top-table-main

29. MacFarquhar N With homicides rising, cities brace for a violent summer. *New York Times*. Published June 1, 2021. Accessed June 17, 2021. https://www.nytimes.com/2021/06/01/us/shootings-in-us.html

30. Bates J. Report: homicides continue to rise slowly in the U.S., while other violent crime rates decline. *Time Magazine*. Published August 4, 2021. Accessed September 14, 2021. https://time.com/6086558/us-homicides-violent-crime-rates/

31. Ganzel BL, Morris PA, Wethington E. Allostasis and the human brain: integrating models of stress from the social and life sciences. *Psychol Rev*. 2010;117(1):134-174. doi:10.1037/a0017773

32. Yong E. Meet the woman without fear. *Discover*. Published December 16, 2010. Accessed April 5, 2021. https://www.discovermagazine.com/mind/meet-the-woman-without-fear

33. Shalev AY, Marmar CR. Posttraumatic stress disorder. In: Sadock BJ, Sadock VA, Ruiz P, eds. *Kaplan & Sadock's Comprehensive Textbook of Psychiatry*. 10th ed. Vol 1. Wolters Kluwer; 2017:1812-1826.

34. Wicking M, Steiger F, Nees F, et al. Deficient fear extinction memory in posttraumatic stress disorder. *Neurobiol Learn Mem*. 2016;136:116-126. doi:10.1016/j.nlm.2016.09.016

35. Bremner JD. Neuroimaging in posttraumatic stress disorder and other stress-related disorders. *Neuroimaging Clin N Am*. 2007;17(4):523-538, ix. doi:10.1016/j.nic.2007.07.003

36. McEwen BS. Stressed or stressed out: what is the difference? *J Psychiatry Neurosci*. 2005;30(5):315-318. PMID: 16151535.

37. FAIR Health. *A Detailed Study of Patients with Long-Haul COVID: An Analysis of Private Healthcare Claims*. Published June 15, 2021. Accessed June 15, 2021. https://s3.amazonaws.com/media2.fairhealth.org/whitepaper/asset/A%20Detailed%20Study%20of%20Patients%20with%20Long-Haul%20COVID--An%20Analysis%20of%20Private%20Healthcare%20Claims--A%20FAIR%20Health%20White%20Paper.pdf

38. Cañas CA. The triggering of post-COVID-19 autoimmunity phenomena could be associated with both transient immunosuppression and an inappropriate form of immune reconstitution in susceptible individuals. *Med Hypotheses*. 2020;145:110345. doi:10.1016/j.mehy.2020.110345

39. Janiri D, Carfì A, Kotzalidis GD, et al. Posttraumatic stress disorder in patients after severe COVID-19 infection. *JAMA Psychiatry*. 2021;75(5):567-569. doi:10.1001/jamapsychiatry.2021.0109

40. Ahmed H, Patel K, Greenwood DC, et al. Long-term clinical outcomes in survivors of severe acute respiratory syndrome and Middle East respiratory syndrome coronavirus outbreaks after hospitalization or ICU admission: a systematic review and meta-analysis. *J Rehabil Med*. 2020;52(5):jrm00063. doi:10.2340/16501977-2694

41. Sekowski M, Gambin M, Hansen K, et al. Risk of developing post-traumatic stress disorder in severe COVID-19 survivors, their families and frontline workers: what should mental health specialists prepare for? *Front Psychiatry*. 2021;12:562899. doi:10.3389/fpsyt.2021.562899

42. Kisley S, Warren N, McMahon L, Dalais C, Henry I, Siskind D. Occurrence, prevention, and management of the psychological effects of emerging virus outbreaks on healthcare workers: rapid review and meta-analysis. *Br Med J*. 2020;369:m1642. doi:10.1136/bmj.m1642

43. Clement S, Pascual C, Ulmanu M. Stress on the front lines of COVID-19. *Washington Post*. Published April 6, 2021. Accessed April 6, 2021. washingtonpost.com/health/2021/04/06/stress-front-lines-health-care-workers-share-hardest-parts-working-during-pandemic/?itid=hp_alert

44. Wan W. Burned out by the pandemic, 3 in 10 health-care workers consider leaving the profession. *Washington Post*. Published April 22, 2021. Accessed June 12, 2021. https://www.washingtonpost.com/health/2021/04/22/health-workers-covid-quit/

45. Mo S, Shi J. The psychological consequences of the COVID-19 on residents and staff in nursing homes. *Work Aging Retire*. 2020;6(4):254-259. doi:10.1093/worker/waaa021

46. Centers for Medicine & Medicaid Services. *COVID-19 Nursing Home Data*. Updated May 30, 2021. Accessed June 12, 2021. https://data.cms.gov/stories/s/COVID-19-Nursing-Home-Data/bkwz-xpvg/

47. Jo S, Kim YJ, Park WK, et al. Association of NO_2 and other air pollution exposures with risk of Parkinson disease. *JAMA Neurol*. 2021;78(7):800-808. Accessed Jun 16, 2021. doi:10.1001/jamaneurol.2021.1335

48. Younan D, Petkus AJ, Widaman KF, et al. Particulate matter and episodic memory decline mediated by early neuroanatomic biomarkers of Alzheimer's disease. *Brain*. 2020;143(1):289-302. doi:10.1093/brain/awaa007

49. Arnold C. The man who warned the world about lead. *NOVA*. Published May 31, 2017. Accessed June 16, 2021. https://www.pbs.org/wgbh/nova/article/herbert-needleman/

50. Borunda A. The origins of environmental justice—and why it's finally getting the attention it deserves. *National Geographic*. Published February 24, 2021. Accessed June 16, 2021. https://www.nationalgeographic.com/environment/article/environmental-justice-origins-why-finally-getting-the-attention-it-deserves?loggedin=true

51. Phillips CM, Perry IJ. Depressive symptoms, anxiety, and well-being among metabolic health obese subtypes. *Psychoneuroendocrinology*. 2015;62:47-53. doi:10.1016/j.psyneuen.2015.07.168

52. Duong M, Cohen JI, Convit A. High cortisol levels are associated with low quality food choice in Type 2 Diabetes. *Endocrine*. 2012;41(1):76-81. doi:10.1007/s12020-011-9527-5

53. Kim H, Rebholz CM, Hegde S, et al. Plant-based diets, pescatarian diets and COVID-19 severity: a population-based case-control study in six countries. *BMJ Nutr Prev Health*. 2021;4(1):bmjnph-2021-000272. doi:10.1136/bmjnph-2021-000272

54. Merino J, Joshi AD, Nguyen LG, et al. Diet quality and risk and severity of COVID-19: a prospective cohort study. Preprint. Posted online June 25, 2021. MedRxiv 06.04.21259283. doi:10.1101/2021.06.24.21259283

55. The National Academies of Sciences, Engineering, and Medicine. *Social Isolation and Loneliness in Older Adults: Opportunities for the Health Care System*. The National Academies Press; 2020.

56. Weissbourd R, Batanova M, Lovison V, Torres E. *Loneliness in America: how The Pandemic Has Deepened an Endemic of Loneliness and What We Can Do About It.* Making Caring Common Project. Accessed June 17, 2021. https://static1.squarespace. com/static/5b7c56e255b02c683659fe43/t/6021776bdd04957c4557c212/1612805995893/ Loneliness+in+America+2021_02_08_FINAL.pdf

57. Ausubel J. *Older People Are More Likely to Live Alone in the U.S. Than Elsewhere in the World.* Pew Research Center; Published March 10, 2020. Accessed June 17, 2021. https://www.pewresearch.org/fact-tank/2020/03/10/ older-people-are-more-likely-to-live-alone-in-the-u-s-than-elsewhere-in-the-world/

58. Kahlon MK, Aksan N, Aubrey R, et al. Effect of layperson-delivered, empathy-focused program of telephone calls on loneliness, depression, and anxiety among adults during the COVID-19 pandemic. *JAMA Psychiatry.* Published online February 23, 2021;78(6):616-622. doi:10.1001/jamapsychiatry.2021.0113

59. *Provisional COVID-19 Deaths by Sex and Age.* Centers for Disease Control and Prevention; Updated June 2, 2021. Accessed June 6, 2021. https://data.cdc.gov/NCHS/ Provisional-COVID-19-Deaths-by-Sex-and-Age/9bhg-hcku/data

60. *Provisional COVID-19 Deaths by Sex and Age.* Centers for Disease Control and Prevention; Updated September 11, 2021. Accessed September 15, 2021. https://data.cdc.gov/NCHS/ Provisional-COVID-19-Deaths-by-Sex-and-Age/9bhg-hcku/data

61. Thompson LW, Breckenridge JN, Gallagher D, Peterson J. Effects of bereavement on self-perceptions of physical health in elderly widows and widowers. *J Gerontol.* 1984;39(3):309-314. doi:10.1093/geronj/39.3.309

62. Feld S, George LK. Moderating effects of prior social resources on the hospitalizations of elders who become widowed. *J Aging Health.* 1994;6(3):275-295. doi:10.1177/089826439400600301

63. Weinberger AH, Gbedemah M, Martinez AM, Nash D, Galea S, Goodwin RD. Trends in depression prevalence in the USA from 2005 to 2015: widening disparities in vulnerable groups. *Psychol Med.* 2018;48(8):1308-1315. doi:10.1017/S0033291717002781

64. American Psychiatric Association. *Diagnostic and Statistical Manual on Mental Disorders.* 5th ed. The American Psychiatric Association; 2013.

65. Panchal N, Kamal R, Cox C, Garfield R. *The Implications of COVID-19 for Mental Health and Substance Use.* KFF website; Published February 10, 2021. Accessed April 5, 2021. https://www.kff.org/coronavirus-covid-19/issue-brief/ the-implications-of-covid-19-for-mental-health-and-substance-use/

66. Michl LC, McLaughlin KA, Shepherd K, Nolen-Hoeksema S. Rumination as a mechanism linking stressful events to symptoms of depression and anxiety: longitudinal evidence in early adolescents and adults. *J Abnorm Psychol.* 2013;122(2):339-352. doi:10.1037/ a0031994

67. Dostoyevsky F. *The House of the Dead.* Trans. McDuff D. Penguin Books; 1985:43.

68. Jamrami H, BaHammam AS, Bragazzi NL, et al. Sleep problems during the COVID-19 pandemic by population: a systematic review and meta-analysis. *J Clin Sleep Med.* 2021;17(2):299-313. doi:10.5664/jcsm.8930

69. McEwen BS. Protective and damaging effects of stress mediators: central role of the brain. *Dialogues Clin Neurosci.* 2006;8(4):367-381. doi:10.31887/DCNS.2006.8.4/bmcewen

70. Nutt D, Wilson S, Peterson L. Sleep disorders as core symptoms of depression. *Dialogues Clin Neurosci.* 2008;10(3):329-336. doi:10.31887/DCNS.2008.10.3/dnutt

71. Ahmad FB, Anderson RN. The leading causes of death in the US for 2020. *J Am Med Assoc.* 2021;325(18):1829-1830. doi:10.1001/jama.2021.5469

6

Psychological Impact of COVID-19 in Children, Young Adults, and Caregivers

This country has been a beacon to the world when it comes to their protection, and our society has always taken pride in championing the welfare of the children. There are clear-cut rules and laws established to protect our children from harm, be it physical, sexual, mental, or another form of trauma. We go to great lengths to educate our teachers, as well as numerous other medical and mental health providers, and have implemented mandatory courses for recognizing and preventing child abuse. Therefore, this should come as no surprise when the issue of child welfare is addressed in the context of dangerous communicable diseases. All children are mandated to receive vaccinations after birth and before attending school. These vaccine mandates have been established not only for the individual but also for the safety and wellbeing of others in our society. There have been numerous instances when certain groups have defied these rules and, consequently, either the children have been refused entrance to school or schools have been shut down. Apart from a small segment of the society who has always challenged the wisdom of the vaccines, most parents have adhered to the vaccination guidelines without much thought or debate. Unfortunately, the politicization of COVID-19 guidelines, including those pertaining to vaccination, has led many to defy the kind of scientific approach one would expect when dealing with a deadly virus about which so much remains unknown.

In addition to worries about contracting the virus or spreading it, children have also had to deal with many of the same psychosocial stressors that have affected adults. This includes social isolation, a myriad of potential family difficulties often arising from the stress of parents or guardians, the indefinite suspension of regularly scheduled activities (especially school), and grief due to the death of family or friends. This chapter is meant to help one navigate through the maze of medical and mental health consequences of COVID-19 among children and to help caregivers have a better understanding of how to make an informed decision for the welfare of their child.

COVID-19 Pathology in Children

Adolescents infected with SARS-CoV-2 typically experience less severe bouts of COVID-19 than adults with rare exceptions. The reason for this remains unclear at this time, but several hypotheses have been postulated to explain the phenomenon. Adults may be especially prone to the illness because of damage to endothelial cells over the course of their lives, increased angiotensin-converting enzyme 2 or transmembrane protease serine expression, higher levels of inflammation, or low levels of vital nutrients. Children may also have enhanced immunity because of more recent exposure to common coronaviruses that do not cause severe illness (HCoV-229E, HCoV-HKU1, HCoV-NL63, or HCoV-OC43), a healthier microbiota, or a stronger and as-of-yet-identified immune system response to specific viral insults.[1] As of September 2021, researchers are still without definitive answers.

What is known is that COVID-19 presents as a relatively minor respiratory illness in most pediatric cases.[2] Common symptoms in pediatric patients include fever, chills, cough, and fatigue.[3] Approximately half of pediatric patients with COVID-19 experience no symptoms or mild symptoms, and only a paucity of the children develop symptoms severe enough to warrant intensive care unit (ICU) admission or hospitalization. Preston and colleagues, who examined the discharge data from 869 medical facilities between March 1 and October 31, 2020, found that only 3.65% (756) of the total pediatric patients (20,714) who tested positive for COVID-19 were hospitalized with severe forms of the illness, that a similar number 3.61% (747) were admitted to ICU, and that only 0.83% (172) became ill enough to warrant the use of mechanical ventilation. Similar to adults, children with underlying chronic illnesses faced an increased risk of developing severe COVID-19.[4]

Leeb and colleagues, meanwhile, found that even fewer children were hospitalized. Their study, which involved over 277,000 students across 47 US states who tested positive for COVID-19 between March 2020 and September 2020, found that only 1.2% (3240) of the students were hospitalized, that 0.1% (404) were admitted to the ICU, and that only 0.02% (51) died. Furthermore, their findings revealed that younger children (5-11 years of age) were less likely to experience severe symptoms than older children (12-17 years of age). Approximately, 1.0% (1021) of the former group (n = 101,503) were hospitalized, 0.14% (145) were admitted to the ICU, and 0.0197% (20) died. Within the older group (n = 175,782), 1.26% (2219) were hospitalized, 0.15% (259) were admitted to the ICU, and 0.0176% (31) died.[5]

Children appear to be at less of a risk for developing long COVID though data on the subject remain scant. Zimmermann and colleagues performed a review involving 14 international studies including 19,426 children and found that, in the majority of studies, symptoms did not typically persist for longer than 12 weeks in those infected with SARS-CoV-2. Despite this seemingly positive conclusion, the authors noted multiple limitations in their study and strongly suggested more studies into the potential effects of long COVID on children to accurately determine the level of risk to children and the implementation of the most prudent policies.[6]

While there is a reduced risk of long COVID among individuals under the age of 18 years, children and very young adults are at an increased risk of developing multisystem inflammatory syndrome in children (MIS-C) (also known as pediatric inflammatory multisystem syndrome), a condition where multiple organs become inflamed following infection. The affected organs can include the kidneys, heart, lungs, spleen, eyes, gastrointestinal tract, skin, and even the brain.[7] Symptoms include fever, vomiting, diarrhea, nausea, abdominal pain, neck pain, rash, bloodshot eyes, and drowsiness.[8] Patients typically present with GI symptoms but can go on to develop myocarditis, cardiac dysfunction, and coronary artery dilation. While it is rare (occurring in 2.1 per 100,000 persons younger than 21 years in the United States), an estimated 60% of individuals who develop MIS-C are admitted to ICUs and most recover with intensive care support.[9] The estimated mortality is 2% to 4%.[10] As of September 14, 2021, a total of 4661 cases have been reported in the United States and 41 (0.9%) have proven fatal.[11]

Age does appear to affect prognosis. Children between 0 and 4 years of age typically have fewer complications and fewer admissions to intensive care, while patients in the age group of 18 to 20 years with recent infection of COVID-19 have been more likely to experience myocarditis, acute respiratory distress syndrome, or pneumonia.[9] Median age for MIS-C is 9 years and 60% of reported patients have been males.[11] Like COVID-19, MIS-C has disproportionately impacted Black and Hispanic children—30% and 32% of cases, respectively.[11,12] Social determinants in health, particularly poverty, housing and employment dynamics within their families, and insurance status, have placed both Hispanic and Black individuals at greater risk of COVID-19 infection and greater risk of severe complications, including MIS-C.[9]

SARS-CoV-2 Transmission in Children

While there appears to be no question that healthy children without preexisting conditions are at less of a risk of developing severe COVID-19 symptoms than adults (especially seniors) or children from struggling communities, the risk of infection even in resource flush communities remains quite high, especially given the increased transmissibility of the Delta variant. In Marin County, California, an unvaccinated teacher read aloud to a classroom of 24 students 2 days after developing symptoms in May 2021. The teacher chose to read without wearing a mask, despite school requirements to mask while indoors. Consequently, 12 of the 24 students in the classroom—all of whom were too young to be vaccinated—received a positive test result for COVID-19. Eight of the 10 students in the two rows closest to the teacher's desk tested positive (attack rate = 80%), while 4 in 14 in the three back rows tested positive (attack rate = 28%). Fourteen additional infections could be traced back to the class, bringing the total to 27 (26 individuals in addition to the teacher). Of the 27 individuals, 3 were fully vaccinated and 22 (81%) reported symptoms.[13]

While children are at risk of infection, the role they play in community and household transmission remains poorly defined. Zhu and colleagues conducted a meta-analysis that examined 213 household SARS-CoV-2 transmission clusters and found that only 8 (3.8%) included a pediatric case, and that secondary attack rates in households with a confirmed pediatric case were significantly lower than secondary attack rates in households with confirmed adult cases.[14] Of course, there were numerous limitations with this study; chief among them was the fact that it was not clear what role, if any, asymptomatic pediatric cases played in secondary attack rates within households.

Far more surprising is the fact that an Ontario study involving more than 6000 households found that younger children (aged 13 years and under) are actually more likely to spread SARS-CoV-2 within a household than older children (between the ages of 14 and 17 years), even if older children were more likely to be primary household case.[15] Moreover, children aged 0 to 3 years were more likely than the study's other three age groups (4-8, 9-13, and 14-17) to transmit SARS-CoV-2 infection.[15] While this seems counterintuitive at first, it could be explained by several factors. Some have hypothesized that younger children carry a larger viral load than older children or adults. Others have noted that younger children are most likely to be asymptomatic than any age group and because younger children are incapable of self-isolating even if symptomatic. Furthermore, as anyone who has had a teenager or can remember being one can tell you older children tend to demand more of their own personal space than younger children.

The Pandemic's Impact on Children

While children infected with COVID-19 may have a favorable prognosis when compared to adults, the same cannot be said for their mental health. Throughout the pandemic, children have faced the same kinds of stresses that adults have been forced to confront, and they have also felt trapped, bored, anxious, or afraid. The data have shown that they have responded in much the same way as adults to these stressors. However, children have also faced unique difficulties that clinicians should appreciate if they are to act with empathy and fully understand the specific circumstances that children have endured throughout the COVID Era.

Anxiety, Depression, and Defiance

The COVID-19 Era is simply not sustainable for the mental health of anyone, children included. As noted throughout Chapter 5, *Psychosocial and Economic Impact of COVID-19—A Nation Under Siege*, humans are not blank slates, and their adaptability can only go so far until their physical and mental health begin to suffer. Children are no different and the elevated rates of symptoms associated with mental health difficulties support this position.

A meta-analysis from the University of Calgary examined 29 individual studies from around the world that included 80,879 children and found that depression and anxiety symptoms had doubled from prepandemic averages among similar cohorts—from 12.9% and 11.6% to 25.2% and 20.5%, respectively. This means approximately one out of every four children globally are experiencing depression symptoms while one in five report clinically elevated anxiety symptoms.[16] A Norwegian study involving 2536 adolescents—1621 of whom were surveyed prior to the pandemic and 915 of whom were surveyed during the pandemic—showed a stronger connection between high pandemic anxiety and not only depression symptoms but also poor physical health. Of the 915 adolescents surveyed during the pandemic, 158 (17.3%) experienced high pandemic anxiety and were significantly more likely to have experienced depressive symptoms and poor physical health.[17]

This should sound reminiscent of the positive feedback loops discussed in previous chapters. Though it may not provide proof of directionality, it does suggest that COVID-19, anxiety, and depressive symptoms, as well as poor physical health, may reinforce one another. Furthermore, these can be compounded by poverty, housing precarity, food insecurity, and other factors common among households of low socioeconomic status. What is important to remember, however, is that these studies suggest that COVID-19 anxiety may be relatively common among children but that it is far from universal. The majority of children will prove to be resilient in the face of COVID-19 stress, and parents and guardians can increase the likelihood that their children will process the experience in an appropriate way by fostering an environment of love and support.

Similar approaches should be taken with children who have developed oppositional defiant disorder. Evidence is starting to emerge that more children are becoming more defiant and aggressive during the pandemic, particularly among younger children. A study involving 5823 children from three age groups (1-6 years, 7-10 years, and 11-19 years) across Germany, Austria, Liechtenstein, and Switzerland revealed that the youngest age group had the most notable increase in defiant behaviors (43% of the group), the middle group showed moderate increases in emotional and behavioral problems, while the oldest group reported higher rates of anxiety than the middle group (but lower than the youngest) and complained of "being overtired, underactive, and nervous."[18]

Yet another Canadian study that surveyed 587 children between 5 and 18 years of age with attention deficit hyperactive disorder also found moderately higher levels of anxiety and depression (14.1% and 17.4%, respectively) among the participants but that 38.6% of participants displayed behaviors indicative of oppositional defiant disorder.[19] Given oppositional defiant disorder is estimated to have a prevalence rate between 1% and 11%, and that DSM-V estimates that the average prevalence to be 3.3%, this seems like a worrisome observation that warrants more study.[20]

There are numerous potential reasons for these kinds of phenomena. While it is certainly a possibility that the child's homelife may have deteriorated, as they may live with a caregiver or relative who is negligent, struggling with substance abuse, or abusive, not all pediatric mental health problems can be traced back to mistreatment. Like many adults, some children may feel socially isolated because their ability to see people from outside of their household has been severely disrupted. Others may not be able to feel comfortable because of the lack of stability in their life or the fact that they have a new awareness of their own mortality, possibly brought on by the death of someone close to them. Still others may simply feel overburdened by the multiple stresses of the pandemic.

Many older children and teenagers will likely also feel they have missed major life milestones and coming of age moments due to pandemic restrictions. They may also be frustrated by the fact that they cannot physically be with their peers for friendship and support or that the pandemic has also severely reduced opportunities for intimacy. Platonic and romantic relationships are integral parts of separation-individualization from the family unit, and the creation of social bonds within peer groups often supplant the family unit as the individual's primary source of social support. As the pandemic has arrested this process, it has likely led to feelings of angst or potentially depression, as well as significant friction between children attempting to assert their independence and parents attempting to maintain their authority at a time when they could expect neither consistency nor predictability from the world outside their homes. Meanwhile, those who stand on the precipice of adulthood but have been unable to leave the proverbial nest due to COVID-19 restrictions may experience an even greater sense of indignation and resentment. Those who obsess over these perceived injustices will likely find themselves searching for a specific culprit to blame for their predicament and may be especially vulnerable to demagogues and social media campaigns designed to exploit this need to assign blame.[21]

It is difficult to speculate how long these types of negative emotions will persist and even the most educated guess about how long rates of anxiety and depression will remain elevated among children and late adolescents cannot account for unforeseen variables. In addition, there is a lack of available data as to how epidemics or pandemics have historically impacted children's growth and development or how widespread masking and social isolation will affect different age groups. For example, some have speculated that widespread masking may interfere with the development of speech and nonverbal language among young children, but there are not enough data to support this claim or to completely refute it.[22]

What one should keep in mind is that humanity's historical record is littered with extended periods of plague, war, and natural disasters, but the vast majority of individuals persevered. The children who endured these difficult periods largely grew into well-adjusted adults. Furthermore, while it has not been easy for families to go through extended periods of quarantine together, this has not always been a torturous experience.

There is evidence to suggest that many fathers are taking a more active role in their children's lives, with one report finding that 43% of the fathers surveyed (n = 534) have discovered new, shared interests with their children; 50% of fathers say they are sharing more about their feelings with their children; and 53% of fathers say their children are more open to sharing their feelings with them.[23]

Obesity and Increases in Body Mass Index

As many adults learned during the most restrictive phases of the pandemic, it can be difficult to remain healthy and active when one has limited access to gyms and many types of activities outside of the home are discouraged. Furthermore, many adults learned that this kind of sedentary lifestyle can lead to accelerated weight gain. In addition, many individuals were experiencing increases in stress, sleep disturbances, irregular mealtimes, and changes in eating habits that were oftentimes for the worse.[24] Especially in the earliest days of the pandemic, it was far more common to cook from the pantry each day rather than make regular stops by the green grocers or their local farmers' market, which necessarily meant fewer fresh fruits and vegetables and more processed foods on the dinner tables of families across the world.

No surprise, the accelerated weight gain reported among adults appears to have impacted children, too.[25] As reported in a cohort study of 432,302 individuals aged 2 to 19 years, children also saw accelerated increases in body mass index (BMI) and rates of obesity became notably higher in the early months of the pandemic.[26] According to the report, the estimated percentage of children with obesity increased from 19.3% to 22.4% between August 2019 and August 2020, as the rate of BMI increase approximately doubled from 0.052 to 0.100 kg/m^2/month. Furthermore, the authors found that individuals who were already overweight or obese were more likely to experience accelerated rates of BMI increase during the most restrictive pandemic months.[26]

Trauma and Abuse

While stresses of the pandemic may have affected both adults and children, the psychosocial effects of the pandemic have certainly impacted the two groups differently. Upward of 22 million jobs in the United States simply vanished in the 4 weeks following the declaration of a national emergency on March 13, 2020.[27] For those who base their worth on their ability to provide for their families, this must have been a tremendous blow to their self-esteem, as well as a constant source of anxiety about retaining the role of provider. This stress was often compounded by additional psychosocial factors tied to the pandemic, including increases in crime rates, disruptions in supply chains, and fears associated with the virus, and then further compounded by substance abuse.

In children and many adults, this kind of stress can lead to anxiety and depression. Unfortunately, this toxic mixture also disrupted otherwise stable living situations and led to skyrocketing rates of domestic abuse for women and children. As Jacky Mulveen, project manager of Women's Empowerment and Recovery Educators (WE:ARE) in Birmingham, England, told Jeffrey Kluger of *Time Magazine*, COVID-19 did not suddenly turn an individual into an abuser. "It gives them more tools, more chances to control you. The abuser says, 'You can't go out; you're not going anywhere,' and the government also is saying, 'You have to stay in.'"[28]

The increase is not just anecdotal. Local police in China's Hubei province reported a 300% increase in reports of domestic violence in February 2020 compared to February 2019, while domestic violence reports during the initial March 2020 lockdowns in France and Argentina increased by 30% and 25%, respectively, while the number of helpline calls related to domestic violence in Singapore and Cyprus increased 33% and 30%, respectively. Similar spikes occurred throughout the US Portland, Oregon, reported a 22% increase in domestic violence arrests in the weeks following stay-at-home orders when compared to prior weeks. Meanwhile, between March 2020 and March 2021, the San Antonio Police Department observed an 18% increase in calls pertaining to violence in the home; the Sheriff's Office in Jefferson County Alabama reported a 27% increase in calls about domestic violence; and the New York Police Department recorded a 10% increase in reports of domestic violence.[29] Preliminary data from emergency rooms paint an equally doleful, though incomplete, picture.[30,31]

What is perhaps most unsettling of all is that reports of child abuse appear to have plummeted. An analysis by the Associated Press (AP) found that there were 400,000 fewer child welfare concerns and 200,000 fewer child abuse and neglect investigations and assessments from the start of March through the end of November 2020 than during the same 9-month period in 2019. This constitutes an 18% decrease in both. The AP report also noted that, while there were many factors contributing to the decline in investigations and reports, the most important was that many children spent months out of the public eye due to school closures. Teachers, administrators, counselors, nurses, coaches, and other school staff receive training to identify the warning signs of abuse or neglect and are required by law to report any potential instances. They are the top reporters of child abuse. Once the United States shifted to virtual learning, abuse and neglect reports from school source declined by 59%.[32]

This suggests that child abuse has been dramatically underreported. Unfortunately, we will likely not have a full understanding of the scope of the problem until the worst of the pandemic has passed nor will we fully understand how life in an unstructured home has impacted the development of children and adolescents until years from now. A relatively small study involving 398 parents from across North America following the H1N1 outbreak in 2009 found that nearly one-third of the children who experienced isolation due to quarantining or social distancing efforts met criteria for posttraumatic stress disorder (PTSD), and that there was a very clear correlation between children who had clinically significant levels of PTSD symptoms and parents who had similar symptoms, suggesting that parents' responses to traumatic experiences can influence how their children process these experiences. Nearly 86% of parents who experienced PTSD symptoms had children who also experienced PTSD symptoms.[33] Once again, this highlights the importance of providing a loving and nurturing environment for children, especially during tumultuous times.

Dangers of Social Media Use

Like adults, older children and adolescents have almost certainly also looked for outlets for their stress and frustrations, thereby leading them to engage in unhealthy behaviors, including excessive social media use.[34] Some have found refuge in online environments that ignore the doom and gloom of the world outside their home, while others have instead wandered into a veritable funhouse where misinformation runs rampant and reality is distorted to exploit individuals' prejudices or insecurities, oftentimes for commercial gain. Data suggest that social media platforms, when used excessively, have a negative impact on people (especially children) who may have body image problems, and researchers have found that excessive use is associated with appearance-related comparisons and dysmorphia concern.[35] In fact, some of the social media companies' own research has found that use of such technology makes body image issues worse for as many as one in three teen girls.[36] As many children (and adults) have experienced increases in BMI and spent a lot of time using social media throughout the pandemic, it stands to reason that the problem has only grown worse. A similar phenomenon, known as "Zoom dysmorphia," has also been reported by those who see themselves on camera for sometimes hours a day.[37]

Numerous social media platforms have also distorted perceptions of the world by allowing users to create hermetic social environments where shared worldviews meet little, if any, opposition. This echo chamber creates a false sense of certainty about one's opinions, even if they are based on misinformation. Given the fact that researchers have found that individual publishers who use specific social media channels to spread misinformation are rewarded by the platform's algorithm, this means that children who lack sufficient knowledge of world events may come to align their beliefs with false narratives that adults who are more well-versed in historical knowledge would not find persuasive.[38] This not only fuels extremist thinking but also belief in falsities about the pandemic, SARS-CoV-2, and public health officials, thereby frustrating attempts to ensure compliance with public health guidelines. Meanwhile, video platforms, which have been accused of promoting conspiracy theories and extremist content through their video-recommending algorithm for several years, have hosted videos that contain misleading information about COVID-19.[39] Li and colleagues found 27.5% of the most watched videos about COVID-19 (accounting for more than 62 million views) contained misleading information.[39]

Grief

Around the world, young children have lost over 1 million parents due to COVID-19.[40] It is too early to say how this will impact the emerging generation. Worries that the COVID-related fatality of relatively young parents will result in more children developing bereavement disorders seem like a warranted concern, but this position remains premature at this time. While no studies have been conducted to support the implantation of specific policies, it would seem most prudent to find ways of offering grief-related services to children who need them sooner rather than later.

Impact on Caregivers

It is difficult to quantify exactly how difficult the COVID-19 pandemic has been on caregivers who need to balance their careers with parenting duties at a time when labor markets are being upended and schools and daycare services are shuttering their door. It has no doubt been the hardest on working class, single parents (most of whom are women) who have oftentimes had to work outside of the home and have struggled to find childcare or prevent virtual truancy, maintain regular doctors' appointments for things like routine vaccinations, perform household chores, and provide well-balanced meals.[41]

An analysis performed by Adams and colleagues on relative stress levels before and during the pandemic has found that caregivers from all walks of life are mostly experiencing more stress and that there are a variety of contributing factors. The study, which involved 433 parents with at least one child aged 5 to 18 years (95% of whom were women), found that the most common stressor was the change in children's daily structure and routines. This should come as no surprise because most children thrive under predictable routines and feel more secure when provided with structure. Similarly, this allows parents to schedule their day in a manner that allows for clear delineations between work and leisure time. Other stressors included worry about COVID-19, demands pertaining to online schooling, and inadequate money or food.[42]

This study, which surveyed parents at two different points in time, April/May 2020 and September 2020, also observed that stress levels decreased between May and September 2020 but that they remained relatively greater than the retrospective, pre–COVID-19 values. This should not come as a surprise. In the spring of 2020, the United States was still largely in lockdown and parents were still attempting to orient themselves to the seismic changes that took place between the prepandemic era and the COVID Era. By September, some children were once again attending school and adults had become more adapt at navigating pandemic-related stresses by employing a number of strategies, including doing more activities as a family, keeping in touch with friends/family virtually, and abiding by a daily routine.[42]

School Policy

One of the most vociferous debates between 2020 and 2021 has concerned school policy. Without question, children need socialization and education. School provides both these things. It also provides caregivers with a chance to earn a living without having to pay for private childcare or leave the child in the care of an older relative who is no longer part of the workforce. Primary school, therefore, serves three vital functions for our society: It teaches children the basic skills they will need to further educate themselves; it gives children the opportunity to learn how to interact with other children outside of their family unit; and it provides adults with more of an opportunity to pursue a career outside of the home. Without schools, our society cannot function properly.

While there is a need for schools, there is also a need to protect both school personnel, the children who attend the school, and the families of those children. Research and clinical data as well as all medical guidelines suggest that the most effective way to do so is through a combination of masking, ventilation, testing, and vaccination.[43] As the FDA has yet to grant emergency use authorization for any COVID-19 vaccine for children under the age of 12 years, many districts have opted to pursue mandatory vaccination policies for school personnel. Mandatory vaccination for students seems likely to occur, as well, and there is legal precedent for this policy in the United States dating back to at least 1809 when Massachusetts began requiring all students be vaccinated for smallpox before attending class.[44] In addition, it is a routine policy for all school-age children to be vaccinated against many communicable diseases to attend school and college.

Like vaccine campaigns in the past, this will likely be met with a great deal of resistance (see Box 6.1), and it would be wrong to characterize everyone who is reluctant to vaccinate their children as being against science. One cannot assume that anyone refusing a vaccine is against science. They are worried parents, and their faith in institutions has been rocked to its core over the course of the pandemic. The appropriate action should be to be an empathic listener to their fears while continuing to provide data-driven information in simple language that is palatable and easily comprehended rather to label them into a certain group, which will only alienate them further. As of August 2021, roughly one in five of those polled who had not had their children vaccinated said their reason for the delay was because they wanted more research to be conducted.[50]

BOX 6.1   A Brief History of Vaccines

Edward Jenner played a pivotal role in the development of vaccines and the eventual eradication of smallpox, though his groundbreaking work did not take place in a vacuum. For at least 500 years, Chinese physicians had known that they could prevent smallpox infections in healthy children by harvesting scabs from the scars of people with relatively mild smallpox infections, treating and grinding them into a powder, and then administering the powder via nasal insufflation. For possibly just as long, physicians from the Indian subcontinent had performed a similar procedure, though the attenuated smallpox material was introduced through subcutaneous administration.[45] The latter technique came to be known as variolation and word of its efficacy spread throughout the Ottoman Empire and eventually into Europe and their colonies in the Western Hemisphere.[46]

Despite being effective at preventing severe smallpox infection, variolation was still a risky procedure because it involved being infected with live smallpox virus. Many people went on to experience inflammation around the site of the incision, as well as the hallmark symptoms of smallpox. In some cases, it could result in severe illness. Despite this, the dangers that smallpox posed to the community were clear enough

BOX 6.1   A Brief History of Vaccines   (Continued)

that variolation grew in popularity even if many in Europe and Britain's North American colonies violently rejected the practice initially. There was even well-documented attempt on the life of Cotton Mather, who had become convinced of the efficacy of inoculation through variolation after learning about the practice from his slave, Onesimus. After trying to spread awareness of variolation to the people of Boston, he had a bomb thrown through his window. Attached was the following note: "Cotton Mather, you dog, dam you: I'll inoculate you with this; with a Pox to you."[47] Luckily for Mather it did not explode. Though it remained controversial (and even illegal in Virginia), there was little question of its efficacy. In fact, when an outbreak of smallpox threatened to derail General George Washington's campaign against the British, he ordered the entire Continental Army be inoculated in 1777, writing that "necessity not only authorizes but also seems to require the measure."[48]

While variolation used an attenuated form of smallpox to confer immunity to patients, the vaccine that ultimately eradicated smallpox in the 20th century relied on the use of the relatively mild cowpox (vaccinia) virus. As the story goes, Edward Jenner recognized that milkmaids rarely suffered severe infection or disfigurement from smallpox but did regularly become infected with minor infections of the hands and arms due to cowpox within their first few months of working with cows and thought that infection with vaccinia (from which we get the word *vaccine*) would provide immunity from smallpox. While Jenner proved his hypothesis in a clinical setting in 1796, it had already been tested in the field more than 20 years previously when Benjamin Jesty, a farmer from Yetminter, decided to follow a hunch during a smallpox outbreak in 1774 and walked his wife and two sons into a Dorset pasture that was home to a herd infected with cowpox, scraped some material from the udder of an infected cow with a stocking needle, and then performed a procedure similar to variolation. While Jenner was heralded as a genius, Jesty's experiment was met with shock by the community. Many feared that the family would turn into horned beasts, and they were subsequently run out of town.[44]

In the Untied States during the 1800s, few jurisdictions or school districts mandated vaccinations, even if there were several major outbreaks around the country, and much of the American population remained unvaccinated. In the United Kingdom, multiple vaccination acts were passed during the 19th century, oftentimes resulting in massive protests where effigies of Jenner were set on fire.[44] By the early 20th century,

(Continued)

> **BOX 6.1 A Brief History of Vaccines (Continued)**
>
> however, vaccination programs had largely eradicated smallpox from the industrialized world and a global effort that began in 1966 led to the elimination of the disease in South America, Asia, and Africa within approximately a decade. The last case of natural infection was documented in Merca, Somalia, on October 26, 1977. On May 8, 1980, the 33rd World Health Assembly officially declared that the world was free of smallpox.[49]

This was the most common reason cited, and it does not suggest that this is solely not only due to them being manipulated by misinformation or disinformation but also due to mistrust. They need to trust that the vaccine is safe and this is part of our duty as clinicians. As mentioned earlier, our system of healthcare has always been a sacred space between the medical provider and the individual, and at this time, it is pertinent that we fulfill this obligation. After all, the word "doctor" comes from the Latin verb *doceo*, which means "to teach" or "to instruct." We should be providing guidance to our patients through science and reason and assuaging their fears about the vaccine by means of conversation. Ultimately, our job is not to convince parents of anything but to provide them with unbiased scientific information so they can make the best-informed decision.

Conclusion

There is certainly cause to be concerned about the mental health of children. This has been an incredibly difficult time for people throughout the world, and many people will struggle to process the experience of the pandemic and any additional traumas they have endured since March 2020. Though the current data on depression and anxiety disorders are very important to provide adequate support and treatment at this point, they do not suggest that these rates will continue to exist or increase if the pandemic begins to wind down. Additionally historic data from prior pandemics do not support the hypothesis that children will continue to struggle with mental health issues. Despite the stark data pertaining to the pandemic and the mental health of children, history has taught us that children tend to overcome such obstacles in time. They will struggle, but they will persevere as we come together to tackle the problems created by the pandemic, and the majority of these kids will eventually grow into thriving adults.

We must remember that children are nothing if not resilient, especially if they feel safe and loved and can rely on their caregivers to promote a nurturing environment. As I have discovered through my research in the remote villages and towns in the Northwestern Frontier Province of Pakistan following the October 8, 2005, earthquake that caused an estimated quarter million casualties and left approximately 3.5 million people without homes, individuals with the strongest social bonds have the best chances of successfully weathering traumatic experiences and extended periods of difficulty.[51] The ultimate lesson that I have taken away from this experience is that adults and especially children are at their strongest when they feel as though they can rely on their family and their community.

REFERENCES

1. Zimmermann P, Curtis N. Why is COVID-19 less severe in children? A review of the proposed mechanisms underlying the age-related difference in severity of SARS-CoV-2 infections. *Arch Dis Child*. 2020;106:429-439. archdischild-2020-320338. doi:10.1136/archdischild-2020-320338

2. Martines RB, Ritter JM, Matkovic E, et al. Pathology and pathogenesis of SARS-CoV-2 associated with fatal coronavirus disease, United States. *Emerg Infect Dis*. 2020;26(9):2005-2015. doi:10.3201/eid2609.202095

3. Shi L, Wang Y, Wang Y, Duan G, Yang H. Dyspnea rather than fever is a risk factor for predicting mortality in patients with COVID-19. *J Infect*. 2020;81(4):647-679. doi:10.1016/j.jinf.2020.05.013

4. Preston LE, Chevinsky JR, Kompaniyets L, et al. Characteristics and disease severity of US children and adolescents diagnosed with COVID019. *JAMA Netw Open*. 2021;4(4):e215298. doi:10.1001/jamanetworkoppen.2021.5298

5. Leeb RT, Price S, Sliwa S, et al. COVID-19 trends among school-aged children—United States, March 1-September 19, 2020. *MMWR Morb Mortal Wkly Rep*. 2020;69(39):1410-1415. doi:10.15585/mmwr.mm6939e2

6. Zimmermann P, Pittet LF, Curtis N. How common is long COVID in children and adolescents. *Pediatric Infect Dis J*. 2021;40(12):e482-e487. doi:10.1097/INF.0000000000003328

7. Duarte-Neto AN, Caldini EG, Gomes-Gouvêa MS, et al. An autopsy study of the spectrum of severe COVID-19 in children: from SARS to different phenotypes of MIS-C. *EClinicalMedicine*. 2021;35:100850. doi:10.1016/j.eclinm.2021.100850

8. *Multisystem Inflammatory Syndrome (MIS-C)*. Centers for Disease Control and Prevention. Updated June 25, 2021. Accessed September 27, 2021. https://www.cdc.gov/mis-c/

9. Belay ED, Abrams J, Oster ME. Trends in geographic and temporal distribution of US children with multisystem inflammatory syndrome during the COVID-19 pandemic. *JAMA Pediatr*. 2021;175(8):837-845. doi:10.1001/jamapediatrics.2021.0630

10. Levin M. Childhood multisystem inflammatory syndrome – a new challenge in the pandemic. *N Engl J Med*. 2020;383(4):393-395. doi:10.1056/NEJM/e2023158

11. Centers for Disease Control and Prevention. *Health Department – Reported Cases of Multisystem Inflammatory Syndrome in Children (MIS-C) in the United States*. Updated August 27, 2021. Accessed September 14, 2021. https://www.cdc.gov/mis-c/cases/index.html

12. Frey WH. *Less than Half of US Children under 15 Are white, Census Shows*. Brookings Institute. Updated July 17, 2019. Accessed September 27, 2021. https://www.brookings.edu/research/less-than-half-of-us-children-under-15-are-white-census-shows/

13. Lam-Hine T, McCurdy SA, Santora L, et al. Outbreak associated with SARS-CoV-2 B.1.617.2 (Delta) variant in an elementary school – Marin county, California, May-June 2021. *MMWR Morb Mortal Wkly Rep*. 2021;70:1214-1219. doi:10.15585/mmwr.mm7035e2

14. Zhu Y, Bloxham CJ, Hulme KD, et al. A meta-analysis on the role of children in severe acute respiratory syndrome coronavirus 2 in household transmission clusters. *Clin Infect Dis*. 2021;72(12):e1146-e1153. doi:10.1093/cid/ciaa1825

15. Paul LA, Daneman N, Schwartz KL, et al. Association of age and pediatric household transmission of SARS-CoV-2 infection. *JAMA Pediatr*. 2021;175:1151-1158. Accessed September 28, 2021. doi:10.1001/jamapediatrics.2021.2770

16. Racine N, McArthur BA, Cooke JE, Eirich R, Zhu J, Madigan S. Global prevalence of depressive and anxiety symptoms in children and adolescents during COVID-19: a meta-analysis. *JAMA Pediatr*. 2021;175:1142-1150. Accessed September 28, 2021. doi:10.1001/jamapediatrics.2021.2482

17. Andreas JB, Brunborg GS. Self-reported mental and physical health among Norwegian adolescents before and during the COVID-19 pandemic. *JAMA Netw Open*. 2021;4(8):e2121934. doi:10.1001/jamanetworkopen.2021.21934

18. Schmidt SJ, Barblan LP, Lory I, Landolt MA. Age-related effects of the COVID-19 pandemic on mental health of children and adolescents. *Eur J Psychotraumatol*. 2021;12(1):1901407. doi:10.1080/20008198.2021.1901407

19. Swansburg R, Hai T, MacMaster FP, Lemay JF. Impact of COVID-19 on lifestyle habits and mental health symptoms in children with attention-deficit/hyperactivity disorder in Canada. *Paediatr Child Health*. 2021;26(5):e199-e207. doi:10.1093/pch/pxab030

20. American Psychiatric Association. *Diagnostic and Statistical Manual on Mental Disorders*. 5th ed. The American Psychiatric Association; 2013.

21. Reich W. *The Mass Psychology of Fascism*. Farrar, Straus & Giroux; 1970.

22. Jacobson L. *Science Shows Mask-Wearing Is Largely Safe for Children*. KHN. Published August 18, 2021. Accessed September 30, 2021. https://khn.org/news/article/science-shows-mask-wearing-is-largely-safe-for-children/

23. Weissbourd R, Batanova M, McIntyre J, Torres ER. *How the Pandemic Is Strengthening Fathers' Relationships with Their Children*. Making Caring Common Project. Harvard Graduate School of Education. Published June 2020. Accessed September 30, 2021. https://static1.squarespace.com/static/5b7c56e255b02c683659fe43/t/5eeceba88f50eb19810153d4/1592585165850/Report+How+the+Pandemic+is+Strengthening+Fathers+Relationships+with+Their+Children+FINAL.pdf

24. American Psychological Association. *Stress in America: One Year Later, a New Wave of Pandemic Health Concerns*. Accessed September 28, 2021. https://www.apa.org/news/press/releases/stress/2021/sia-pandemic-report.pdf

25. Woolford SJ, Sidell M, Li X, et al. Changes in body mass index among children and adolescents during the COVID-19 pandemic. *J Am Med Assoc*. 2021;326(14):1434-1436. Accessed September 28, 2021. doi:10.1001/jama.2021.15036

26. Lange SJ, Kompaniyets L, Freedman DS, et al. Longitudinal trends in body mass index before and during the COVID-19 pandemic among persons aged 2-19 years—United States, 2018-2020. *MMWR Morb Mortal Wkly Rep*. 2021;70:1278-1283. doi:10.15585/mmwr.mm7037a3

27. Long H. U.S. now has 22 million unemployed, wiping out a decade of job gains. *Washington Post*. Published April 16, 2020. Accessed June 16, 2021. https://www.washingtonpost.com/business/2020/04/16/unemployment-claims-coronavirus/

28. Kluger J. Domestic violence is a pandemic within the COVID-19 pandemic. *Time*. Published February 3, 2021. Accessed September 28, 2021. https://time.com/5928539/domestic-violence-covid-19/

29. Boserup B, McKenney M, Elkbuli A. Alarming trends in US domestic violence during the COVID-19 pandemic. *Am J Emerg Med*. 2020;38(12):2753-2755. doi:10.1016/j.ajem.2020.04.077

30. Holland KM, Jones C, Vivolo-Kantor AM, et al. Trends in US emergency department visits for mental health, overdose, and violence outcomes before and during the COVID-19 pandemic. *JAMA Psychiatry*. 2021;78(4):372-379. doi:10.1001/jamapsychiatry.2020.4402

31. Piquero AR, Jennings WG, Jemison E, Kaukinen C, Knaul FM. Domestic violence during the COVID-19 pandemic – evidence from a systematic review and meta-analysis. *J Crim Justice*. 2021;74:101806. doi:10.1016/j.crimjus.2021.101806

32. Ho S, Fassett C. Pandemic masks ongoing child abuse crisis as cases plummet. *AP News*. Published March 29, 2021. Accessed September 28, 2021. https://apnews.com/article/coronavirus-children-safety-welfare-checks-decline-62877b94ec68d47bfe285d4f9aa962e6

33. Sprang G, Silman M. Posttraumatic stress disorder in parents and youth after health-related disorders. *Disaster Med Public Health Prep*. 2013;7(1):105-110. doi:10.1017/dmp.2013.22

34. Zhao N, Zhou G. COVID-19 stress and addictive social media use (SMU): mediating role of active use and social media flow. *Front Psychiatry*. 2021;12:635546. doi:10.3389/fpsyt.2021.635546

35. Senín-Calderón C, Perona-Garcelán S, Rodríguez-Testal JF. The dark side of Instagram: predictor model of dysmorphic concerns. *Int J Clin Health Psychol*. 2020;20(3):253-261. doi:10.1016/j.ijchp.2020.06.005

36. Criddle C. Facebook grilled over mental-health impact on kids. *BBC News*. Published September 30, 2021. Accessed September 30, 2021. https://www.bbc.com/news/technology-58753525

37. Rice SM, Siegel JA, Libby T, Graber E, Kourosh AS. Zooming into cosmetic procedures during the COVID-19 pandemic: the provider's perspective. *Int J Womens Dermatol*. 2021;7(2):213-216. doi:10.1016/j.ijwd.2021.01.012

38. Dwoskin E. Misinformation on Facebook got six times more clicks than factual news during the 2020 election, study says. *Washington Post*. Published September 4, 2021. Accessed September 30, 2021. https://www.washingtonpost.com/technology/2021/09/03/facebook-misinformation-nyu-study/

39. Li HO, Bailey A, Huynh D, Chan J. YouTube as a source of information on COVID-19: a pandemic of misinformation? *BMJ Glob Health*. 2020;5(5):e002604. doi:10.1136/bmjgh-2020-002604

40. Dube R, Magalhaes L. Covid's hidden toll: one million children who lost parents. *Wall St J*. Published September 26, 2021. Accessed September 28, 2021. https://www.wsj.com/articles/covid-children-orphans-parent-deaths-million-11632675021

41. Bateman N, Ross M. *Why Has COVID-19 Been Especially Harmful for Working Women?* Brookings Institute. Published October 2020. Accessed September 30, 2021. https://www.brookings.edu/essay/why-has-covid-19-been-especially-harmful-for-working-women/

42. Adams EL, Smith D, Caccavale LJ, Bean MK. Parents are stressed! Patterns of parent stress across COVID-19. *Front Psychiatry*. 2021;12:626456. doi:10.3389/fpsyt.2021.626456

43. MacIntyre CR, Kelly G, Seale H, Holden R. *From Vaccination to Ventilation: 5 Ways to Keep Kids Safe from COVID When Schools Reopen*. The Conversation. Published September 1, 2021. Accessed September 30, 2021. https://theconversation.com/from-vaccination-to-ventilation-5-ways-to-keep-kids-safe-from-covid-when-schools-reopen-166734

44. Kinch M. *Between Hope and Fear: A History of Vaccines and Human Immunity*. Pegasus Books, Ltd; 2018

45. Flemming A. *The Origins of Vaccination*. Nature Portfolio. Published September 28, 2020. Accessed September 30, 2021. https://www.nature.com/articles/d42859-020-00006-7

46. Boylston A. The origins of inoculation. *J R Soc Med*. 2021;105(7):309-313. doi:10.1258/jrsm.2012.12k044

47. McHugh J. A Puritan minister incited fury by pushing inoculation against a smallpox epidemic. *Washington Post*. Published March 8, 2020. Accessed September 22, 2021. https://www.washingtonpost.com/history/2020/03/07/smallpox-coronavirus-antivaxxers-cotton-mather/

48. Lawler A. *How a Public Health Crisis Nearly Derailed the American Revolution*. National Geographic. Published April 16, 2020. Accessed October 1, 2021. https://www.nationalgeographic.com/history/article/george-washington-beat-smallpox-epidemic-with-controversial-inoculations

49. Strassburg MA. The global eradication of smallpox. *Am J Infect Control*. 1982;10(2):53-59. doi:10.1016/0196-6553(82)90003-7

50. Hamel L, Lopes L, Kearney A, et al. *KFF COVID-19 Vaccine Monitor: Parents and the Pandemic*. KFF. Published August 11, 2021. Accessed September 30, 2021. https://www.kff.org/coronavirus-covid-19/poll-finding/kff-covid-19-vaccine-monitor-parents-and-the-pandemic/

51. Ahmad S, Feder A, Lee EJ, et al. Earthquake impact in a remote South Asian population: psychosocial factors and posttraumatic symptoms. *J Trauma Stress*. 2010;23(3):408-412. doi:10.1002/jts.20535

7

Pandemic Ethics—How We Ought to Respond

In this chapter, I plan to focus on four fundamental ethical questions that can apply not only to ethics during the COVID Era but also ethics that can be applied during other pandemics. These questions are as follows:

1. How ought nonmedical professionals respond?
2. How ought medical professionals respond?
3. How ought medical professionals and policymakers engage with the public?
4. How ought we strive to control the disease?

The chapter will also examine some public health questions that emerged during the pandemic, especially those that centered around masking and vaccinations. Though these topics are often presented as being strictly scientific, the reality is that they border on a fine line between medicine, ethics, law, and politics. This constant change in policy decisions regarding masking or vaccination is driven by the fact that it is largely based on data that evolve over time. While unsavory and the type of thing that is routinely questioned by pundits playing Monday morning quarterback, these decisions were often deemed preferable to the passive act of waiting for more data to become available while the virus was given free rein to spread. This is not to applaud every decision that was made; rather, it puts them into context. These are sensitive issues that each of us view through a different lens, and my approach is not to validate or defend any particular point of view but to be objective and present both sides of the coin for the reader to understand how difficult it is for legislatures, clinicians, and scientists to make policies that consider how to balance saving lives with respecting individual freedoms.

The Foundations of Ethics

Ethics are foundational principles that guide decision-making processes and help individuals determine how to act. Within the world of public health, ethical systems are integral, especially when dealing with an emerging disease where there are significant gaps in knowledge among scientists. As Lawrence Gostin, a law professor at Georgetown University who specializes in public health law, wrote in 2004, "There is no way to avoid the dilemmas posed by acting without full scientific knowledge, so the only safeguard is the adoption of ethical values in formulating and implementing public health decisions."[1] These ethical systems help guide policymakers and experts to make calculated decisions about how to allocate resources, triage patients, and engage with the public.

There are multiple approaches to ethics, including deontology (or duty-based ethics), consequentialism (maximizing "the good" and/or minimizing harm), virtue ethics, and theories, that center on the concept of rights. While these approaches are distinct, they frequently overlap, and multiple systems may ultimately prescribe the same solutions when agents are faced with ethical decisions. Conversely, similar theoretical approaches may oftentimes lead to different conclusions about how one ought to act since definitions of core objectives may diverge.

For example, consequentialism, in its most rudimentary form, typically defines "the good" as life and would therefore dictate that one ought to save the most people in a scenario where there are two groups of people and one can only save one of those groups. For example, if a person is forced to make a choice between saving 5 people (and allowing 10 people to die), saving 10 people (and allowing 5 people to die), or failing to choose, in which case all 15 people die, then the moral choice would be to save the 10 people. Things, of course, get more difficult as one assigns moral values to things beyond life. For example, if a consequentialist ethic is combined with a chauvinistic form of nationalism, then one might claim that "the good" is not just saving the most people, but the most people of a certain type. Consequently, this would alter the calculus that is used to determine what is the moral response. In other words, how different individuals define "the good" can drastically alter our decisions, even if we are adhering to the same frameworks.

Consequentialism stands in contrast to other systems, particularly deontological ethics, which champion moral behavior that is less concerned with consequences and more concerned with refusing to violate certain categorical imperatives. For example, if the scenario above were modified in a way so that the agent actively had to murder five to let ten live, the consequentialist might maintain that killing the five is the correct course of action. A deontological approach would likely refute that by claiming that killing five people would violate the categorical imperative to never murder anyone. In scenarios such as these, any attempt to find common ground (let alone synthesis) between the two schools of thought breaks down.

Schools of thought similarly opposed to one another emerged during the pandemic. At the most elemental, the question revolved around the degree to which one should amend their habits to prevent the spread of the virus. If one says that some amendments are necessary and ethical, while others claim that all amendments are supererogatory, then there is no possible way to harmonize the disagreement. This was further complicated by the fact that the power of the state was employed to discourage or prevent individuals from engaging in behavior deemed too risky as a means to promote public health. This does have legal precedent in the United States (see *Jacobson v. Massachusetts*[i]).[2] However, given the political climate of 2020, it supercharged the initial argument about what changes to one's routine are ethical in the time of a pandemic and became an issue of personal freedom versus state authority—a philosophical/political/ legal debate rather than one about public health. The question ultimately became: Is it more important to take steps to mitigate risk and thereby save lives or is there a higher duty that precludes taking steps to mitigate loss of life? This leads to additional questions. Where is the threshold of acceptable risk? What can the state reasonably ask citizens to do in a time of crisis? What is the line between an assault on one's personal freedom and an inconvenience that arises because one must share space with others during ordinary times compared to times of crisis? To say that no risk is acceptable is untenable or a straw man argument as is the position that we must never make concessions to others in shared public space. The former is the premise on which the ham-fisted of dystopian stories are based. The latter would be akin to a Hobbesian state of warfare involving all against all.

Still, exploring these premises can lead to profound questions that strike to the heart of political science and what people believe about the

---

[i] In Jacobsen, the plaintiff appealed the issuance of a $5 fine and presented a constitutional challenge to a local ordinance enacted by the city of Cambridge, Massachusetts, which required individuals be vaccinated for smallpox to stem an outbreak. He argued that mandatory vaccination was arbitrary, unreasonable, oppressive, and violated the liberties guaranteed to him via due process. The Court rejected this appeal, writing that the Constitution "does not import an absolute right in each person to be, at all times and in all circumstances, wholly freed from restraint. There are manifold restraints to which every person is necessarily subject for the common good."

relationship between the individual, the community, and the state, and an individuals' position cannot be taken lightly or written off as just a tribalistic allegiance devoid of moral reasoning. Everyone must balance their willingness to accept restrictions on their actions and livelihood with the risk of being a link in a chain of transmission that could potentially make thousands of others sick and lead to dozens of deaths. In many cases, these are questions that require risk calculation, not just ethical considerations, and these are decisions that must be made by organizations, as well as individuals. As Spanish philosopher Jose Ortega y Gasset wrote in his 1939 essay, *The Self and The Other*, "Without a strategic retreat into the self, without vigilant thought, human life is impossible."[3]

I would add to Ortega y Gasset's sentiment by saying that this retreat into the self, this act of vigilant thought (and, transitively, human life), is impossible without truth. Valorizing truth is fundamental to ethics since ethics is impossible without an earnest desire to search out the truth. More importantly, that search is impossible without trust. If we are to let ethics be our guide, we will need to emerge from this pandemic with the ability to trust one another again and promote more civil discourse rather than the kind of tribal bickering that masquerades as discussion. As Leonardo di Vinci long ago observed, "Dove si grida non è vera scienza" (*where there is shouting there is no true knowledge*).

Mitigation Strategies

For scientists and policymakers, one of the greatest difficulties of the pandemic has been the lack of information about the SARS-CoV-2 virus and the pathology of COVID-19. As outbreaks were occurring with increasing regularity throughout the United States in early 2020 (possibly even the very end of 2019[4]), a lot of guesswork was involved in trying to implement regulations and processes to protect the public from widespread infection. Unfortunately, when the science of a disease is not clear because of its novelty, this can make consistent messaging difficult and, without a question, there was often dissonance in guidelines, as well as open disagreement among elected officials and public health officials about how to proceed.[5]

The ethical motivation of elected officials is understandable. While a cynical approach would be to claim that they are only after reelection, a more empathetic reading of their situation would recognize that they are bound by duty to protect their constituents' life, liberty, economic interests, and social wellbeing. They did not want to incite a panic or take preventative measures that would ultimately cause more harm than good.

To what degree it was prudent to remain skeptical and risk-adverse was also difficult to ascertain since it depended upon the risks associated with inaction, which they could not have known.

The motivation of public health officials, meanwhile, is often more straightforward and focuses solely on preventing deaths and illness.

In some countries, these two groups butted heads. In others, the two recognized that there was far more overlap between their concerns than their differences, and so they managed to cooperate. They recognized that significant disruptions to daily life and the economy would undoubtedly occur but had the prescience to understand that these disruptions would be relatively minor if community transmission were to be squelched out quickly or prevented entirely. While rigid infection control procedures were enforced during periods of lockdown, the underlying principle was that they were warranted because they would allow the economy to quickly resume normal function and would mean more resources could be dedicated to containment, establishing a perimeter, and monitoring that perimeter. This was the model that Taiwan followed from the beginning of the pandemic. Australia and New Zealand eventually also followed the same model though the latter initially attempted to "flatten the curve."[6]

A "flatten the curve" approach is more of a mitigation strategy. The goal is not merely to blunt the sharpest spike in cases and prevent the complete breakdown of national health care systems due to a tsunami of patients demanding emergency care but to buy researchers time to devise improved treatments.[7] In the United States and many European countries, this strategy was preferred but imperfectly implemented.

As of September 14, 2021, Taiwan, which has a population of approximately 23.5 million, has had 16,093 confirmed cases of COVID-19 (67.5 per 100,000) and 839 total deaths (3.5 per 100,000).[ii] It should be noted that, as of May 1, 2020, there had only been 1132 reported cases and 12 confirmed deaths and that the numbers were inflated by an outbreak that occurred between early May 2021 and early July 2021 that has been responsible for the vast majority of all reported cases and deaths.[8]

As of September 14, 2021, Australia, which has a population of over 25 million, has reported 78,544 confirmed cases of COVID-19 (304.6 per 100,000) and 1116 total deaths (4.3 per 100,000).[9] The biggest spike in 2020 occurred in late July and early August when daily new confirmed cases topped 700, and (though it may seem counterintuitive) approximately, 53% of infections have occurred in less vulnerable individuals, those

---

[ii] For additional country by country information, see Appendix A.

between the ages of 20 and 50 years, while just over 12% of cases were reported in individuals over the age of 70 years.[10] It should be noted that Australia's response has not been flawless. While lockdowns have kept many Australians safe, the country's leaders started to receive a great deal of criticism in the middle of 2021 because of their failure to procure enough doses of vaccine, thus delaying a full reopening of the country. This failure has muted the applause for the nation's initial response to the pandemic.[11] Additionally, cases began rising in July 2021 due to the spread of the Delta variant. While this has led to more lockdowns and more complaints, vaccination efforts have progressed quickly and there is currently hope for a springtime reopening, even if it may not be complete.[12]

As of September 14, 2021, New Zealand, which has a population of just under 5 million, had reported 3982 confirmed cases of COVID-19 (81.9 per 100,000) and confirmed its highest spike in cases on April 5, 2020, when 75 new cases were reported. As of September 2021, 27 people (<1 per 100,000) in New Zealand have died due to COVID-19. Since the beginning of May 2020, only seven have died.[13]

As of September 14, 2021, the total number of confirmed cases in the United States is 41.37 million (12,425.1 per 100,000) and there have been 663,929 confirmed deaths (199.4 per 100,000).[14]

To challenge the efficacy of these three nations' strategies and competencies is a difficult position to take, especially if the argument rests on the presumption that economic vitality needs to be considered in conjunction with the raw data point of number of lives lost. If our goal is to reduce death and illness, then there is no question that these are the countries that we should choose to emulate, even if no system was perfect.[15] On the other hand, if our goal is to reduce death and illness and provide economic vitality, once again the Taiwanese, Australian, and Kiwi models are favorable. Taiwan's economy grew by 3.11% in 2020 and was forecast to grow by 4.64% in 2021.[16] While Australia had its first economic contraction in 30 years in 2020, the nation's economy, as June 2021, is 1.1% bigger than at the beginning of the pandemic.[17] The New Zealand economy shrank by 2.9% in 2020, but economic growth was estimated to be close to 0.8% above prepandemic levels.[18,19] Though GDP in the United States fell by 2.9% in 2020, it has since returned to nearly prepandemic levels and is expected to continue to grow for the foreseeable future.[20] This is comparable to the other models, but the number of people who became sick and the number of people who died of COVID-19 are several orders of magnitude larger.

One of the reasons that these countries had low infection and mortality rates is that all three of them are island nations, which certainly makes it easier to screen and prevent infected individuals from entering the community and spreading the contagion. However, this misses the larger point that especially New Zealand and Taiwan were able to launch a coordinated national response in the early stages of the pandemic that mandated the screening of airline passengers from high-risk areas and quarantining them for 14 days upon returning to their native country. In Taiwan, widespread masking, early delays to the start of the school year, and bans on large gatherings played a crucial role in preventing the early spread of the virus. On the other hand, in New Zealand, once the number of cumulative cases exceeded 100, a full lockdown was implemented on March 23, 2020.[13]

While this is a very broad analysis that does not examine the nuances of each country or the myriad of specific factors, it does reveal that democratic nations where more stringent public health measures were quickly and effectively put into place fared better than the United States Flattening the curve may be an effective strategy for combatting infectious diseases that are less transmissible than SARS-CoV-2, but it was not an effective means of fighting COVID-19.

Individual Ethical Duties

Within the United States, literature about the ethics of pandemics created prior to 2020 focused on the potential challenges of operating with limited resources and questions about how to allocate medicines, ventilators, and personal protective equipment in an ethical or just manner. Writers also spent a great deal of time pondering about our ethical duties to other countries. To read older documents about pandemic ethics that date back well before SARS-CoV-2 can be a bit of a shock, since there seems to be an unspoken presumption that the United States would be able to manage its own affairs and that most policy discussions would center on the logistical challenges and moral imperatives of providing assistance to other countries or resource-starved parts of the United States.[21]

This debate has largely been coopted by the question about how one ought to behave with respect to social distancing protocols and mask wearing, and then about whether to get vaccinated. Frankly, most of the arguments revolving around social distancing protocols and masking in public do not represent ethical quandaries. No one should be losing sleep over these kinds of questions. If you have the option of preventing the spread of a deadly pathogen or not preventing the spread while out in public, you try to prevent it by making some concessions. To rule all voluntary concessions out because they are examples of "authoritarianism" is to brand basic civics as a form of tyranny. While there is a legitimate argument against the government mandating these kinds of measures, this is a political question and not one of ethics. Furthermore, the claim that social distancing and mask wearing do not prevent the spread of the virus is simply incorrect, even if it is accurate to say that they are not 100% effective.

The various protocols set in place to prevent the spread of the coronavirus helped to reduce the number of COVID-19 cases, and there is now evidence that they also prevented the spread of influenza. Due to decreases in mass gatherings and travel, on the one hand, and social distancing measures, mask wearing, and better hand sanitation, on the other, the 2020 to 2021 flu season more or less disappeared. There were fewer than 2000 laboratory-confirmed cases (down from around 200,000 in an average year).[22] Deaths were significantly down, too. In the United States, where an estimated average of 38,750 individuals have died of the flu each season from 2012-2013 to 2019-2020, preliminary reports estimate that only 600[iii] died of the flu this past season.[23,24] That is about 1.55% of the deaths in an average year. Assuming that these same protocols reduced COVID-19 deaths by a comparable rate through the spring of 2021, one can argue that the approximately 600,000 deaths that occurred as of June 2021 due to COVID-19 represent 1.55% of the possible 38.75 million deaths that could have occurred without these measures. While this is not a valid argument for a variety of reasons, there is no doubt that there would have been a far greater number of fatal cases of COVID-19 without regular masking. Based on statistical data, continued skepticism on the matter of masking seems unfounded and has become more of a personal belief that is rooted in politics rather than science.

No doubt, public health guidelines have been a serious encumbrance throughout the pandemic. Masking is inconvenient and keeping a safe distance apart made it difficult and even impossible for some people to earn a living. Shutting down states and cities hurt people financially and psychologically. Not seeing family members for months at a time except through Zoom calls was emotionally harmful. If we were not still recovering from the difficulties of living through the pandemic, this book would not have been written. Despite all the hardship and tragedies, these actions saved countless lives and prevented the collapse of local hospital systems that, even years into the pandemic, continue to show signs of extreme

---

[iii] As noted in a footnote in Chapter 1, the Centers for Disease Control and Prevention (CDC) estimates the number of influenza deaths each year and tends to add significant padding to the number, only to lower it significantly when a more accurate count is available later and the CDC's flu numbers include pneumonia deaths. In other words, the figure of 600 deaths is an estimate. Furthermore, there were far more cases of the flu than 2000. That was just the number of laboratory-confirmed cases.

distress from being overburdened by patients with COVID-19, which has consequently led to the rationing of care and unnecessary deaths.

If we presume that saving lives is the primary objective of ethical behavior, then following proven health guidelines that prevent infection with SARS-CoV-2 and reduce the strain on health care systems would be ethical and shunning them would be unethical. As discussed before and mentioned in the media, the CDC at times did not effectively communicate about masking and social distancing measures and at times provided contradictory and confusing guidelines. However, if we are to constantly vindicate our criticism based on bad messaging by the CDC and overlook the scientific guidelines, then we are once again putting politics ahead of science. To throw out these live-saving guidelines because of bad messaging is like throwing out the baby with the bathwater.

The idea that the impermanence of protocols is evidence of voluntary caprice is unfounded, as well. As the French philosopher and scientist Blaise Pascal is purported to have said: "There is no such thing as the truth, we can only deliver the best available evidence and calculate a probability."[25] *Information about the virus is constantly being updated based on new data and as more studies are conducted. It would be far more concerning if protocols did not evolve as more information was obtained about the transmission dynamics of the virus and other issues like vaccine efficacy. Medicine is a constantly evolving field, and questions about proper treatment and recommendations are dynamic and not static. This may be confusing and frustrating for the public, but this is not a failure of science. Rather, it is a failure of messaging and communication.*

In the future, the CDC should consider coordinating their messaging with pillars of the community, including religious leaders, members of civic organizations, elected local officials, and the like. Many people are often skeptical of government officials as a rule and may be loath to respond to recommended guidelines that may be extremely inconvenient or harmful to their livelihood. Meanwhile, individuals are less likely to want to "shoot the messenger" if they have a long-standing relationship with them.

Vaccines

The case for getting vaccinated is slightly different than wearing a mask. There are risks associated with vaccination (specifically the Pfizer/BioNTech, Moderna, or Janssen [Johnson & Johnson] vaccines) that do not exist with mask wearing or social distancing. Common side effects include fever, chills, aches, injection-site soreness, nausea, and tiredness. Instances of Bell palsy have been reported, but the increased risk is small

(an estimated additional 2 people for every 100,000 people given the Pfizer/
BioNTech vaccine), and the condition is usually temporary.[26] Approximately
100 instances of Guillain-Barré syndrome (GBS) have occurred among the
12.5 million Americans who have received the Johnson & Johnson vaccine.
Of those 100 cases, 95 were serious enough to require hospitalization.
So far, one fatality has been reported as of September 2021.[27] While an
association appears to exist between the vaccine and GBS, the Food and
Drug Administration (FDA) has not yet said that this is sufficient evidence
to establish a causal relationship.[28] Meanwhile, a study that examined the
risk of relapse in patients with a previous history of GBS among those
who received Comirnaty, the Pfizer/BioNTech vaccine, showed that only 1
individual out of the 702 patients required brief medical care for relapse of
previous syndrome but quickly recovered.[29]

Other severe adverse reactions have also been reported. The
most concerning specific side effects are anaphylaxis, thrombosis with
thrombocytopenia syndrome, and myocarditis or pericarditis. Anaphylaxis
has occurred in approximately 2 to 5 people per million vaccinated in the
United States,[30] though it should be noted that rates of anaphylaxis from
any vaccine is estimated to be 1.3 per million.[31] As of September 7, 2021:

- 45 confirmed reports of thrombosis with thrombocytopenia syndrome
  have been reported following the administration of 14.3 million doses of
  Janssen vaccine and tend to occur in women under the age of 50 years;
- 1404 confirmed cases of myocarditis or pericarditis have been reported
  following the administration of approximately 365 million mRNA
  vaccines (Pfizer-BioNTech or Moderna[32]) and tend to occur in male
  adolescents or young adults; and
- The Vaccine Adverse Event Reporting System has been notified of 7439
  deaths following vaccination following a total of approximately 380
  million doses and that health care providers are directed to report these
  instances of death following vaccination even if it is unclear if the vaccine
  played a role in cause of death.[33]

As is the case with all vaccines, long-term side effects are extremely
rare and typically occur within 2 months of vaccination.[34]

As of this writing, only Comirnaty, the vaccine developed by Pfizer/
BioNTech, has been approved by FDA for use in individuals 12 years of
age and older though several vaccines have been given Emergency Use
Authorization (EUA) (see Table 7.1).[38] The difference between EUA and
FDA approval is that, in the midst of a public health emergency, the FDA
may grant EUA before FDA approval.[39] All vaccines have gone through the
three phases of clinical trials and have been shown to be highly effective
(see Table 7.2) at preventing infection and the spread of the virus though
breakthrough cases can and do occur. Still, virus-naïve individuals who

TABLE 7.1 Vaccine Approval Status as of September 15, 2021

Vaccine	Emergency Use Authorization (Adults)	Emergency Use Authorization (Adolescents)	FDA Approval (Adults)	FDA Approval (Adolescents)
Pfizer/ BioNTech[35] (Comirnaty)	December 11, 2020 (Ages 16+)	May 10, 2021 (Ages 12-15)	August 23, 2021	August 23, 2021 (Ages 12+)
Moderna[36]	December 18, 2020 (Ages 18+)	Not at this time	Not at this time	Not at this time
Janssen (Johnson & Johnson)[37]	February 27, 2021 (Ages 18+)	Not at this time	Not at this time	Not at this time

TABLE 7.2 Vaccine Efficacy—Prior to Delta Variant

Vaccine	Clinical Efficacy	Real-World Efficacy	Doses	Timeline
Pfizer/ BioNTech (Comirnaty)	95%[40]	90%[41]	2	Full efficacy 1 wk after second dose, which is ideally administered 21 d after first dose.
Moderna	94.1%[40]	90%[41]	2	Full efficacy 2 wk after second dose, which is ideally administered 28 d after first dose.
Janssen (Johnson & Johnson)	72%[40]	76.7%[42] (preprint study)	1	2 wk after administration of single dose.

received a full vaccine series have been found to have a risk of breakthrough infection of between 1 in 5000 and 1 in 10,000.[43] In these rare cases of infection, symptoms are typically mild but an experience on par with a very bad flu is not out of the question. Individuals may experience more severe symptoms and complications, especially if their immune system is compromised. This is preferable to not being vaccinated since an examination of cases, hospitalizations, and deaths among Americans 18 years of age or older across 13 states between April 4 and July 17, 2021, found that unvaccinated individuals, when compared to fully vaccinated individuals, were 4.5 times more likely to become infected with SARS-CoV-2, approximately 10 times more likely to be hospitalized with COVID-19, and had 10 times the mortality risk.[44]

To be clear, vaccines reduce the risk of severe COVID-19 by training the body's adaptive immune system to recognize SARS-CoV-2 antigens. This translates into less severe infections and less risk of transmission. Vaccines do not eliminate all risk of infection, and there is evidence that they may be less effective at preventing infection by variants, particularly the Delta variant (see Table 7.3). However, less effective does not mean ineffective. The Israeli government's report from early July found that the efficacy of the Pfizer/BioNTech vaccine (BNT162b2) fell from 94% to 64% once the Delta variant became the dominant strain in the country; the vaccine's efficacy then fell further in late July and was estimated to be only 39% effective in preventing infection.[48] While this is discouraging, other studies have not observed such precipitous falls. Public Health Scotland reported a similar decline in protection against symptomatic infection as the Alpha variant was supplanted by the Delta variant for both the Pfizer/BioNTech and Oxford AstraZeneca (AZD1222) vaccines—from 92% to 79% and from 73% to 60%, respectively.[49] Bernal and colleagues, meanwhile, reported that a single dose of either the Oxford AstraZeneca or Pfizer/BioNTech vaccines was 30.7% effective at preventing symptomatic disease, while two doses offered effectiveness against the Delta variant of 67% and 88%, respectively.[50]

There is some indication that vaccine effectiveness may erode over time—possibly in as little as just a few months—which could help explain why the Israeli study was so different from the others. Keehner and colleagues found that the University of California San Diego Health

TABLE 7.3 Preliminary Estimates of Vaccine Efficacy—Delta Variant

Vaccine	Efficacy
Pfizer/BioNTech (Comirnaty)	39%-88%; 52.4%[45]
Moderna	50.6%-76%[45,46]
Janssen (Johnson & Johnson)	Insufficient data[a]

[a]The J&J vaccine has been shown to be 71% effective against hospitalization and 95% effective against death, but not enough information exists as of September 2021 to estimate its efficacy at preventing infection.[47]

workforce declined from March 1 to July 31, 2021, from over 90% to 65.5%. While the increasing dominance of the Delta variant over the spring and summer of 2021 certainly played a role in the decline of efficacy, the attack rate was 6.7 per 1000 persons for those who completed the vaccination series in January or February 2021, while those who completed the vaccination series between March and May saw an attack rate of 3.7 per 1000 persons (and among unvaccinated individuals the attack rate was 16.4 per 1000 persons).[51]

Researchers have also found that patients with immune-mediated diseases that are taking medications, specifically disease-modifying antirheumatic drugs, may experience a less robust vaccine response. A study published in May by Scher and colleagues found that 98.1% of healthy controls experienced an antibody response after receiving two doses of the Pfizer/BioNTech vaccine, and that antibody response dipped to 91.9% in patients with immune-mediated disease who were not on methotrexate, while patients with immune-mediated diseases who were taking methotrexate experienced only a 62.2% antibody response.[52] The Delta variant's impact on these figures remains unclear.

Given the data, there is no doubt that vaccination is an effective tool at preventing severe COVID-19 infection. However, there are risks, even if those risks are small and the most severe adverse reactions are exceptionally rare. This would seem to give credence to the argument that vaccination is an individual's choice. While true, the individual is not the only one who is affected by the decision. They can become infected more easily than those who are vaccinated, and then infect others who have not yet been vaccinated or who may not be able to get the vaccine. Furthermore, continued community spread of the virus can lead to more mutations, which can lead to more variants. There is concern that significant mutations could render natural immunity and vaccines unable to prevent severe infection (or reinfection), thereby resulting in yet another cycle of pandemic. Therefore, the argument against getting the vaccine is not akin to a decision that solely affects the agent, as would be the case with wearing a seatbelt, but would be more like deciding to drive drunk. In other words, the behavior not only puts the agent at risk; it also puts members of the community at risk and is, consequently, not ethical. As with the case of masking, whether or not vaccines can be mandated is a political or legal question and beyond the scope of discussion.

That said, there is an argument to be made about vaccine exceptions for individuals who have been infected with the virus since initial studies have shown that they are comparably protected from infection to individuals who have been vaccinated. Still, emerging evidence that has not been peer reviewed at this time suggests that individuals who developed antibodies following natural infection and received a full series of vaccine have demonstrated better immunity than individual who were infected without vaccination or individuals who received vaccination but were never infected.[53] This should be considered in any risk-benefit analysis, especially given the increasing probability that COVID-19 will become an endemic disease.

Boosters

A far more interesting ethical question concerns the issue of vaccine boosters. While the FDA has granted EUA on August 12, 2021, for some immunocompromised individuals to receive additional doses of either the Moderna or Pfizer/BioNTech (Comirnaty) vaccine as little as 28 days following their second dose, it is unclear how necessary a booster shot is for individuals with healthy immune systems.[54] There are also insufficient data to support getting a second dose of the Johnson & Johnson vaccine. Therefore, there does not seem to be strong evidence to support booster vaccines from a public health perspective, even if evidence that has yet to be peer reviewed does show that third and even fourth jabs do offer increased protection to individuals.[55]

This may seem like a contradiction. The efficacy of the vaccine appears to be waning in individuals after only a few months, and preliminary studies suggest that booster shots do improve protection. Why would they not be approved for the use in all adults? Many have argued that this is an ethical problem. While people in wealthier countries have had the opportunity to receive a full series of vaccines, the vast majority of individuals in poorer countries have yet to receive a single dose. If you had the option of giving a coat to two people who were forced to weather a trek through a snowstorm, one of whom was dressed for a day at the beach and the other who was dressed for a moderately cold day, it would seem unreasonable and morally abominable to give the latter person the coat. They are already protected, however, imperfectly. This is a humanitarian concern. There is also an epidemiological one. Giving third doses of vaccine to people who are already protected means that more people in poor nations will become ill with COVID-19 and that there is also a risk that more widespread transmission will lead to more variants that make the vaccines less effective.

That said, if the question were simply whether one had the option of taking an additional dose of vaccine to improve one's protection at a time when billions around the world have no access to their initial vaccine doses and are therefore completely unprotected, then the answer would be simple: The act is not ethical for individuals with healthy immune systems.

Unfortunately, wealthier countries have enacted policies that have led to the hoarding of vaccine, and there appears to be no mechanisms that private citizens can employ to get more of these doses to poorer countries where the vaccine is in short supply. If the vaccine is not used by its expiration date, it is discarded.[56] Consequently, the question for individuals in wealthier nations becomes one of letting the vaccine go to waste or receiving a booster that has been shown to significantly reduce one's risk of infection, thereby providing the individual and the community with increased protection against the virus. Though the best-case scenario, from an ethical standpoint, would be to share the vaccine with the countries who need it most, the harsh realities of federal policy make questions about booster shots more complicated than they initially seem.

Infodemic

Conspiracy theories became extremely common during the pandemic for several reasons. Individuals often perceive cataclysmic events as being part of a larger narrative or plan because we project our own rational mind onto the world. Philosophers refer to this as teleology—the study of design and purpose. It is something we all do on occasion, even if we do not earnestly believe that there is an overarching reason why seemingly commonplace events occur. Anyone who has felt as though they have hit every red light when in danger of running late knows this feeling; it is belief that some force is *actively trying* to make you late. Most of us, when pressed on this belief, will acknowledge that it is not sincere. We do not actually believe that there is a conscious force or agents from *The Adjustment Bureau* acting behind the scenes to ensure some grand (potentially sinister) plan come to fruition.

With larger, more monumental events, the belief may become a bit more difficult to shake. There is a sense that these things do not just happen. One of the peculiarities of the English language is that the very word to describe two incidents happening simultaneously contains an inherent subtext of incredulity. To ask, "You think it is a coincidence?" is a less direct way of asking someone if they are stupid or gullible. The answer is always undoubtedly, "No."

Many of these theories initially suggested that either there was no virus or doubted its severity. In late March 2020, many amateur reporters began filming empty parking lots of local hospitals as "proof" that the pandemic was being sensationalized in the press or that it was just a global plot to tar the image of prominent politicians and purposefully hurt the economy in an election year.[57] When stay-at-home orders and other preventative measures to "flatten the curve" were implemented, these same individuals began openly flouting public health measures and even holding demonstrations around and even in state Capitol Buildings. While no demonstration is safe during a pandemic with an airborne virus, many antilockdown demonstrators seemed to take perverse delight in flouting the rules concerning masks and social distancing. It should also be noted that many of them later got sick and tried to dissuade others from similar acts of temerity.

Politics played an outsized role in the spread of misinformation, especially as one's impression of the US response to the pandemic became seen through party affiliation. A poll by Pew Research Center conducted through June and August of 2020 found that support or opposition to the ruling political party clearly colored attitudes about how those surveyed believed their government had been handling the virus and the economic fallout caused by social distancing measure. The survey involved 13 advanced economies and those who supported the governing party were more likely to say that their country had done a good job dealing with the coronavirus outbreak, while those who opposed the governing party were less likely to say their country had done a good job (see Figure 7.1). In Denmark and Austria, for example, 98% of those who supported the governing party approved of their handling of the outbreak, while only 93% of those who opposed the governing party approved of how their government had responded during the pandemic. The difference between the two was 5%. Across the 13 countries, the average difference was 20%. The greatest difference was in the United States, where only 29% of those who said they did not support the ruling party thought the United States was adequately handling the pandemic, while 76% of those who supported the ruling party thought the government was doing a good job—a difference of 47%.[58]

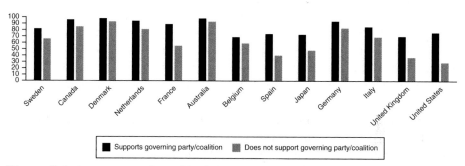

Supports governing party/coalition   Does not support governing party/coalition

Figure 7.1 A survey conducted in July and August 2020 asked individuals in 13 counties if they believed their country has done a good job dealing with the pandemic. Political affiliation was shown to color their opinion.

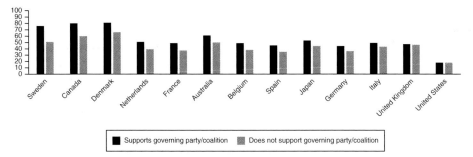

Figure 7.2 A survey conducted in July and August 2020 asked individuals in 13 counties if they believed their country was more united or less united since the start of the pandemic.

The same survey found similar biases with respect to how individuals believed their countries' economies were performing, with the disparity between those who supported the ruling party in the United States and those who did not being greater than any of the other nations polled. 52% of supporters said the economic situation in the United States was good, while only 16% of nonsupporters said the economic situation was good. The closest level of division was observed in Canada, with 50% of supporters believing that the economic situation was good compared to only 32% of nonsupporters. That difference (18%) was half the difference observed in the United States (36%).[58] The only thing that those in the United States seemed to be in agreement on concerned how divided they were. 18% of supporters said the country was more united than before the coronavirus outbreak. An identical percentage of nonsupporters said the same (see Figure 7.2).

The lens through which one judged their nation's response to the pandemic and economic fallout was often applied to their feelings about masking and vaccines, as well as the efficacy of medications that were backed by insufficient or oftentimes dubious science. While it would be inaccurate to claim that all vaccine skeptics and people who have doubted the efficacy of masks are cut from the same cloth, the most vocal opponents of these kinds of public health policies have typically relied on cherry-picked data to give their arguments about personal liberty a scientific artifice. There is some evidence to suggest that vaccine skepticism is on the decline, especially following the FDA approval of the Pfizer/BioNTech (Comirnaty) on August 23, 2021, for individuals 12 years of age and older, but it is too early to tell. What is certain is that vaccine skepticism will continue as it has done since the 1800s[59] and that the only new feature will be that it will be fueled by misinformation campaigns through social media.

Considerations for Clinicians

The point to take away from this is that misinformation and conspiracy theories pervert discourse in a way so that we are no longer having a difference of opinion about policy or morality; individuals end up believing that those who disagree with them are either voluntarily or involuntarily participating in a larger conspiracy or at least somehow duplicitous in it. This applies even to medical professionals, and it is not just trust in authority that has eroded but medicine and science itself. Even in cases where our personal motives may not be suspect, our professional opinions are often perceived as being tainted by our association with the government, pharmaceutical companies, or international, nongovernmental organizations.

As noted in the above, valorizing truth is fundamental to ethics, since ethics is impossible without an earnest desire to search out the truth and that search cannot occur without trust—in data, in reports, in observations. How we restore that trust will be one of the most pressing questions of the post-COVID Era.

For clinicians who are struggling with patients who do not want to be forced to wear a mask or have eschewed vaccination whether because they believe that it was developed too quickly or because they worry about vaccines in general or because they believe that COVID-19 has become endemic and so there is no point to get the vaccine, it is always important to simply present the facts to them and to ask if you have ever steered them wrong in the past. It is also important to be knowledgeable and to address their questions, even if they place the risks associated with the vaccine out of context, even if they sound accusatory, even if they may rest of premises that rest outside established science. The fact is that no vaccine is perfect, but that the alternative, contracting the illness, is far more dangerous than being vaccinated and that one has a far higher likelihood of both contracting the virus and subsequently transmitting the virus to others within the community if they are not vaccinated. Again, one must valorize truth to establish trust, and the only way we will extricate ourselves from the pandemic era is by rebuilding trust between the public and the medical community.

Conclusion

At the beginning of this chapter, four questions were posed. The answer to the first (How ought nonmedical professional respond during a pandemic?) is to follow guidelines as they are updated. While this may be frustrating because they have evolved over the course of the pandemic and may evolve still, they are recommended to keep the community safe. Simply put get vaccinated and wear a mask as often as possible when in an indoor setting with individuals who may not be vaccinated. The answer to the second (How ought medical professionals respond?) and the third (How ought medical professionals and policymakers engage with the public?) are intimately tied together and undergird the response to the fourth (How ought we strive to control the disease?): In a way that fosters trust, truth, and community solidarity. We are at our strongest when we unite, and we are at our weakest when we fight among ourselves. As we emerge from the COVID Era, this lesson will apply to everything from rebuilding our economy to helping one another as we process the social and psychological effects of the pandemic.

REFERENCES

1. Gostin LO. Pandemic influenza: public health preparedness for the next global health emergency. *J Law Med Ethics*. 2004;32(4):565-573. doi:10.1111/j.1748-720x.2004.tb01962.x
2. The Centers for Law and the Public's Health: A Collaborative at Johns Hopkins and Georgetown Universities. *Tuberculosis Control Law and Policies: A Handbook for Public Health and Legal Practice*. CDC website; Published October 1, 2009. Accessed September 14, 2021. https://www.cdc.gov/tb/programs/tblawpolicyhandbook.pdf
3. y Gasset JO. *The Dehumanization of Art: And Other Essays on Art, Culture, and Literature*. Princeton University Press; 1968.
4. Roy M. Five U.S. states had coronavirus infections even before the first reported cases – study. *Reuters*. Published June 15, 2021. Accessed June 18, 2021. https://www.reuters.com/business/healthcare-pharmaceuticals/five-us-states-had-coronavirus-infections-even-before-first-reported-cases-study-2021-06-15/
5. Interlandi J. Can the C.D.C. be fixed? *New York Times*. Published June 16, 2021. Accessed June 20, 2021. https://www.nytimes.com/2021/06/16/magazine/cdc-covid-response.html
6. Summers J, Cheng HY, Lin HH, et al. Potential lessons from the Taiwan and New Zealand health responses to the COVID-19 pandemic. *Lancet Reg Health West Pac*. 2020;4:100044. doi:10.1016/j.lanwpc.2020.100044
7. Roberts S. Flattening the coronavirus curve. *New York Times*. Published March 27, 2020. Accessed June 20, 2021. https://www.nytimes.com/article/flatten-curve-coronavirus.html
8. Ritchie H, Ortiz-Ospina E, Beltekian D, et al. *Taiwan: Coronavirus Pandemic Country Profile*. Our World in Data; Updated September 15, 2021. Accessed September 15, 2021. https://ourworldindata.org/coronavirus/country/taiwan#citation
9. Ritchie H, Ortiz-Ospina E, Beltekian D, et al. *Australia: Coronavirus Pandemic Country Profile*. Our World in Data; Updated September 15, 2021. Accessed September 15, 2021. https://ourworldindata.org/coronavirus/country/australia
10. Department of Health of Australia. *Coronavirus (COVID-19) Current Situation and Numbers*. Updated June 18, 2021. Accessed June 19, 2021. https://www.health.gov.au/news/health-alerts/novel-coronavirus-2019-ncov-health-alert/coronavirus-covid-19-current-situation-and-case-numbers
11. Dewan A. Sydney in lockdown, borders shut and hardly anyone vaccinated. How long can Australia go on like this? *CNN*. Published June 28, 2021. Accessed June 28, 2021. https://www.cnn.com/2021/06/27/australia/sydney-lockdown-australia-covid-pandemic-intl-cmd/index.html
12. Zhuang Y. Australia starts vaccinating children as young as 12. *New York Times*. Published September 13, 2021. Accessed September 13, 2021. https://www.nytimes.com/2021/09/13/world/australia/australia-vaccinate-children.html

13. Ritchie H, Ortiz-Ospina E, Beltekian D, et al. *New Zealand: Coronavirus Pandemic Country Profile*. Our World in Data; Updated September 15, 2021. Accessed September 15, 2021. https://ourworldindata.org/coronavirus/country/new-zealand

14. Ritchie H, Ortiz-Ospina E, Beltekian D, et al. *United States: Coronavirus Pandemic Country Profile*. Our World in Data; Updated September 15, 2021. Accessed September 15, 2021. https://ourworldindata.org/coronavirus/country/united-states

15. Mao F. COVID: why Australia's 'world-class' quarantine system has seen breaches. *BBC News*. Published February 8, 2021. Accessed June 19, 2021. https://www.bbc.com/news/world-australia-55929180

16. Lee YN. Asia's top-performing economy in 2020 could grow even faster this year. *CNBC*. Published February 22, 2021. Accessed June 19, 2021. https://www.cnbc.com/2021/02/23/taiwan-asias-top-performing-economy-in-2020-could-grow-faster-in-2021.html

17. Janda M, Chalmers S. Australia's economy 1.1 per cent bigger than at the start of the COVID pandemic, GDP data shows. *ABC News*. Updated June 2, 2021. Accessed June 19, 2021. https://www.abc.net.au/news/2021-06-02/gdp-march-quarter-economic-growth-covid-rebound/100184004

18. Withers T. New Zealand economy surges out of recession in V-shaped recovery. *Bloomberg*. Updated on December 16, 2020. Accessed June 19, 2021. https://www.bloomberg.com/news/articles/2020-12-16/new-zealand-economy-surges-out-of-recession-amid-spending-spree

19. Menon P. NZ economy surges as housing, retail drive post-COVID recovery. *Reuters*. Published June 16, 2021. Accessed June 19, 2021. https://www.reuters.com/world/asia-pacific/nz-economy-surges-housing-retail-drive-post-covid-recovery-2021-06-16/

20. Guilford G, Cambon SC. The economic recovery is here. It's unlike anything you've seen. *Wall Street Journal*. Published June 2, 2021. Accessed June 19, 2021. https://www.wsj.com/articles/the-economic-recovery-is-here-rebound-jobs-stock-market-unemployment-biden-aid-package-11622642152

21. Institute of Medicine (US) Forum on Microbial Threats. *Ethical and Legal Considerations in Mitigating Pandemic Disease*. National Academies Press; 2007.

22. Dunn L. After year with virtually no flu, scientists worry the next season could be a bad one. *NBC News*. Published May 9, 2021. Accessed June 19, 2021. https://www.nbcnews.com/health/health-news/after-year-virtually-no-flu-scientists-worry-next-season-could-n1266534

23. McCarthy N. How many Americans die from the flu each year? [Infographic]. *Forbes*. Published October 7, 2020. Accessed June 19, 2021. https://www.forbes.com/sites/niallmccarthy/2020/10/07/how-many-americans-die-from-the-flu-each-year-infographic/?sh=7ba6ee5913ea

24. Faust JS. Comparing COVID-19 deaths to flu deaths is like comparing apples to oranges. *Scientific American*. Published April 28, 2020. Accessed June 19, 2021. https://blogs.scientificamerican.com/observations/comparing-covid-19-deaths-to-flu-deaths-is-like-comparing-apples-to-oranges/

25. Shah M. The failure of public health messaging about COVID-19. *Scientific American*. Published September 3, 2020. Accessed June 21, 2021. https://www.scientificamerican.com/article/the-failure-of-public-health-messaging-about-covid-19/

26. Wan EYF, Chui CSL, Lai FTT, et al. Bell's palsy following vaccination with mRNA (BNT162b2) and inactivated (CoronaVac) SARS-CoV-2 vaccines: a case series and nested case-control study. *Lancet Infect Dis*. Published online August 16, 2021. doi:10.1016/S1473-3099(21)00467-9. Accessed August 20, 2021.

27. FDA News Release. *Coronavirus (COVID-19) Update: July 13, 2021*. U.S. Food and Drug Administration; Published July 13, 2021. Accessed August 20, 2021. https://www.fda.gov/news-events/press-announcements/coronavirus-covid-19-update-july-13-2021

28. FDA News Release. *Coronavirus (COVID-19) Update: July 13, 2021*. U.S. Food and Drug Administration; Published July 13, 2021. Accessed September 16, 2021. https://www.fda.gov/news-events/press-announcements/coronavirus-covid-19-update-july-13-2021

29. Shapiro Ben David S, Potasman I, Rahamin-Cohen D. Rate of recurrent Guillain-Barré syndrome after mRNA COVID-19 vaccine BNT162b2. *JAMA Neurol.* 2021;78(11):1409-1411. doi:10.1001/jamaneurol.2021.3287

30. Centers for Disease Control and Prevention. *Selected Adverse Events Reported After COVID-19 Vaccination.* Updated June 14, 2021. Accessed June 21, 2021. https://www.cdc.gov/coronavirus/2019-ncov/vaccines/safety/adverse-events.html

31. Ledford H. Six months of COVID vaccines: what 1.7 billion doses have taught scientists. *Nature.* 2021;594(7862):164-167. doi:10.1038/d41586-021-01505-x

32. Centers for Disease Control and Prevention. *Reporting COVID-19 Vaccinations in the United States.* Updated August 26, 2021. Accessed September 13, 2021. https://covid.cdc.gov/covid-data-tracker/#vaccinations_vacc-total-admin-count-total

33. Centers for Disease Control and Prevention. *Selected Adverse Events Reported After COVID-19 Vaccination.* Updated September 7, 2021. Accessed September 13, 2021. https://www.cdc.gov/coronavirus/2019-ncov/vaccines/safety/adverse-events.html

34. Parents PACK. *Featured Article: Long-Term Side Effects of COVID-19 Vaccine? What We Know.* Children's Hospital of Philadelphia; Published February 4, 2021. Accessed June 22, 2021. https://www.chop.edu/news/long-term-side-effects-covid-19-vaccine

35. U.S. Food and Drug Administration. *Pfizer-BioNTech COVID-19 Vaccine.* Updated August 23, 2021. Accessed September 14, 2021. https://www.fda.gov/emergency-preparedness-and-response/coronavirus-disease-2019-covid-19/pfizer-biontech-covid-19-vaccine

36. U.S. Food and Drug Administration. *Moderna COVID-19 Vaccine.* Updated April 1, 2021. Accessed June 21, 2021. https://www.fda.gov/emergency-preparedness-and-response/coronavirus-disease-2019-covid-19/moderna-covid-19-vaccine

37. U.S. Food and Drug Administration. *Janssen COVID-19 Vaccine.* Updated June 16, 2021. Accessed June 21, 2021. https://www.fda.gov/emergency-preparedness-and-response/coronavirus-disease-2019-covid-19/janssen-covid-19-vaccine

38. U.S. Food and Drug Administration. *FDA Approves First COVID-19 Vaccine.* Published August 23, 2021. Accessed September 12, 2021. https://www.fda.gov/news-events/press-announcements/fda-approves-first-covid-19-vaccine

39. U.S. Food and Drug Administration. *Emergency Use Authorization of Vaccines Explained.* Updated November 20, 2020. Accessed June 21, 2021. https://www.fda.gov/vaccines-blood-biologics/vaccines/emergency-use-authorization-vaccines-explained

40. Katella K. Comparing the COVID-19 vaccines: how are they different. *Yale Medicine.* Published June 16, 2021. Accessed June 21, 2021. https://www.yalemedicine.org/news/covid-19-vaccine-comparison

41. Thompson MG, Burgess JL, Naleway AL, et al. Interim estimates of vaccine effectiveness of BNT162b2 and mRNA-1273 COVID-19 vaccines in preventing SARS-CoV-2 infection among health care personnel, first responders, and other essential and frontline workers – eight U.S. locations, December 2020-March 2021. *MMWR Morb Mortal Wkly Rep.* 2021;70:495-500. doi:10.15585/mmwr.mm7013e3

42. Corchad-Garcia J, Puyraimond-Zemmour D, Hughes T, et al. Real-world effectiveness of Ad2.COV2.S adenoviral vector vaccine for COVID-19. Preprint. Posted online April 30, 2021. medRxiv. doi:10.1101/2021.04.27.21256193

43. Leonhardt D. One in 5,000. *New York Times.* Published September 7, 2021. Accessed September 12, 2021. https://www.nytimes.com/2021/09/07/briefing/risk-breakthrough-infections-delta.html

44. Scobie HM, Johnson AG, Suthar AB, et al. Monitoring incidence of COVID-19 cases, hospitalizations, and deaths, by vaccination status – 13 U.S. jurisdictions, April 4 – July 17, 2021. *MMWR Morb Mortal Wkly Rep.* 2021;70(37):1284-1290. doi:10.15585/mmwr.mm7037e1

45. Nanduri S, Pilishvili T, Derado G, et al. Effectiveness of the Pfizer-BioNTech and Moderna vaccines in preventing SARS-CoV-2 infection among nursing home residents before and during widespread circulation of the SARS-CoV-2 B.1.617.2 (Delta) variant – National

Healthcare Safety Network, March 1 – August 1, 2021. *MMWR Morb Mortal Wkly Rep.* 2021;70:1163-1166. doi:10.15585/mmwr.mm7034e3

46. Reuters. *Moderna May Be superior to Pfizer Against Delta; Breakthrough Odds Rise with Time*. Published August 9, 2021. Accessed September 14, 2021. https://www.reuters.com/business/healthcare-pharmaceuticals/moderna-may-be-superior-pfizer-against-delta-breakthrough-odds-rise-with-time-2021-08-09/

47. Schwartz F. J&J vaccine highly effective against delta variant in South African trial. *Wall Street Journal.* Published August 6, 2021. Accessed September 16, 2021. https://www.wsj.com/articles/j-j-vaccine-highly-effective-against-delta-variant-in-south-african-trial-11628292645

48. Lovelace BJr. Israel says Pfizer COVID vaccine is just 39% effective as delta spreads, but still prevents severe illness. *CNBC.* Updated July 23, 2021. Accessed August 19, 2021. https://www.cnbc.com/2021/07/23/delta-variant-pfizer-covid-vaccine-39percent-effective-in-israel-prevents-severe-illness.html

49. Sheikh A, McMenamin J, Taylor B, Robertson C, Public Health Scotland and the EAVE II Collaborators. SARS-CoV-2 Delta VOC in Scotland: demographics, risk of hospital admission, and vaccine effectiveness. *Lancet.* 2021;397(10293):2461-2462. doi:10.1016/S0140-6736(21)01358-1

50. Bernal JL, Andrews N, Gower C, et al. Effectiveness of COVID-19 vaccines against the B.1.617.2 (Delta) variant. *N Engl J Med.* 2021;385(7):585-594. doi:10.1056/NEJMoa2108891

51. Keehner J, Horton LE, Binkin NJ, et al. Resurgence of SARS-CoV-2 infection in a highly vaccinated health system workforce. *N Engl J Med.* 2021;385(14):1330-1332. doi:10.1056/NEJMc2112981. Accessed September 10, 2021.

52. Walsh N. Methotrexate impairs COVID vax response. *Medpage Today.* Published May 25, 2021. Accessed May 26, 2021. https://www.psychiatryadvisor.com/home/topics/general-psychiatry/in-pandemic-health-related-socioeconomic-risks-related-to-mental-health-problems/

53. Gazit S, Schlezinger R, Perez G, et al. Comparing SARS-CoV-2 natural immunity to vaccine-induced immunity: reinfections versus breakthrough infections. Preprint. MedRxiv. 2021.08.24.21262415. doi:10.1101/2021.08.24.21262415

54. U.S. Food and Drug Administration. *Coronavirus (COVID-19) Update: FDA Authorizes Additional Vaccine Dose for Certain Immunocompromised Individuals.* Published August 12, 2021. Accessed September 14, 2021. https://www.fda.gov/news-events/press-announcements/coronavirus-covid-19-update-fda-authorizes-additional-vaccine-dose-certain-immunocompromised

55. Bar-On YM, Goldberg Y, Mandel M, et al. BNT162b2 vaccine booster dose protection: a nationwide study from Israel. Preprint. MedRxiv 2021.08.27.21262679. doi:10.1101/2021.08.27.21262679

56. Levin D. The U.S. is wasting vaccine doses, even as cases rise and other countries suffer shortages. *New York Times.* Updated August 2, 2021. Accessed September 12, 2021. https://www.nytimes.com/2021/08/01/us/covid-us-vaccine-wasted.html

57. Adler B. Conservative amateur sleuths deny New York hospital crisis. *City & State.* Published April 1, 2020. Accessed March 5. 2021. https://www.cityandstateny.com/articles/opinion/commentary/conservative-amatuer-sleuths-deny-new-york-hospital-crisis.html

58. Mordecai M, Connaughton A. *Public Opinion about Coronavirus Is More Politically Divided in U.S. Than in Other Advanced Countries.* Pew Research Center; Published October 28, 2020. Accessed May 20, 2021. https://www.pewresearch.org/fact-tank/2020/10/28/public-opinion-about-coronavirus-is-more-politically-divided-in-u-s-than-in-other-advanced-economies/

59. Kinch M. *Between hope and Fear: A History of Vaccines and Human Immunity.* Pegasus Books; 2018.

8

Extended Social Impact

The COVID-19 pandemic will have lasting social impacts that we are only beginning to fully recognize. These societal influences will be informed by the economic and psychological effects of COVID-19, and they will likely alter conventions, customs, and social life in the United States for years to come, especially if the virus becomes endemic. One could engage in an endless amount of speculation on the many potential changes to society, but this chapter will focus on how many Americans will likely experience lasting feelings of vulnerability that may make any return to "normal" extremely challenging and how tectonic cultural and economic shifts may affect crime rates, demographics, and even specific industries. Of particular concern is the exodus of highly skilled personnel from the medical field due to extreme physical and psychological fatigue brought on by long hours, witnessing innumerable deaths, and the sense of there being no respite in the near future. Additionally, loneliness may be a major problem for many in the short- and long-term, as they remain homebound for myriad reasons or otherwise struggle to adapt to the postpandemic world. There is no doubt that though the rift created by the pandemic between our past and the present will be difficult for many to bridge, many others may find it easy to adapt to the new world, or they may have even experienced positive changes in their individual circumstances. Sometimes being placed in a difficult situation forces us to make decisions that we would not otherwise choose out of comfort or fear of the unknown, but many may have finally forged ahead with a decision they had been unwilling to make prior to the pandemic, like moving to a new city, starting a new career, or ending a toxic relationship.

No Longer Impervious

There is a sense of unity and belief among most Americans that the events of 9/11 were a kind of wakeup call. The events that day reminded us that we are not invulnerable. For those of us in New York City, it was a harrowing experience akin to suddenly being tossed into a warzone. For those of us who worked in the hospitals that day, and the following weeks, it was the kind of thing for which no amount of training can ever prepare you. Even months later, colleagues were still struggling to make sense of what happened that day, as were Americans from thousands of miles away.

This is not to say that previous events had not shocked us to our core. The Oklahoma City bombing in 1996 and the Columbine school shooting 3 years later were both truly horrific events, but the impact that 9/11 had on the national psyche was different. The sense that the United States was somehow impervious to the hostilities engulfing many parts of the world disappeared overnight, leaving many of us feeling vulnerable, confused, and scared. People who watched the events unfold on their television screens and far away from the carnage in Lower Manhattan still experienced what are, according to DSM-5, the hallmark symptoms of trauma- and stress-related disorders: hypervigilance, avoidant behavior, reexperiencing the traumatic moment, and negative changes in thinking or mood.[1] It was a traumatic event and we walked away from the experience irrevocably altered. Some went on to be diagnosed with conditions like posttraumatic stress disorder (PTSD) or generalized anxiety disorder, but the vast majority of Americans eventually ceased to feel the persistent unease of existential dread and emerged into a new-normal.

The changes caused by the COVID-19 pandemic will no doubt be of similar magnitude because we have endured a consistent needling of our collective psyche for such an extended period of time. It already has created a paradigmatic shift in the way millions of Americans think of illness, and it is likely to change the way we think and talk about mental illness because the psychosocial and economic impacts, as well as the long-term effects of the disease, will be felt by a large segment of the population for years to come. Millions of people remained largely cloistered in their homes for over a year. As noted previously at the start of the second part of this book, adults and children have no doubt developed sleep problems, anxiety disorders, affective disorders, and trauma- and stress-related disorders throughout this time. Furthermore, to cope with these issues and disorders, many may have indulged in unhealthy habits that then turned into substance use disorders. Others may have developed health problems associated with excessive weight loss or weight gain. More importantly, there is also the fact that an enormous number of people died and that there have been multiple individual days when more than 3000 people lost their lives due to complications from COVID-19. In mid-January 2021, the average number of people dying per day swelled to over 3400,[2] and by spring of 2021, it was estimated that more than 37,000 children lost at least one parent to COVID-19.[3]

In addition to its psychological impact, the lingering effects of the pandemic will also have wide-ranging economic implications. A World Economic Forum held 2 years prior to the pandemic estimated that mental health problems would cost $16 trillion in lost economic output between 2010 and 2030 globally.[4] Again, these projections were made *before* the crippling, once-in-a-lifetime nightmare scenario that has now lasted for over 2 years and might persist far longer. Proposing an estimate to reflect the new reality is beyond my expertise, but I can say with certainty that avoiding the problem will only make it worse, and that "worse," in this context, means a lower quality of life for millions of people and a greater burden to taxpayers, since public spending as a percentage of total spending for mental health services has held fairly constantly for the past decade at around 60% but was expected to increase even before the pandemic.[5] The fact that Medicaid currently covers 74 million Americans, a figure that increased by 9.7 million between February 2020 and January 2021, would suggest that these costs will be even higher.[6]

It would be wrong to pathologize national experience in the wake of trauma, but it would also be wrong to simply ignore these issues and pretend like everyone is going to eventually wake up one day and be capable of going back to normal. Many of the old ideas we had about "normal" have been washed away by the pandemic, and we will emerge from this cataclysm[i] with the need to create a new definition of normal. This is not something that we can individually shape or purposefully influence. It will gradually come into its own as new conventions, new mores, and new limitations on what constitutes acceptable behavior become adopted and people express how comfortable or uncomfortable they are with certain activities.

To venture a guess as to what these conventions will look like come 2023 or even late 2022 would be analogous to the science fiction writer from 1950 imagining what 2021 might be like. I am certain that most of it would be comically wrong, especially given the misplaced optimism of spring 2021, the impact of the Delta variant over the course of that summer, and the increasingly common belief that SARS-CoV-2 has become

---

[i] Cataclysm comes from the Greek *kata* "down" and *klyzein* "to wash," and is frequently used to describe the Great Deluge of the Bible.

an endemic virus. However, what I have noticed is that many people are recognizing in the pandemic not a newfound sense of vulnerability but a newfound sense of agency. Like Noah's flood, and like all cataclysms, the pandemic destroyed the old world but has given birth to a new one. This is not to make light of the amount of death and pain and suffering that have taken place since the SARS-CoV-2 virus began spreading throughout our communities but to acknowledge that we are on the precipice of something new.

As I have said elsewhere, the pandemic has been kind of like a protracted night. Many of us spent this time cocooned in our thoughts and maybe reconsidered how we were living our lives and planned to make changes once the worst of it had passed. For some, this may have been a thought exercise akin to dreaming about how they might spend millions of dollars should they ever win the lottery. For others, these dreams are now turning into concrete action as they quit their jobs, start new businesses, leave behind stagnant relationships, and move to new homes. While there is no doubt that the COVID-19 pandemic has been a tragedy of Biblical proportions, and that millions of Americans will struggle with psychological and physiological postacute COVID-19 sequelae, as well as trauma- and stress-related disorders, many may see the aftermath as a time to make a new start and to take this as an opportunity to break out of old patterns and explore opportunities that may not have arisen otherwise.

It is worth bearing in mind that, prior to the pandemic, 83% of people in the United States were estimated to have gone through an experience that would satisfy criteria within DSM-5 for a traumatic event. However, PTSD prevalence for those individuals is a little over 8% or around 1 in 12.[7] Many Americans may no doubt be awkward in their behavior, slightly avoidant, or even haunted by the experience of the pandemic. Similarly, many more may be vigilant, moody, or more anxious than they were before the pandemic. This does not mean that they have PTSD.

As psychiatrists, we need to avoid the urge to pathologize these symptoms and to help our patients recognize that these are common behaviors after stressful events and may not be indicative of mental illness. We need to stress the importance of talking about these feelings and processing them in a healthy way so that patients can emerge from the pandemic humbled but ultimately more well-adjusted. It has never been clearer that shutting oneself up and walling oneself in from the world can have deleterious consequences to mental health. We need to encourage patients and otherwise reluctant members of the public that now is the time to open up and talk about the difficulties they faced while coping with the effects of the pandemic.

The Return

It is impossible to say how quickly individuals will fully recover from the COVID-19 pandemic or when the majority of people will feel safe returning to public life without cumbersome restrictions on behavior. Still, it is worth noting that humans can be exceptionally resilient, even in the face of tremendous adversity, but this has been a truly novel event. Trying to estimate the number of people who will immediately bounce back and be able to resume somewhat normal social activities or, conversely, those who will not be comfortable resuming these activities is a matter of conjecture and not science.

Similarly, there simply have not been enough data accumulated to make more than an educated guess about how the pandemic and social distancing efforts will impact the prevalence of substance use disorders, anxiety, depressive, or trauma- and stressor-related disorders. Though these statistics from the American Psychological Association have already been mentioned, they bear repeating: During the pandemic, 23% of adults reported drinking more, 61% said that they have experienced undesired changes in weight, and 67% said their sleep patterns had been negatively impacted by the pandemic.[8] While there is most certainly overlap between these three groups (excessive alcohol consumption can lead to weight gain and sleep problems), what is far more troubling is that these are not conditions that one heals from overnight. Alcoholism is not a phase that one casually wanders in and out of. For far too many people throughout the world, they will emerge from COVID-19 not only with anxiety disorders or depression but also trapped in a cycle of substance abuse, as well.

What is certain is that the process of acclimatizing to social situations is going to take more time for some people than others and that differences in comfort levels is perfectly natural. Some people have already fallen right back into the swing of things with minimal discomfort or awkwardness or changes to their prepandemic behaviors. Others are going to struggle to feel comfortable in social situations even if they live in a community with extremely high-vaccination rates and an extremely low number of COVID-19 cases. I do not think it is wise to try to put a limit on what constitutes a normal amount of time to readjust. We just need to show patience and encourage people to go at their own pace for the foreseeable future.

That said, we need to be empathetic to those who need support and who are struggling with anxiety disorders, affective disorders, and trauma- and stress-related disorders. An Italian study has found that

30% of patients with severe COVID-19 infection met criteria for PTSD,[9] while a network cohort study using data from 69 million individuals, 62,354 of whom were diagnosed with COVID-19, found that as many as a third of patients are reporting neurological or psychiatric conditions between 14 and 90 days after COVID-19 diagnosis and that 5.8% of those patients received a first recorded diagnosis of a psychiatric disorder.[10] For comparison, psychiatric disorder incidence during the same time period following diagnoses of other medical issues was far lower; this includes influenza (2.8%), other respiratory diseases (3.4%), skin infections (3.3%), cholelithiasis (3.2%), urolithiasis (2.5%), and fractures (2.5%).[11] A separate Italian study screened 402 adults with COVID-19 for psychiatric symptoms with clinical interviews and self-report questionnaires 1 month following hospital treatment for COVID-19 and found that 56% of those screened scored in the pathological range in at least one clinical dimension. This included reports of PTSD (28%), depression (31%), anxiety (42%), obsessive-compulsive disorder (20%), and insomnia (40%).[12]

Increases in psychiatric disorders have purportedly risen across the board, regardless of whether one was diagnosed with COVID-19 or not. Since late spring of 2020, the average share of adults reporting symptoms of anxiety or depressive disorder has averaged close to 38% while during the first half of 2019, only 11% of adults were experiencing these symptoms.[13] There is also anecdotal evidence that the challenges associated with quarantine led women, who have historically consumed less alcohol than men, to drink as much as their male counterparts. No surprise, this phenomenon is driven largely by the need to cope with the stresses of juggling professional, social, and familial obligations simultaneously and without reprieve while also experiencing the novel stresses of the pandemic.[14]

Resiliency is a finite resource and people can only take so much stress before their mental health begins to suffer. For most people, this is not going to lead to some kind of overdramatic nervous breakdown. Instead, one may notice that they are more irritable than they once were, that they are not sleeping particularly well, or that they have a nagging sense of discomfort and stress when doing activities that they used to think of as normal (eg, a trip to the grocery store, meeting up with friends, going to work). We also need to avoid the urge to treat those who feel a little awkward or self-conscious about going back to the office or seeing friends and family again for the first time since the prepandemic era as if there is something wrong with them or that they are poorly adjusted. However, we also have to balance this with a show of concern when individuals are failing to adjust to the new-normal.

Demographic Changes, Changes to Labor Markets, and Crime

Speaking from experience, one of the clearest changes that occurred in urban centers during the pandemic was the change in demographics. It is far too early to jump to conclusions on this matter, but there could be a significant change in urban demographics as trends reverse and college-educated individuals begin to look for large spaces to call home and the premium that had once been put on urban living dissipates. This has the potential to be one of the most transformative aspects of COVID-19. New York City, Los Angeles, San Francisco, and other superstar cities have pulled human resources from the hinterlands of this nation in addition to being a cultural magnet that has attracted the world's most talented artists for year. That living in these cities is no longer a requirement for gaining access to their job markets suggests that there will be a significant drop in the number of college-educated individuals who remain in these cities, and that rural areas in the surrounding environs will see property values explode in both housing markets and commercial/retail markets. The clinical significance of these demographic changes is that many individuals may attempt to maintain their relationship with their physicians and, consequently, may continue to rely on telemedicine well after the pandemic.

Another issue that has arisen as vaccine rates have risen and the economy has begun to fire on all cylinders is that demand for goods and services is increasing, but employers are struggling to keep up with this demand because workers can afford to be picky about the jobs they take. Even into the late summer of 2021, many positions are going unfilled and many low-wage, high-stress jobs are being abandoned.[15]

Rather than providing higher wages, which will then be cemented into place, employers believe that waiting for the more generous unemployment benefits that were offered during the pandemic to lapse will allow them to once again offer wages that are only desirable if the alternative is complete and total penury. Many of these benefits have begun to expire as of the time of this writing in September 2021. It is unclear if the elimination of the supplemental benefits will lead more strenuous competition for low-wage positions or if employers will be forced to raise wages.

Yet another consequence of the pandemic has been increases in crime and violent incidents.[16] At this time, there is no consensus as to the specific reasons behind this phenomenon but the jump in violent crime, particularly in homicides, following decades of downward trends is no doubt linked in some way to the pandemic since people are more "on edge" in general, and that is likely why seemingly minor incidents can escalate into overt displays of aggression and violence.[17] The stress that is making anger management ostensibly impossible for some people is likely tied to the myriad stresses of the pandemic and will have clinical relevance because these psychosocial stressors do have physiological correlates (hypertension, weakened immune system, enteric symptoms, etc.) and may be associated with additional symptoms like sleep problems, headaches, and sexual dysfunction, to name a few.[18] Meanwhile, rises in crime rates in one's neighborhood or city are associated with increases in psychological stress, even if one is not directly the victim of a criminal act. What is deeply concerning is that the relationship may be bidirectional, meaning crime feeds stress and stress feeds crime. This would suggest yet another self-sustaining cycle of stress and disease mirroring those discussed in *Chapter 5: Psychosocial and Economic Impact of COVID-19—A Nation Under Siege.*

Changes in Careers and the Exodus From Medicine

In addition to moving to different areas, many patients may seek new career opportunities. In some cases, this may be fueled by necessity due to the collapse of an industry in their region. Less tragically, it may be because of a newfound sense of possibility in their own abilities or the belief that they have been granted a second chance. To call it is an existential crisis would be perhaps to cheapen this recognition that there is much to be explored in the limited time that we are each allotted. The proverbial angel of death has passed over their bed but opted to leave them unmolested. What people decide to do with this new sense of agency remains to be seen. Some may decide that they want to make positive changes in their lives. Some may decide to take more risks or satisfy hedonistic appetites that have been starved during the most oppressive months of lockdown. Still others may decide that they simply cannot handle the stresses that they have been forced to endure, oftentimes for years, and that the pandemic has afforded them an ideal time to make a change.

This latter sentiment is currently very common among people who work in the field of medicine. In the spring of 2021, just under 3 in 10 health care workers admitted to thinking about leaving the profession entirely, while over half reported feeling burned out, and 60% said that pandemic stress had adversely impacted their mental health.[19] This is not a uniquely American phenomenon, either. In the United Kingdom, similar numbers have been reported. In fact, 17% of participants in one survey said that they would rather work in a different country.[20]

There is a laundry list of reasons why different health care workers feel particularly burnt out. For some, the COVID-19 pandemic was the straw that broke the camel's back after years of complaints about long hours and difficult working conditions. For others, the sheer volume of death and sickness to which they were exposed during the most difficult months of the pandemic have had a powerful effect on them. For still others, they feel a sense of betrayal from the community at large for refusing to take vaccination, masking, social distancing guidelines seriously, even if it meant that they would ultimately get sick and have to be treated at a hospital that was struggling to ensure that staff had sufficient resources to treat the sick and to stay safe while doing so. "You feel expendable," an emergency room doctor in Pennsylvania told *The Washington Post*. "You cannot help thinking about how this country sent us to the front lines with none of the equipment needed for the battle."[19]

Psychiatrist Jessica (Jessi) Gold characterized this kind of "compassion fatigue" as a combination of exhaustion, sadness, and frustration that comes from being empathetic people working in a field that requires one witness a great deal of pain and suffering.[21] While many clinicians may often be thought of as rather cold people who robotically dispense medical services, even those of us who have practiced for years and have learned how to insulate ourselves from the worst elements of the job still have our limits. While this is largely conjecture at this point in time and there is hope that those who have worked in the field for years will stay and that a sense of duty to help the sick will be more salient to younger generations, it is certainly possible that many people may leave medicine because their limits were reached during the pandemic. The level of stress of fighting COVID-19, combined with a sense of open hostility to pandemic protocols and in some cases medical professionals themselves, may have been too much for many to bear. Whether or not this exodus occurs is yet to be seen, and it will only ensure that we are even less prepared for future medical crises.

Loneliness

Loneliness and social isolation are two peas in a pod, unfortunately. According to a consensus study report published by The National Academies of Sciences, Engineering, and Medicine, social isolation is defined as, "The objective state of having few social relationships or infrequent social contact with others," while loneliness is defined as, "a subjective feeling of being isolated."[22] The two are distinct, since individuals may be socially isolated without being lonely and people can be lonely without being socially isolated, but it appears as though the COVID-19 pandemic made both phenomena worse, particularly among seniors. Many seniors have experienced extended periods of isolation to maintain social distancing protocols, even if an estimated 24% of community-dwelling Americans over the age 65 years were already considered socially isolated before the pandemic.[22] At least 27% of adults over the age of 60 years lived by themselves prior to the pandemic—a larger percentage than anywhere else in the world.[23] Loneliness appears to be more pronounced among seniors with lower socioeconomic statuses.[24]

Even before the pandemic began, this was extremely concerning. Loneliness is associated with worse overall mental health, as well as specific symptoms like depression and anxiety, as well as cardiovascular diseases, stroke, and pain disorders like fibromyalgia.[25-27] In addition, people who are lonely may be far worse at coping with trauma than those who perceive themselves as being connected to a social network,[28,29] including for elders who have become widowed. There is no question that during the height of a pandemic people felt less connected and that a lot of seniors became widowed, particularly women, since COVID-19 was more fatal in older men.[30] The Global Fund for Widows characterized the disease as "a widow-making machine" in a report published in May 2020.[31]

There is no doubt that the stresses of the COVID Era have been more onerous for all people, including seniors, and surveys have found that the pandemic has made older Americans lonelier.[32,33] This is not said to cast doubt on the necessity of social distancing during times of rampant community spread but to acknowledge that being with family and friends over Zoom during a pandemic or in the wake of a tragedy is a poor substitute for their physical presence, and that this kind of virtual existence may only exacerbate one's sense of alienation.

Apart from being the age group least likely to quickly adopt and use new technologies, studies and surveys have repeatedly found that seniors are also the least likely age group to voluntarily seek out psychiatric care. As Conner and colleagues wrote, they found "critically low intention to seek and engage in professional mental health services" among the study's senior participants.[34] This was especially pronounced among the study's Black participants. Meanwhile, Ghafoori and colleagues found a negative association between the use of mental health services and individuals who lived in urban areas, were recent immigrants, lived below the poverty line, and/or were exposed to trauma. If they had limited social support from family, significant others, or friends, the negative correlation was even more salient.[35]

There is no question that loneliness will continue to be an issue long after the worst of the COVID-19 pandemic has passed, but what is more alarming is deteriorations in mental health, catalyzed by the experience of loneliness during the pandemic, may be most pronounced in the populations that are the most underserved, the least likely to reach out for help, and from the communities that suffered the worst outbreaks during the worst days of the pandemic: those among the urban working class. Resources will need to be dedicated to outreach in these communities and will likely be most successful if done in partnership with community groups, houses of worship, and other local and trusted organizations.

Conclusion

There is no doubt that many may see the end of the pandemic as a time of rebirth. As they emerge from the COVID-19 cocoon, they may opt to make significant lifestyle changes to improve their mental health and overall sense of wellness by making a career change, leaving behind a toxic relationship, or finding novel ways to prioritize what is ultimately important (family, friends, health) to their quality of life.

However, others will struggle to emerge from the initial stages of the pandemic era and may feel stuck in a kind of purgatory from which they cannot easily extricate themselves. Data are still emerging about how widespread the lingering psychological and neurological effects of COVID-19 will be and the same is true for the lingering effects of dealing with the initial stresses of the pandemic era. What is clear is that the stresses of enduring an event of this magnitude will leave an indelible mark on the psyche of every American, even those who never became sick, and that many may experience a deterioration in mental health that simply cannot be undone by a shot (or two) in the arm. They will need to take proactive steps to make improvements and we need to mobilize outreach efforts to ensure those who seek help can obtain it and destigmatize the act of seeking help for mental health issues. It is vital that we remember that the longer these disorders are allowed to fester, the more entrenched they will become. If we are to emerge from the COVID-19 Era successfully as a nation, we will have to strive to make sure that the most vulnerable among us are free to seek the care they need to become healthier and do not feel judged or belittled when they ask for help.

REFERENCES

1. American Psychiatric Association. *Diagnostic and Statistical Manual on Mental Disorders*. 5th ed. The American Psychiatric Association; 2013.
2. Ritchie H, Ortiz-Ospina E, Beltekian D, et al. *United States: Coronavirus Pandemic Country Profile*. Our World in Data. Updated June 19, 2021. Accessed June 19, 2021. https://ourworldindata.org/coronavirus/country/new-zealand
3. Kidman R, Margolis R, Smith-Greenaway E, et al. Estimates and projections of COVID-19 and parental death in the US. *JAMA Pediatr*. 2021;175(7):745-746. doi:10.1001/jamapediatrics.2021.0161. Accessed June 19, 2021.

4. London E, Varnum P. *Why This Is the Year We Must Take Action on Mental Health*. World Economic Forum. Published January 2, 2019. Accessed June 22, 2021. https://www. weforum.org/agenda/2019/01/lets-make-2019-the-year-we-take-action-on-mental-health/

5. Levit K, Richardson J, Frankel S, et al. *Projections of National Expenditures for Treatment of Mental and Substance Use Disorders, 2010-2020*. Substance Abuse and Mental Health Services Administration. Accessed June 22, 2021. https://store.samhsa.gov/sites/default/ files/d7/priv/sma14-4883.pdf

6. Goldstein A. Medicaid enrollment swells during the pandemic, reaching a new high. *Washington Post*. Published June 21, 2021. Accessed June 22, 2021. https://www.washingtonpost.com/health/medicaid-enrollment-during-the-pandemic/2021/06/21/8ee670d6-d27e-11eb-9f29-e9e6c9e843c6_story.html

7. Koenen KC, Ratanatharathorn A, Ng L, et al. Posttraumatic stress disorder in the world mental health surveys. *Psychol Med*. 2017;47(13):2260-2274. doi:10.1017/ S0033291717000708

8. American Psychological Association. *Stress in America: One Year Later, a New Wave of Pandemic Health Concerns*. Accessed June 6, 2021. https://www.apa.org/news/press/ releases/stress/2021/sia-pandemic-report.pdf

9. Janiri D, Carfì A, Kotzalidis GD, et al. Posttraumatic stress disorder in patients after severe COVID-19 infection. *JAMA Psychiatry*. 2021;78(5):567-569. doi:10.1001/ jamapsychiatry.2021.0109

10. Taquet M, Luciano S, Geddes JR, Harrison PJ. Bidirectional associations between COVID-19 and psychiatric disorder: retrospective cohort studies of 62,354 COVID-19 cases in the USA. *Lancet Psychiatry*. 2021;8(2):130-140. doi:10.1016/S2215-0366(20)30462-4

11. Taquet M, Geddes JR, Husain M, Luciano S, Harrison PJ. 6-month neurological and psychological outcomes in 236379 survivors of COVID-19: a retrospective study using electronic health records. *Lancet Psychiatry*. 2021;8:416-427.

12. Mazza MG, De Lorenzo R, Conte C, et al. Anxiety and depression in COVID-19 survivors: Role of inflammatory and clinical predictors. *Brain Behav Immun*. 2020;89:594-600. doi:10.1016/j.bbi.2020.07.037

13. Panchal N, Kamal R, Cox C, Garfield R. *The Implications of COVID-19 for Mental Health and Substance Use*. KFF website; Published February 10, 2021. Accessed April 5, 2021. https://www.kff.org/coronavirus-covid-19/issue-brief/ the-implications-of-covid-19-for-mental-health-and-substance-use/

14. Pattani A. *Women Now Drink as Much as Men—Not So Much for Pleasure, But to Cope*. NPR; Published June 9, 2021. Accessed June 9, 2021. https://www.npr.org/sections/health-shots/2021/06/09/1003980966/ women-now-drink-as-much-as-men-and-suffer-health-effects-more-quickly

15. Romans C. *American Workers Don't Want to Go Back to Normal, and That Makes Sense*. CNN; Updated June 22, 2021. Accessed June 22, 2021. https://www.cnn.com/2021/06/22/ economy/job-shortage-workers/index.html

16. Witte G, Berman M. As homicides soar nationwide, mayors see few options for regaining control. *Washington Post*. June 22, 2021. Accessed June 22, 2021. https://www. washingtonpost.com/national/homicides-up-nationwide-mayors/2021/06/21/13e5aa46-d058-11eb-9b7e-e06f6cfdece8_story.html

17. Prose F. *What Is Causing Outbursts of Rage on Planes and Grocery Checkout Lines?* The Guardian; Published June 22, 2021. Accessed June 22, 2021. https://www.theguardian. com/commentisfree/2021/jun/22/rage-planes-grocery-stores-hidden-pandemic-trauma

18. American Psychological Association. *Stress Effects on the Body*. APA.org; Published November 1, 2018. Accessed June 22, 2021. https://www.apa.org/topics/stress/body

19. Wan W. Burned out by the pandemic, 3 in 10 health-care workers consider leaving the profession. *Washington Post*. Published April 22, 2021. Accessed June 22, 2021. https:// www.washingtonpost.com/health/2021/04/22/health-workers-covid-quit/

20. Gilchrist K. *COVID Has Made It Harder to Be a Health-Care Worker. Now, Many Are Thinking of Quitting*. CNBC; Updated June 1, 2021. Accessed September 12, 2021. https:// www.cnbc.com/2021/05/31/covid-is-driving-an-exodus-among-health-care-workers.html

21. Gold J. The cost of compassion fatigue during COVID. *MedPage Today*. Published August 31, 2021. Accessed September 12, 2021. https://www.medpagetoday.com/publichealthpolicy/generalprofessionalissues/94304

22. The National Academies of Sciences, Engineering, and Medicine. *Social Isolation and Loneliness in Older Adults: Opportunities for the Health Care System*. The National Academies Press; 2020.

23. Ausubel J. *Older People Are More Likely to Live Alone in the U.S. Than Elsewhere in the World*. Pew Research Center; Published March 10, 2020. Accessed June 17, 2021. https://www.pewresearch.org/fact-tank/2020/03/10/older-people-are-more-likely-to-live-alone-in-the-u-s-than-elsewhere-in-the-world/

24. Kahlon MK, Aksan N, Aubrey R, et al. Effect of layperson-delivered, empathy-focused program of telephone calls on loneliness, depression, and anxiety among adults during the COVID-19 pandemic. *JAMA Psychiatry*. 2021;78(6):616-622. doi:10.1001/jamapsychiatry.2021.0113

25. Banerjee D, Rai M. Social isolation in COVID-19: the impact of loneliness. *Int J Soc Psychiatr*. 2020;66(6):525-527. doi:10.1177/0020764020922269

26. Valtorta NK, Kanaan M, Gilbody S, Ronzi S, Hanratty B. Loneliness and social isolation as risk factors for coronary heart disease and stroke: systematic review and meta-analysis of longitudinal observational studies. *Heart*. 2016;102(13):1009-1016. doi:10.1136/heartjnl-2015-308790

27. Wolf LD, Davis MC. Loneliness, daily pain, and perceptions of interpersonal events in adults with fibromyalgia. *Health Psychol*. 2014;33(9):929-937.

28. Feder A, Ahmad S, Lee EJ, et al. Coping and PTSD symptoms in Pakistani earthquake survivors: purpose in life, religious coping and social support. *J Affect Disord*. 2013;147(1-3):156-163. doi:10.1016/j.jad.2012.10.027

29. Lee JS. Perceived social support functions as a resilience in buffering the impact of trauma exposure on PTSD symptoms via intrusive rumination and entrapment in firefighters. *PLoS One*. 2019;14(8):e0220454. doi:10.1371/journal.pone.0220454

30. Peckham H, de Gruitjer NM, Raine C, et al. Male sex identified by global COVID-19 meta-analysis as a risk factor for death and ITU admission. *Nat Commun*. 2020;11(1):6317. doi:10.1038/s41467-020-19741-6

31. Onofrio J, Ibrahim-Leathers H. *COVID-19 & Widowhood: The Virus' Invisible Victim*. Global Fund for Widows; Published May 2020. Accessed June 22, 2021. https://uploads-ssl.webflow.com/5fce889a3c0f6e35f56692ce/5fce889a3c0f6e0e0f669306_COVID-and-Widowhood-MAY-2020.pdf

32. Kotwal AA, Holt-Lunstad J, Newmark RL, et al. Social isolation and loneliness among San Francisco Bay Area older adults during the COVID-19 shelter-in-place orders. *J Am Geriatr Soc*. 2021;69(1):20-29. doi:10.1111/jgs.16865

33. Piette J, Solway E, Singer D, Kirch M, Kullgren J, Malani P. *Loneliness Among Older Adults Before and During the COVID-19 Pandemic*. University of Michigan National Poll on Healthy Aging; Published September 2020. Accessed June 22, 2021. https://www.healthyagingpoll.org/report/loneliness-among-older-adults-and-during-covid-19-pandemic

34. O'Connor KO, Copeland VC, Grote NK, et al. Mental health treatment seeking among older adults with depression: the impact of stigma and race. *Am J Geriatr Psychiatry*. 2010;18(6):531-543. doi:10.1097/JGP.0b013e3181cc0366

35. Ghafoori B, Fischer DG, Koresteleva O, Hong M. Factors associated with mental health service use in urban, impoverished, trauma-exposed adults. *Psychol Serv*. 2014;11(4):451-459. doi:10.1037/a0036954

9

Implications for Psychiatric Patients

Psychiatric patients faced unique challenges during the worst of the COVID-19 pandemic. This includes those who were presented with psychiatric emergencies or struggled with severe and persistent mental illnesses (SPMI), some with substance use disorders (SUDs), and lastly those with preexisting or new-onset psychiatric disorders that are not chronic psychotic and mood disorders.

Psychiatric Emergencies

In the early days of the pandemic, colleagues noted a major reduction in the number of individuals arriving in emergency departments. What were initially anecdotal observations from people who work in these parts of the hospital was soon validated by a study from the Centers for Disease Control and Prevention, which reported a precipitous drop in emergency room visits during the first weeks of the pandemic.
The most pronounced decline was during the 4 weeks from March 29 to April 25, 2020, when emergency room visits across the United States plummeted by 42% compared to the same 4-week period the previous year.[1]

This finding did not just apply to people who suffered minor injuries or traumas. In the 10 weeks after March 13, 2020, when COVID-19 was declared a national emergency, emergency departments saw declines in the number of patients presenting with myocardial infarction, stroke, and hyperglycemic crisis of 23%, 20%, and 10%, respectively, when compared to the 10 weeks prior to the declaration.[i] Meanwhile, surgeries, routine screenings, and clinical trials for new therapies were cancelled and oncologists tried to revise chemotherapy protocols to reduce the frequency of visits and the level of immunosuppression for those receiving treatment.[2]

While these numbers have since rebounded and are close to their prepandemic levels as of the middle of 2021,[3] the trajectory for psychiatric emergencies is slightly different. While there were fewer psychiatric patients arriving in the hospital in the weeks following the declaration of the national emergency,[4] numbers have since risen back to prepandemic levels though the types of emergencies have changed. Data from December 2020 through January 2021 show that emergencies due to feeding and eating disorders have been and remain relatively low, while more adults and children are seeking emergency care pertaining for behavioral or mental health concerns related to socioeconomic or psychosocial issues.[5] What remains a question is if these are symptoms associated with COVID-19 or long COVID. Secondly, did these symptoms arise due to pandemic-related stressors or did they occur independently of COVID-19?

As noted throughout several chapters thus far, even those who have not been infected with SARS-CoV-2 have suffered psychological strain due to a multitude of factors and may have developed worsening symptoms or new-onset psychiatric disorders. This is confounded by the fact that anxiety and depression are common symptoms associated with COVID-19; moreover, many of those who were hospitalized with COVID-19 have been diagnosed with posttraumatic stress disorder , and many long haulers have reported psychiatric symptoms that extend beyond anxiety and depression and include difficulty concentrating, malaise, sleep problems, and adjustment disorders.[6] It should come as no surprise, therefore, that a growing number of patients seeking emergency care report behavioral or mental health concerns related to socioeconomic or psychosocial issues but a full understanding of common etiologies remains unknown.

---

[i] The 10-week period prior to the declaration is technically January 5 through March 14, 2020, and the 10-week period following the declaration is technically March 15 through May 23, 2020.

Impact on Patients with SPMI[ii]

The pandemic has altered the way that many of us live our daily lives and will likely continue to have an impact on social behaviors going forward. For outpatient psychiatric patients, these issues have been compounded by unique challenges that can make maintaining treatment regimens especially difficult. Nonadherence is common in patients with mental illnesses, particularly in schizophrenia where partial or total nonadherence may reach 75%,[7] and the dissolution of support networks during the pandemic adversely impacted this figure though data has not revealed to what extent. Long-acting injections may have attenuated these effects but, again, no studies have been released on the subject as of this time.

These were not the only hardships that patients with SPMI (schizophrenia and related disorders, bipolar disorder, and severe depression) experienced.[8] A systematic review and meta-analysis published in July 2021 that involved 16 observational studies from seven countries found patients with mental health disorders were at risk for higher COVID-19–related mortality and that individuals with schizophrenia and/or bipolar disorder were at an even higher risk of mortality.[9] There are multiple factors contributing to this association, as individuals with SPMIs oftentimes suffer from poor self-care, comorbid SUDs, poor overall health, and the kinds of chronic inflammatory conditions that make one more vulnerable to severe COVID-19, while also being more likely to experience homelessness or reside in shared housing facilities.[10] Preliminary reports suggest that infection was extremely common in these shelters and that individuals who experienced homelessness during the pandemic were at a far higher risk of dying of COVID-19.[11] An analysis published in June 2020 by Coalition for the Homeless, an advocacy group based in New York City, reported that the COVID-19 mortality rate for sheltered homeless New Yorkers was 61% higher than the overall New York City rate.[12] Individuals with SPMIs are also overrepresented in prison populations, where an estimated 14.5% of men and 31.0% of women are believed to have at least one SPMI, and those in prison were estimated to have been infected with the coronavirus

---

[ii] Though some ambiguity exists with respect to this term, I refer to the original definition introduced by the National Institute of Mental Health in 1987, which consists of three dimensions: diagnosis, disability, and duration. "Diagnosis" is self-explanatory. Those considered to have a "disability" must satisfy at least two of the following criteria: (1) be unemployed, employed and in supportive housing, or have a poor work history; (2) require public financial assistance; (3) lack established social support systems; (4) be incapable of fulfilling basic domestic duties unassisted; or (5) behave in a manner that results in frequent interactions with mental health professionals and/or the judicial system. To meet the "duration" criteria, patients must have undergone intensive psychiatric treatment more than once in their lifetime or experienced a chronic episode severe enough to require supportive residential care and preclude living independently.

at almost four times the rate of those in the United States overall (9% vs 34%).[13,14]

Compliance with preventative measures and public health directives may be more difficult for individuals with SPMIs due to impaired decision-making abilities, which may be compounded by comorbid SUDs. Prophylactic regimens (frequent hand washing, confinement, social distancing, wearing a mask, etc) may also be difficult to follow as patients with these disorders often suffer from delusions, hallucinations, poor insight, and paranoid thinking, which can make public health directives sound sinister or even part of larger plot to harm them. Given the rise of misinformation and conspiracies about both the virus in general and the vaccine in particular, efforts to convince patients about the benefits of vaccination may prove especially difficult.

Concerns about superspreading events within inpatient and residential facilities led to polymerase chain reaction testing for all new admissions and restricted access for nonessential personnel. These efforts were warranted to ensure a contagion-free facility that would allow patients free access to communal areas and free exchange with other patients. Creating an atmosphere of increased isolation would not be conducive to providing treatment since group work is often integral for patients in these facilities. Furthermore, placing patients in virtual isolation to protect them from infection would have been less than ideal as these conditions could potentially lead to symptom deterioration. Additionally, masking may not be possible for all individuals within inpatient psychiatric facilities, as there have been reports of some patients using the masks provided to commit acts of self-harm.[15]

How long these policies will need to remain in place remains an open question.

Impact on Individuals with SUDs

Like patients with SPMIs, individuals with SUDs often lack access to health care, confront socioeconomic headwinds, and have several comorbidities, including cardiovascular, pulmonary, and metabolic diseases. Consequently, patients with SUDs often have a greater risk of developing severe COVID-19. This appears to be particularly true among Black Americans.[16] Wang and colleagues reported: "COVID-19 patients with SUD had significantly worse outcomes (death: 9.6%, hospitalization: 41.0%) than general COVID-19 patients (death: 6.6%, hospitalization: 30.1%) and African Americans with COVID-19 and SUD had worse outcomes (death: 13.0%, hospitalization: 50.7%) than Caucasians (death: 8.6%, hospitalization: 35.2%)." The study also found that patients with opioid use disorder (OUD) were at the greatest risk of infection and that there was no significant difference in risk between patients with OUD who were receiving medications (methadone, buprenorphine, or naltrexone) compared to those who were receiving no medications.[16]

Patients in recovery for SUDs very frequently rely on in-person meetings and group work through 12-step programs networks like Alcoholics Anonymous or Narcotics Anonymous to maintain sobriety, and the sudden disappearance of these anchors almost certainly fueled instances of relapse, though it is still too early to tell how widespread the problem has been. There is significant anecdotal evidence suggesting that the problem is immense and will continue to linger on well after the worst of the pandemic has passed, especially if SARS-CoV-2 becomes endemic and fear of infection can be used as a reason to forego participation in group work.[17]

Changes in social dynamics have also played a major role in the exacerbation of the problem. One of the hallmarks of addiction is isolation. As one's life begins to revolve around the use of a substance, other elements of their life are cast off. Work-related responsibilities go by the wayside, as do social obligations. Those struggling with addiction often end up keeping secrets from friends, loved ones, and family members either because they are embarrassed of how much they are struggling and/or because they are worried that someone might intervene and prevent the appeasement of the addiction. That pandemic stress led many to cope with drugs and alcohol and social distancing measures actively encouraged isolation, which not only created a perfect storm for relapses but also led to the cultivation of novel addictions that could be hidden from prying eyes.

While there is no data to confirm this hypothesis, given the fact that many people were in relative isolation for over a year and anecdotal evidence indicates that rampant binge drinking and drug use was extremely common, it seems likely that the pandemic led many to develop SUDs.

Impact on Psychiatric Outpatients

For existing psychiatric patients who required routine treatment rather than emergency services or support for SUDs, telemedicine offered an ideal solution (for further discussion, see *Chapter 10: Implications for Clinicians— Telemedicine and the Virtual Clinic*). Though certain procedures (ketamine infusions, electroconvulsive therapy, transcranial magnetic stimulation, etc) require patients to be onsite, many services can *temporarily* be delivered virtually without serious degradations in quality of care.[18] Psychotherapy was one of the most common telemedicine services throughout 2020 and into 2021 and mental health conditions made up 51.3% of telemedicine diagnoses as of January 2021 (up from 30% in January 2020).[19] As of March 2021, generalized anxiety disorder and major depressive disorder made up over 50% of all mental health diagnoses nationwide. In all regions but the Western United States, generalized anxiety disorder was more common than major depressive disorder, while the inverse is true for states west of the Great Plains.[20]

The extent to which telemedicine attenuated or even prevented psychiatric crises is unknown. However, it seems very reasonable to assume a significant degree of efficacy through telemedicine that is comparable to in-person consultations. Given the available options and the need to take preventative steps to avoid spreading the virus, this was and still remains the best available method. The same can also be said of new patients who, overwhelmed by the stresses of the pandemic, have sought out mental health professionals as a means for support, as well as to improve their mental health. It is too early to tell if the convenience of telemedicine will convince them to continue with treatment as social distancing measures are eased, but the fact that it is often more affordable and does not require patients worry about traveling or seeking childcare during an appointment may make it a popular tool to be used when meeting in person is not an option.[21] It should be stressed here that in-person counseling is the superior option because it allows clinicians to discern certain nonverbal cues that may not be salient in a virtual setting.

A far more common criticism of telemedicine is that some patients may struggle to use or lack access to devices that allow for these types of communication. While the telephone can offer a potential solution, particularly for older patients who may struggle or simply not want to use video or mobile platforms, this medium is less effective than video or, to reiterate, in-person appointments.[22] Then again, the telephone is not a silver bullet, since some patients may not have access to a mobile phone, may only use a phone with a limited number of minutes, or may not have a single, regular phone that they use, thereby meaning communication is oftentimes a one-way street.

New Onset Psychiatric Conditions

What remains perhaps the biggest question mark in the field at present is the number of undiagnosed cases of psychiatric conditions that have emerged since the start of the pandemic. As has been mentioned several times, anxiety, mood, substance use, and trauma- and stressor-related disorders are intertwined with the pathology of COVID-19 and its psychosocial effects. Similarly, extremely stressful situations may also trigger first episode psychosis.

Data on these conditions is limited, but it is safe to assume that the same fear that kept those who suffered a heart attack out of the emergency room may have also deterred individuals who were already scared and confused because they were experiencing symptoms of mental illness from seeking help for the first time. If these individuals did not have strong support networks or were living independently, they may have had to endure this event alone and may not have been encouraged to seek help. One study based in Milan, Italy, that examined patients who were hospitalized for first episode psychosis between March 8, 2020, and July 8, 2020, and compared the same 4-month period from 2019, observed a 32% jump between the 2 years (n = 27 in 2019 and n = 35 in 2020) and saw a far later age of onset in 2020 (43.5 years) than in 2019 (34.0 years).[23]

Whether or not this is a universal finding remains to be seen. The study of the psychiatric effects of the COVID-19 pandemic on this population remains in its infancy and our understanding will evolve as more data becomes available.

Going Forward

Studies are still emerging that reveal exactly how severe the mental health crisis following the initial phase of the pandemic will be. To put it bluntly, the consensus is that it will be bad. Delays in treatment, increased use of substances, and a host of other problems have certainly contributed to the erosion of many individuals' mental health, even among those who were the paragons of mental hygiene prior to the pandemic. Telemedicine offers many solutions for outpatient care, particularly among patients with sufficient resources and the technological know-how to fully exploit new platforms, monitoring devices, and other technologies. Additionally, growing destigmatization, as discussed in *Chapter 8: Extended Social Impact*, should be encouraged as much as possible to ensure that those who need help seek it.

Several questions remain, however. For starters, there is limited data on the interaction of vaccines with medications that are commonly prescribed to psychiatric patients. Secondly, exactly how badly the stresses of COVID-19 impacted psychiatric patients and led to new onset symptoms remains to be elucidated. Finally, it remains to be seen how patients who typically struggle with compliance with treatment regimens responded to the pandemic and if there were any strategies that were found to improve adherence.

REFERENCES

1. Lange SJ, Ritchey MD, Goodman AB, et al. Potential indirect effects of the COVID-19 pandemic on use of emergency department for acute life-threatening conditions – United States, January-May 2020. *MMWR Morb Mortal Wkly Rep*. 2020;69:795-800. doi:10.15585/mmwr.mm6925e

2. Rosenbaum L. The untold toll—the pandemic's effects on patients without COVID-19. *N Engl J Med*. 2020;382(24):2368-2371. doi:10.1056/NEJMms2009984

3. Carbajal E. *Emergency Heart Care Returns to Pre-COVID-19 Levels, Kaiser Study Finds*. Becker's Hospital Review. 2021. Accessed June 18, 2021. https://www.beckershospitalreview.com/cardiology/emergency-heart-care-returns-to-pre-covid-19-levels-kaiser-study-finds.html

4. Holland KM, Jones C, Vivolo-Kantor A, et al. Trends in US emergency department visits for mental health, overdose, and violent outcomes before and during the COVID-19 pandemic. *JAMA Psychiatry*. 2021;78(4):372-379. doi:10.1001/jamapsychiatry.2020.4402

5. Adjemian J, Hartnett KP, Kite-Powell A, et al. Update: COVID-19 pandemic—associated changes in emergency department visits—United States, December 2020 - January 2021. *MMWR Morb Mortal Wkly Rep*. 2021;70:552-556. doi:10.15585/mmwr.mm7015a3

6. FAIR Health. *A Detailed Study of Patients with Long-Haul COVID: An Analysis of Private Healthcare Claims*. Published June 15, 2021. Accessed June 15, 2021. https://s3.amazonaws.com/media2.fairhealth.org/whitepaper/asset/A%20Detailed%20Study%20of%20Patients%20with%20Long-Haul%20COVID--An%20Analysis%20of%20Private%20Healthcare%20Claims--A%20FAIR%20Health%20White%20Paper.pdf

7. Ifteni P, Dima L, Teodorescu A. Long-acting injectable antipsychotics treatment during COVID-19 pandemic—a new challenge. *Schizophr Res*. 2020;220:265-266. doi:10.1016/j.schres.2020.04.030

8. Shields-Zeeman L, Petrea I, Smit F, et al. Towards community-based and recovery-oriented care for severe mental disorders in Southern and Eastern Europe: aims and design of a multi-country implementation and evaluation study (RECOVER-E). *Int J Ment Health Syst*. 2020;14:30. doi:10.1186/s13033-020-00361-t

9. Fond G, Nemani K, Etchecopar-Etchart D, et al. Association between mental health disorders and mortality among patients with COVID-19 in 7 countries: a systematic review and meta-analysis. *JAMA Psychiatry*. 2021;e212274. Accessed August 19, 2021. doi:10.1001/jamapsychiatry.2021.2274

10. Morgan VA, Waterreus A, Carr V, et al. Responding to challenges for people with psychotic illness: updated evidence from the survey of high impact psychosis. *Aust N J Psychiatry*. 2017;51(2):124-140. doi:10.1177/0004867416679738

11. Aponte CI, Choi A, Durán HA. *COVID Tore through NYC Homeless Shelters. But Residents Were Kept in the Dark*. The City. June 15, 2020. Accessed June 18, 2021. https://www.thecity.nyc/2020/6/15/21292127/covid-tore-through-new-york-homeless-shelters-but-residents-were-kept-in-the-dark

12. Routhier G, Nortz S. *COVID-19 and Homelessness in New York City: Pandemic Pandemonium for New Yorkers without Homes*. Coalition for the Homeless. June 2020. Accessed June 18, 2021. https://www.coalitionforthehomeless.org/wp-content/uploads/2020/06/COVID19HomelessnessReportJune2020.pdf

13. Steadman HJ, Osher FC, Robbins PC, Case B, Samuels S. Prevalence of serious mental illness among jail inmates. *Psychiatr Serv*. 2009;60(6):761-765. doi:10.1176/ps.2009.60.6.761

14. Burkhalter E, Colón I, Derr B, et al. Incarcerated and infected: how the virus tore through the U.S. prison system. *New York Times*. Published April 10, 2021. Accessed June 18, 2021. https://www.nytimes.com/interactive/2021/04/10/us/covid-prison-outbreak.html

15. Katato HK, Guatam M, Akinyemi EO. The danger of face masks on an inpatient psychiatric unit: new protocol to prevent self-harm. *Prim Care Companion CNS Disord*. 2021;23(5):20br03017. doi:10.4088/PCC.20br03017

16. Wang QQ, Kaelber DC, Xu R, Volkow ND. COVID-19 risk and outcomes in patients with substance use disorders: analyses from electronic health records in the United States. *Mol Psychiatry*. 2021;26(1):30-39. doi:10.1038/s41380-020-00880-7

17. Tingley K. How bad is our pandemic drinking problem? *New York Times*. April 21, 2021. Accessed June 20, 2021. https://www.nytimes.com/2021/04/21/magazine/covid-drinking-alcohol-health.html

18. Ongur D, Perlis R, Goff D. Psychiatry and COVID-19. *J AM Med Assoc*. 2020;324(12):1149-1150. doi:10.1001/jama.2020.14294

19. Grant K. Psychotherapy now the most common telehealth procedure. *Medpage Today*. Published April 9, 2021. Accessed June 19, 2021. https://www.medpagetoday.com/special-reports/exclusives/92029

20. *Monthly Telehealth Regional Tracker*. FAIR Health. Accessed June 19, 2021. https://www.fairhealth.org/states-by-the-numbers/telehealth

21. Rogers K, Spring B. *Mental Health Professionals Are in High Demand as the Pandemic Enters a Second Year*. CNBC. Updated April 2, 2021. Accessed June 19, 2021. https://www.cnbc.com/2021/04/02/mental-health-professionals-are-in-high-demand-as-the-pandemic-enters-a-second-year.html

22. Ennis L, Rose D, Denis M, Pandit N, Wykes T. Can't surf, won't surf: the digital divide in mental health. *J Ment Health*. 2012;21(4):395-403. doi:10.3109/09638237.2012.689437

23. Esposito CM, D'Agostino A, Dell Osso B, et al. Impact of the first COVID-19 pandemic wave on first episode psychosis in Milan, Iltay. *Psychiatry Res*. 2021;298:113802. doi:10.1016/j.psychres.2021.113802

10

Implications for Clinicians—Telemedicine and the Virtual Clinic

As the COVID-19 pandemic struck in the spring of 2020, most hospitals, outpatient facilities, doctor's offices, and many other facilities that offer medical and mental health services came to a grinding halt. Needless to say, though this was necessary in the short-term, it is not a viable option for the health care industry or public hospitals, as they provide critical resources to the community and provide essential and necessary services. This abrupt loss of some services required an immediate shift in thinking and an innovative approach to find solutions to continue providing essential health care services to those in need. Consequently, telehealth and telemedicine became necessary during the COVID-19 pandemic. Telehealth allowed some health care workers a means of working remotely during the pandemic, while telemedicine allowed clinicians to safely meet with patients and comply with social distancing guidelines, especially when providing nonemergency care. In March 2020, the federal government eased many restrictions that had previously made the use of telemedicine cumbersome. These changes, in conjunction with the need to avoid unnecessary interactions to reduce the spread of SARS-CoV-2, accelerated the adoption of the telemedicine platforms during 2020 and into 2021, and this was particularly true in the field of mental health. While there are major benefits to the use of telemedicine, critics are justified in noting that it remains an untested medium and that issues of accessibility, privacy concerns, and quality of care remain among the most notable reasons why it should be considered one tool among many rather than a panacea.

COVID-19 and Telemedicine

Though the words "telemedicine" and "telehealth" may sometimes be used interchangeably, they are not the same. Introduced by Thomas Bird in the 1970s, the word "telemedicine" refers to the use of telecommunication technologies to allow clinicians to provide "healing at a distance."[1] Beyond allowing a more convenient means of communication between patients and their doctors, telemedicine also cuts down on travel, can reduce wait time, and allows doctors to monitor patients' vital signs or behaviors. At its most sophisticated, telemedicine can facilitate the virtual presence of medical personnel through wearable technology or allow a surgeon to use a semiautonomous robot during a procedure even when the two are hundreds of miles away from one another.[2,3] At its least sophisticated, it can mean picking up the phone and calling a patient. "Telehealth" is broader and refers to the delivery of health or health-related services via telecommunication or digital communication technologies and includes all services or activities pertaining to health care—including not just medical care to patients but also health care education, provider-to-provider communication, and the use of wearable devices to monitor one's own health.[4]

No surprise, telemedicine and telehealth have become extremely popular during the COVID-19 pandemic. With respect to telehealth, administrative staff from hospitals as well as health care administrators have mirrored trends in other industries with respect to working remotely. With respect to telemedicine, more patients have sought consultations and nonurgent care through the use of telemedicine and even some forms of artificial intelligence. Social distancing protocols during the height of the pandemic made telemedicine the best option for many patients, particularly seniors and individuals with weakened immune systems. Because millions of Americans had been placed in lockdown and were unable or unwilling to leave their homes, pivoting to telemedicine was not just driven by expediency; it was driven by necessity.

The surge in usage was aided by a federal response. Recognizing that eliminating regulations regarding telemedicine would make it easier for clinicians to evaluate patients and provide care to patients from the safety of their homes, Congress authorized the U.S. Department of Health and Human Services (HHS) to temporarily waive "certain Medicaid restrictions and requirements regarding telehealth services during the coronavirus public health emergency" by passing H.R. 6074—Coronavirus Preparedness and Response Supplemental Appropriations Act, 2020, which was signed into law on March 6, 2020.[5] Despite extreme partisanship in Washington, only three members of Congress voted against the bill.

HHS later announced it would temporarily ease the enforcement of some regulations created by the Health Insurance Portability and Accountability Act (HIPAA) of 1996.[6] These rules were waived for patients covered by private insurers, as well as all beneficiaries of Medicare and Medicaid. Previously, they were typically only waived for beneficiaries living in rural areas who often lacked access to specialists.[7] As of March 17, 2020:

1. Patients are allowed to receive telemedicine from clinicians based anywhere in the country.
2. Patients can receive care from clinicians without an established patient-physician relationship.
3. Penalties for using non-HIPAA–compliant telecommunications platforms have been waived.

As of the summer of 2021, many states have begun to roll back these waivers, but they do remain in effect in some states and regulations will likely be frequently updated so long as the pandemic continues.

Benefits of Telemedicine for Mental Health Services

While there have been numerous criticisms of how the United States responded to the pandemic, few have expressed misgivings about the decision to temporarily ease restrictions and regulations on telemedicine and telehealth. Particularly among clinicians who work in the field of mental health, telemedicine has not only allowed us to interface with patients in a safe manner; it has allowed us to potentially mitigate the effects of social isolation and to monitor patients' health states from a distance. As mentioned in *Chapter 8: Extended Social Impact*, social isolation and loneliness will continue to be major issues among individuals from all backgrounds, including those with no history of mental illness. This may be compounded by a reluctance to leave their homes, which both causes and exacerbates feelings of anxiety. Having a means of communicating and providing care will certainly be a part of the solution to this issue.

Psychotherapy has also proven to be a popular telemedicine service through the COVID-19 pandemic, and the majority of diagnoses made through telemedicine for the earliest months of 2021 have concerned mental health conditions.[8] As noted in *Chapter 9: Implications for Psychiatric*

Patients, generalized anxiety disorder and major depressive disorder made up over 50% of all mental health diagnoses nationwide for the first half of 2021.[9] Similarly, Nordh and colleagues recently reported that children and adolescents with social anxiety disorder may benefit from therapist-guided, internet-delivered cognitive behavioral therapy.[10] Additionally, telemedicine also affords potential promise for patients for whom adherence is often problematic, particularly those who suffer from severe and persistent mental illnesses (SPMIs) (schizophrenia and related disorders, bipolar disorder, or major depressive disorder).[11] Finally, clinicians have positive experiences using telemedicine, and they have reported that they tend to find these platforms easy to use.[12]

Criticisms of Telemedicine for Mental Health Services

There are several criticisms of telemedicine. The first is that some patients may struggle to use or lack access to devices that allow for these types of communication and that widespread adoption may exclude these individuals or at the very least make it more difficult for them to access care. While the telephone can offer a potential solution, particularly for older patients who may struggle or simply not want to use video or mobile platforms, this medium is less effective than video or, to reiterate, in-person appointments.[13] Additionally, the telephone should not be considered a silver bullet, since many patients may not have access to a mobile phone, may only use a phone with a limited number of minutes, or may not have a regular phone that they use, thereby meaning communication is oftentimes a one-way street. For individuals with SPMIs who may live on the street, telemedicine services are effectively worthless.

Yet another issue is that we do not know how effective these services are yet. While the technology to allow these platforms to exist is not novel by any means, it was not widely adopted prior to the pandemic, and very few studies have been conducted to examine how telemedicine holds up when compared to the traditional clinic. We have evolved to interact in three dimensions, and flattening the experience can cause clinicians to miss things that we would otherwise observe. For those of us in the field of mental health, this not only includes nonverbal means of communication but also the capacity to establish a sense of trust and safety. This is a fundamental component of psychiatric care, and developing a solid relationship with a patient can often take weeks to months. If telemedicine is not conducive to creating an atmosphere of trust, then it is unclear how effective it can be as a treatment medium.

For clinicians working in nonpsychiatric specialties and general medical care, there are clear roadblocks to successful diagnoses. Writing in the *New York Times*, former emergency room physician Elisabeth Rosenthal noted, "An internist depresses the tongue and looks for pus on the tonsils to detect possible strep throat. A surgeon suspects appendicitis by pushing on the belly to see if there is pain with rapid release."[14] Without the ability to perform these rudimentary tests, it seems extremely unlikely that clinicians will be able to make a correct diagnosis as quickly as when they are in the same room as the patient.

Diagnostic problems can exist in psychiatric care, as well, since it may be difficult to observe signs that would be instantly discernible in a clinical setting, but the patient may be able to obfuscate when suing a telehealth platform.

Finally, and perhaps most troublingly, is the business side of things. Some platforms vying to enter the market may be more concerned with their bottom lines than offering patients better care, and the general level of inexperience with respect to telemedicine may lead to serious lapses in security and sensitive patient information may be exposed. Instances of fraud due to overcharging for appointments have also been reported, as have conflicts between out-of-state and in-state health providers.[15] For these reasons, one should be extremely scrupulous when adopting new technologies.

Conclusion

Telemedicine offered an ideal solution during the first months of the pandemic and clinicians should continue to make use of these applications whenever and wherever they can be safely and effectively implemented. However, telemedicine simply cannot replace the exchange between two people in the same room with one another. As we cautiously go through the dips and surges with constantly shifting policy, we should recognize that telemedicine can be a useful tool but that it is just one among many in our utility belts. We owe it to our patients to only use these services if they advance and promote better care.

REFERENCES

1. Matamala-Gomez M, Bottiroli S, Realdon O, et al. Telemedicine and virtual reality at time of COVID-19 pandemic: an overview for future perspectives in neurorehabilitation. *Front Neurol*. 2021;12:646902. doi:10.3389/fneur.2021.646902

2. Manusamy T, Karuppiah R, Bahuri NFA, Sockalingam S, Cham CY, Waran V. Telemedicine via smart glasses in critical care of the neurosurgical patient—COVID-19 pandemic preparedness and response in neurosurgery. *World Neurosurg*. 2021;145:e53-e60. doi:10.1016/j.wneu.2020.09.076

3. Metz C. The robot surgeon will see you now. *New York Times*. April 30, 2021. Accessed June 19, 2021. https://www.nytimes.com/2021/04/30/technology/robot-surgery-surgeon. html

4. New England Journal of Medicine Catalyst. *What Is Telehealth?* NEJM Catalyst. Published February 1, 2018. Accessed June 19, 2021. https://catalyst.nejm.org/doi/full/10.1056/ CAT.18.0268

5. *H.R. 6074—Coronavirus Preparedness and Response Supplemental Appropriations Act, 2020*. Congress.gov. Updated March 6, 2020. Accessed June 21, 2021. https://www. congress.gov/bill/116th-congress/house-bill/6074?q=%7B%22search%22%3A%5B%22coro navirus+preparedness+and+response+supplemental+appropriations+act%22%5D%7D&r =1&s=2

6. U.S. Department of Health & Human Services. *Notification of Enforcement Discretion for Telehealth Remote Communications during the COVID-19 National Public Health Emergency*. hhs.gov. Updated January 20, 2021. Accessed June 21, 2021. https://www. hhs.gov/hipaa/for-professionals/special-topics/emergency-preparedness/notification-enforcement-discretion-telehealth/index.html

7. Centers for Medicare & Medicaid Services. *Medicare Telemedicine Health Care Provider Fact Sheet*. cms.gov. Published March 17, 2020. Accessed June 21, 2021. https://www.cms. gov/newsroom/fact-sheets/medicare-telemedicine-health-care-provider-fact-sheet

8. Grant K. Psychotherapy now the most common telehealth procedure. *Medpage Today*. Published April 9, 2021. Accessed June 19, 2021. https://www.medpagetoday.com/ special-reports/exclusives/92029

9. *Monthly Telehealth Regional Tracker*. FAIR Health. Accessed June 20, 2021. https://www. fairhealth.org/states-by-the-numbers/telehealth

10. Nordh M, Wahlund T, Jolstedt M, et al. Therapist-guided internet-delivered cognitive behavioral therapy vs internet-delivered supportive therapy for children and adolescents with social anxiety disorder. *JAMA Psychiatry*. 2021;78(7):705-713. doi:10.1001/ jamapsychiatry.2021.0469

11. Basit SA, Matthews N, Kunik ME. Telemedicine interventions for medication adherence in mental illness: a systematic review. *Gen Hosp Psychiatry*. 2020;62:28-36. doi:10.1016/j. genhosppsych.2019.11.004

12. Schinasi DA, Foster CC, Bohling MK, Barrera L, Macy ML. Attitudes and perceptions of telemedicine in response to the COVID-19 pandemic: a survey of naïve healthcare providers. *Front Pediatr*. 2021;9:647937. doi:10.3389/fped.2021.647937

13. Ennis L, Rose D, Denis M, Pandit N, Wykes T. Can't surf, won't surf: the digital divide in mental health. *J Ment Health*. 2012;21(4):395-403. doi:10.3109/09638237.2012.689437

14. Rosenthal E. Telemedicine is a tool. Not a replacement for your doctor's touch. *New York Times*. Published April 29, 2021. Accessed June 22, 2021. https://www.nytimes. com/2021/04/29/opinion/virtual-remote-medicine-covid.html

15. Volz M. *The Boom in Out-of-State Telehealth Threatens in-State Providers*. KHN. Published March 15, 2021. Accessed June 22, 2021. https://khn.org/news/article/ the-boom-in-out-of-state-telehealth-threatens-in-state-providers/

11

Professional Didactic Framework: Planning for the Future

No doubt, changes to medical professionals' didactic framework may incorporate some forms of virtual learning that were developed out of necessity during the most perilous phase of the COVID-19 pandemic when most, if not all, of classroom activities were conducted online.[1] While some of these innovations may or may not be permanent, medical schools and training programs for medical professionals should consider making permanent changes to the curriculum to better prepare students for the next pandemic and future waves of pandemics that involve more virulent variants of the SARS-CoV-2 virus. This includes lessons on crisis management, palliative care, and the use of algorithms to predict postacute sequelae. Additionally, medical workers in all fields should be encouraged to regularly utilize mental health services to prevent burnout, anxiety, depression, posttraumatic stress disorder (PTSD), or substance use disorders, especially in times of crisis. This will require not only changes to the curriculum but cultural changes, as well.

Pandemic Training

For clinicians and medical professionals, some of the most infuriating and upsetting images from the COVID-19 pandemic were those showing emergency department workers fashioning personal protective equipment

(PPE) out of garbage bags during the height of the first wave of the pandemic in spring 2020. Though this situation was not universal in every state/city and hospital setting, it is still important to discuss this issue so as to prevent this serious lack of safety standards in the future. While one can applaud the ingenuity of the personnel on the frontlines during a time of scarcity, the absence of sufficient amounts of PPE was abominable. Every medical professional is a highly trained and highly specialized individual whose well-being and safety should be respected. Though our work often places us in extremely perilous environments, and we voluntarily chose this profession knowing quite well that we could potentially be exposed to dangerous pathogens and situations, very few would find it controversial to say that this does not mean that we should be expected to obsequiously agree to operate in these environments without proper protective equipment. Looking back, every effort should be made to make sure that there should never be a nationwide shortage of this kind of equipment even in the most extenuating of circumstances. It would be like sending an entire army to the frontlines without any form of armor or camouflage.

Of course, material support is not the only thing that clinicians need in the time of crisis. They also need training to keep themselves and patients safe. Without this training, medical professionals are similarly walking into a situation without proper protection. Consequently, crisis resource management (CRM) should be a necessary part of any medical professional's training. CRM focuses on improving nontechnical skills like interpersonal communication, problem-solving, situational awareness, team coordination, and resource management.

It has been estimated that 40,000 to 100,000 Americans die annually due to medical errors.[2] The majority of these errors do not arise because of a lack of knowledge on the part of medical professionals or even poor judgment on the part of one clinician but rather due to miscommunications and dysfunctional team dynamics. Ensuring that students learn practical skills to prepare them for a career that is heavily reliant on being part of a team will go a long way to improving coordination during emergency situations, especially novel ones that require ingenuity and the ability to follow and respond to ad hoc protocols.

While didactic teaching is necessary for medical professionals, it can be supplemented by simulation-based active learning and team-building exercises, including some that can be conducted virtually when in-person options are unavailable.[3] A meta-analysis found that the expanded use of team training exercises for medical professionals optimized team outcomes.[4] However, this kind of training can also improve CRM among students, thereby better preparing them for real-world scenarios. Saravana-Bawan and colleagues found that a single session of low-fidelity simulation-based noncontextual active learning improved students' CRM performance when compared to students who were only given instruction via didactic teaching. When compared to a group that was provided didactic teaching, the active learning group scored significantly better (6.7 points higher on a scale of 42). However, these effects became statistically insignificant 4 months after follow-up, suggesting that active learning exercises should be regularly employed to improve retention.[5]

Yet another facet of training that is often overlooked in medical school is palliative care. Personally, I have often found that hospital chaplains are far better equipped to offer guidance to patients who are in need of end-of-life care and to their grieving families who often feel unmoored by the loss of their loved one. Gaining communication competencies often requires first-hand experience, but simulation-based learning exercises could be utilized to supplement didactic teaching to better prepare medical professionals to offer comfort and empathy to those who struggling with existential anxiety or grief.[6] One need not be deeply religious to learn to speak the language of compassion.

Predictive Algorithms

Predictive algorithms and machine learning have been put to use to predict outcomes for emergency departments and intensive care units with some success. This can help medical professionals better allocate resources during times of crisis, as well as assess whether a patient may be more susceptible to postacute sequelae through the use of psychometric and biomarker data collected through electronic medical records. Given the well-established existence of postacute sequelae of SARS-CoV-2 (see *Chapter 4, Neuropsychiatric Symptoms and Postacute Sequelae of SARS-CoV-2—The Long Haulers*), a predictive algorithm for what is being called long COVID would be beneficial to many patients, especially if it is later discovered that early intervention can mitigate symptom severity or even eliminate the syndrome entirely.

This is an extremely important point since many patients who experience long COVID may not even develop acute symptoms of the disease and may only develop postacute sequelae. A study involving approximately 2 million people who had COVID-19 found that only 5% of those who reported lingering symptoms were hospitalized, while 55% were asymptomatic and another 40% experienced mild symptoms and recovered at home.[7] What this suggests is that only a minority of patients with COVID-19 will seek out medical attention, making such interventions relatively ineffective.

However, medical personnel in emergency departments are in a unique position to collect psychometric and biological data directly following a traumatic event, including recovery from severe COVID-19, to assess the potential for posttraumatic psychiatric disorders. Such predictive algorithms, if utilized during either a large-scale traumatic event like a natural disaster or yet another pandemic, could help mitigate subsequent psychopathology, particularly PTSD.

Emergency departments in the United States discharge an estimated 30 million patients who have experienced a traumatic event as defined by criteria A for PTSD in Diagnostic and Statistical Manual of Mental Disorders, 5th Edition (DSM-5).[8] This includes the following:

- Direct experience: Military combat, physical assault, automobile accident, sexual assault, natural disaster, terrorist attack, kidnapping, incarceration as prisoner of war or in concentration camp, catastrophic medical event.
- Witnessed: Unnatural or gruesome death, serious injury, physical or sexual assault, catastrophic medical event.
- Indirect experience: Learning that a close friend or relative has committed suicide or has been involved in either a very serious accident or an assault and has suffered severe injuries or unnatural death.
- Repeated exposure to the consequences of traumatic events. Examples include police officers documenting details of child abuse, first responders arriving on scenes of carnage, and medical personnel treating patients in a warzone.[9]

Of these 30 million patients, an estimated 10% to 20% will go on to be diagnosed with anxiety, depression, or PTSDs.[10] Unfortunately, strategies to identify susceptibility to these disorders, particularly PTSD, are lacking, which makes it difficult to implement intervention strategies to prevent the development of PTSD. The U.S. National Institute of Mental Health is currently funding a large, multisite consortium to collect data and evaluate the reliability of predictive models of PTSD symptom development.

Recently, Schultebraucks and colleagues have demonstrated the efficacy of their cross-validated algorithm that can predict the manifestation of nonremitting PTSD symptoms up to 12 months after the traumatic event with a high degree of accuracy. Their study relied on two independently collected prospective cohorts of trauma survivors who were recruited from two level 1 emergency trauma centers—one in Atlanta ($n = 377$), one in New York City ($n = 377$). The team performed 12 months of follow-ups on the Atlanta cohort to design the predictive algorithm involving 70 variables, and then externally validated it by performing 12 months of follow-ups on the New York City cohort. According to this study, "With these data, the algorithm achieved high discriminatory accuracy (area under the curve [AUC] = 0.84) to classify ED [emergency department] patients on a nonremitting symptom trajectory versus resilient ED patients in the model development sample. The high discriminatory performance was reproduced (AUC = 0.83) on the external validation dataset."[10] By using this model, the team correctly predicted which patients would go on to develop nonremitting PTSD symptoms 90% of the time, and only 5% of patients who were predicted to manifest nonremitting PTSD symptoms showed signs of resiliency after 12 months. Conversely, of those who were predicted to follow a resilient trajectory, 29% went on to develop nonremitting PTSD symptoms through 12 months.[10]

What this paper demonstrates is that data acquired by clinicians in an emergency setting, especially in the direct aftermath of a traumatic event, can offer crucial insights into the trajectory of patients' mental health months or even years down the line. Students should be learning how to utilize these kinds of algorithms to better predict and prevent posttraumatic sequelae, whether in a pandemic setting or not.

Clinicians and Mental Health Services

Medical professionals notoriously work long hours under grueling conditions and regularly witness events that people from outside the field of medicine would likely find deeply horrifying. For many, the fact that we continue to work diligently to help our patients despite these challenges is a source of pride. We appreciate being the empathetic rock whom others rely on during times of crisis while also projecting an aura of impenetrable stoicism when asked to open up about our own struggles. Even if we repeatedly tell our patients to seek out mental health services following trauma or tragedy and advise them not to feel ashamed for needing help, we ignore this advice when we hear it from a friend, family member, or colleague. We internalize the very stigma we are so wont to criticize in public.

For those of us who worked through the darkest days of the COVID-19 pandemic, the stress of being on the frontlines and worrying about potentially endangering our families, friends, and patients is something we will likely never forget. Whether or not one was infected with SARS-CoV-2, the experience was deeply harrowing. It was not just the magnitude of the pandemic weighing down upon emergency departments in places as disparate as New York City or South Dakota but the sense of helplessness and lack of agency that follows as a corollary. This is really one of the crucial elements of traumatic distress—not just feeling scared or shocked but feeling incapable of stopping the traumatic event from occurring.[11]

That the surges in COVID-19 cases have been so relentless, that they often inundated specific facilities with sick and dying patients for months on end, has made it difficult to feel as though one is in control. There have been days when it felt like we were trying to put out an inferno with water pistols.

To simply shrug off this overwhelming sense of helplessness or the fact that one had to witness such a wealth of human misery and chalk it up to being one of the drawbacks of practicing medicine is to ignore the severity of the situation. While it has been stated elsewhere in this book that pandemics should not be considered anomalous, no one should ever expect to see global death tolls in the millions when there is a novel infectious disease. No one can prepare to go through months where the world is completely turned upside down, while seeing friends and colleagues regularly stricken ill and the deaths of dozens of patients every day. To not at least occasionally feel psychologically crushed by the scope of the tragedy would require a callusing of the soul.

As many as 60% of medical professionals in the United States claim that pandemic stress has been detrimental to their mental health, and the figure is almost certainly higher among those who worked in emergency departments or hospitals located in areas where the pandemic has pushed the limits of what facilities can handle.[12] Distress levels among health care staff who cared for patients during outbreaks of novel viruses like severe acute respiratory syndrome in 2003, Middle East respiratory syndrome in 2012, and Ebola in 2014 have been found to be significantly higher than baseline for upward of 3 years following the outbreaks, and that staff was almost twice as likely to experience acute or posttraumatic stress compared with controls in a typical health care environment.[13] A meta-analysis of 65 studies involving over 97,000 health care workers from across 21 countries who worked during the COVID-19 pandemic found rates of depression, anxiety, and PTSD to be 21.7%, 22.1%, and 21.5%, respectively.[14] One online survey involving 1091 medical workers from Hubei Province found equally troubling figures, with rates of depression, anxiety, and PTSD being 56%, 53%, and 11%, respectively. Almost 80% of respondents said they were suffering from insomnia.[15]

Medical professionals, especially those who are regularly on the frontlines fighting against infectious diseases need more than just commendation for their service; they need to be given the tools to practice self-care and to know when they risk burnout. They need to learn to step back. This is not to say that we should avoid going the extra mile for the sake of our patients or that we should be far more risk adverse. Working as a medical professional entails a higher probability of risk than other occupations. However, we need to accept that there is a point where it is okay and even necessary to seek help when the stresses of the job have made it difficult for us to continue functioning at our best. Analogous to the need for rules regarding how many hours a resident works,[i] medical professionals should be trained to know when they are too stressed out to think clearly rather than being lionized for trudging their way from one shift to another.

This is largely a cultural phenomenon within the field of medicine, and it is something that can only be changed if we stop normalizing behaviors that encourage burnout early on—in residency and medical school. If one is taught that it is a sign of weakness to be unable to brush off the stresses of working in a hospital setting and that the valorized behavior is to be the strong and silent type, then this is going to discourage clinicians from seeking out mental health services for themselves. Even in normal circumstances, this can lead to burnout and anxiety, depressive, or substance use disorders. The latter is particularly common, and studies have repeatedly shown that medical professionals suffer from a higher rate of substance use disorder compared to all U.S. adults. As of 2014, substance use disorder was believed to affect 20.2 million adults in the United States (8.4% prevalence rate).[16] The lifetime rate among all medical professionals has been found to range between 10% and 15%.[17] For nurses, the prevalence rate may be as high as 20%.[18]

What these figures indicate is that medical professionals often prioritize their careers and providing patient care and that they may oftentimes neglect their own psychological well-being. This can lead to a lamentable case of tragic irony characterized by burnout and an inability to offer an optimal level of care. Seen in this light, self-care is an absolute necessity if the best patient care possible is our priority and our ethical duty, which it is.[19] Medical professionals typically have easy access to mental health services through their work. It is highly recommended they start using them to cope with the stresses of the COVID-19 Era and beyond.

Conclusion

Medical professionals should be given all the resources they need to do their jobs as effectively as possible, even during a pandemic. To accomplish this, their curriculum should include lessons on crisis management,

---

[i] As a consequence of the infamous Libby Zion case, New York State prevents residents from working more than 80 h/wk or 24 consecutive hours. Similar regulations were implemented by the Accreditation Council for Graduate Medical Education. These laws stem from a highly publicized case from 1984 involving two residents who were operating on very little sleep made and several critical errors that ultimately led to Zion's death.

palliative care, and the use of algorithms to predict postacute sequelae. Furthermore, the culture within the larger medical industry must recognize that widespread cases of burnout, excessive substance use, and psychiatric disorders are not necessarily occupational hazards but the consequences of a culture that does not prioritize self-care. To prepare the next generation of nurses and physicians to be better equipped to handle crisis scenarios, they need to also learn to recognize the utility of mental health services. Veteran medical professionals could encourage this behavior by leading by example.

REFERENCES

1. Cheng SO. Using online medical education beyond the COVID-19 pandemic—a commentary on "The coronavirus (COVID-19) pandemic: adaptions in medical education." *Int J Surg*. 2020;84:159-160. doi:10.1016/ijsu.2020.11.010
2. Brindley PG. Patient safety and acute care medicine: lessons for the future, insights from the past. *Crit Care*. 2010;14(2):217. doi:10.1186/cc8858
3. Takizawa PA, Honan L, Brissette D, Wu BJ, Wilkins KM. Teamwork in the time of COVID-19. *FASEB Bioadv*. 2020;3(3):175-181. doi:10.1096/fba.2020-00093
4. Hughes AM, Gregory ME, Joseph DL, et al. Saving lives: a meta-analysis of team training in healthcare. *J Appl Psychol*. 2016;101(9):1266-1304. doi:10.1037/apl0000120
5. Saravana-Bawan BB, Fulton C, Riley B, et al. Evaluating best methods for crisis resource management education: didactic teaching or noncontextual active learning. *Simul Healthc*. 2019;14(6):366-371. doi:10.1097/SIH.0000000000000388
6. Smith MB, Macieira TGR, Bumbach MD, et al. The use of simulation to teach nursing students and clinicians palliative care and end-of-life communication: a systematic review. *Am J Hosp Palliat Care*. 2018;35(8):1140-1154. doi:10.1177/1049909118761386
7. FAIR Health. *A Detailed Study of Patients With Long-Haul COVID: An Analysis of Private Healthcare Claims*. Published June 15, 2021. Accessed June 20, 2021. https://s3.amazonaws.com/media2.fairhealth.org/whitepaper/asset/A%20Detailed%20Study%20of%20Patients%20with%20Long-Haul%20COVID--An%20Analysis%20of%20Private%20Healthcare%20Claims--A%20FAIR%20Health%20White%20Paper.pdf
8. DiMaggio CJ, Avraham JB, Lee DC, Frangos SG, Wall SP. The epidemiology of emergency department trauma discharges in the United States. *Acad Emerg Med*. 2017;24(10):1244-1256. doi:10.1111/acem.13223
9. American Psychiatric Association. *Diagnostic and Statistical Manual on Mental Disorders*. 5th ed. The American Psychiatric Association; 2013.
10. Schultebraucks K, Shalev AY, Michopoulos V, et al. A validated predictive algorithm of post-traumatic stress course following emergency department admission after a traumatic stressor. *Nat Med*. 2020;26(7):1084-1088. doi:10.1038/s41591-020-0951-z
11. Volpicelli J, Balaraman G, Hahn J, Wallace H, Bux H. The role of uncontrollable trauma in the development of PTSD and alcohol addiction. *Alcohol Res Health*. 1999;23(4):256-262. PMCID:PMC6760386.
12. Wan W. Burned out by the pandemic, 3 in 10 health-care workers consider leaving the profession. *Washington Post*. Published April 22, 2021. Accessed June 22, 2021. https://www.washingtonpost.com/health/2021/04/22/health-workers-covid-quit/
13. Kisley S, Warren N, McMahon L, Dalais C, Henry I, Siskind D. Occurrence, prevention, and management of the psychological effects of emerging virus outbreaks on healthcare workers: rapid review and meta-analysis. *Br Med J*. 2020;369:m1642. doi:10.1136/bmj.m1642
14. Li Y, Scherer N, Felix L, Kuper H. Prevalence of depression, anxiety and post-traumatic stress disorder in health care workers during the COVID-19 pandemic: a systematic review and meta-analysis. *PLoS One*. 2021;16(3):e0246454. doi:10.1371/journal.pone.0246454

15. Guo WP, Min Q, Gu WW, et al. Prevalence of mental health problems in frontline healthcare workers after the first outbreak of COVID-19 in China: a cross-sectional study. *Health Qual Life Outcomes*. 2021;19:103. doi:10.1186/s12955-021-01743-7

16. Lipari RN, Van Horn SL. *Trends in Substance Use Disorders Among Adults Aged 18 or Older*. Substance Abuse and Mental Health Services Administration (SAMHSA); Published June 29, 2017. Accessed June 29, 2021. https://www.samhsa.gov/data/sites/default/files/report_2790/ShortReport-2790.html

17. Bohigian GM, Croughan JL, Sanders K. Substance abuse and dependence in physicians: an overview of the effects of alcohol and drug abuse. *Mo Med*. 1994;91(5):233-239. PMID:8041352.

18. Monroe T, Kenaga H. Don't ask don't tell: substance abuse and addiction among nurses. *J Clin Nurs*. 2011;20(3-4):504-509. doi:10.1111/j.1365-2702.2010.03518.x

19. Posluns K, Gall TL. Dear mental health practitioners, take care of yourselves: a literature review on self-care. *Int J Adv Couns*. 2020;42(1):1-20. doi:10.1007/s10447-019-09382-w

12

Moving Forward—How to Prepare for the Next Pandemic

Though the COVID-19 has been cataclysmic and led to an unthinkable number of deaths and created widespread havoc, we will have to decide how to move forward. This chapter reexamines some of the larger points made throughout the book and offers guidance as to how we can better prepare for the next pandemic.

Assessing the Damage

The COVID-19 pandemic did not just introduce new social problems; it also exacerbated existing ones that were already nearing a breaking point when the virus began to spread throughout the United States in late 2019 and early 2020. Apart from the fact that social isolation among seniors has been identified as a major problem,[1] there has been a steady increase in the prevalence of anxiety, mood, and substance use disorders, which were already known problems.[2] In addition, deaths due to suicides, overdoses, and out of despair have been on the rise.[3-5] Even metrics like average lifespan were on the decline in the United States.[6] More than half of US adults (51.8%) had at least one of ten of the following chronic conditions: arthritis, asthma, cancer, chronic obstructive pulmonary disease, coronary heart disease, diabetes,

234

hepatitis, hypertension, stroke, or weak/failing kidneys; and 27.2% of US adults had more than one of these conditions, up from 21.8% in 2001.[7]

To blame political affiliations, let alone a few individual politicians, for these psychosocial ills is misguided since these problems have been developing for at least a generation and cannot be resolved overnight by even the most expedient political solution. While many of these problems do relate to a persistent refusal to pay for regular maintenance of existing infrastructure (medical or otherwise) at the federal, state, and local levels, the overarching problem is that leaders of organizations both public and private share a tendency to see redundancy as waste because it is injurious to the bottom line and because the bottom line is given primacy over all other objectives. When one is dealing with issues related to the field of medicine, this means, ipso facto, that saving dollars often takes priority over preparing for pandemics, which is why hospitals were unable to rely on their own stockpiles of supplies when circumstances radically changed as they did in March and April 2020.[8] As discussed earlier (see *Chapter 5: Psychosocial and Economic Impact of COVID-19—A Nation Under Siege*), similar efforts to make supply chains more efficient rather than more adaptive and resilient to crisis left grocery stores' shelves barren.[9] Even in the second half of 2021, there are still shortages of a wide variety of consumer goods and manufacturing components.[10]

Similarly, many social problems are the results of sweeping structural changes that have roots in the reshaping of the American economy due to long-term trends like globalization and deindustrialization. Alterations to how supply chains are routed and how goods are manufactured go back over 60 years and, again, there is no one villain to blame for this process. Similarly, no one tech guru can be blamed for introducing new information technologies that have radically altered how we interface with one another and how we read and digest information.

Suffice to say, a thorough examination of all these factors is well beyond the scope of this book, but I believe that it is important to at least keep them in mind as we consider what steps we need to take moving forward to create more resilient social structures and to adopt or encourage healthier behaviors and lifestyles. Our goal should not be to return to a deeply flawed and untenable baseline but a new and improved world that is stronger and ultimately better for everyone.

Flattening the Curve

I would have hoped that as of this writing (September 2021) the worst aspects of the COVID-19 pandemic would have faded away in time. True, more people have been vaccinated or developed natural immunity following infection, case numbers have dropped (especially in areas with high vaccination rates), strict social distancing efforts have become unnecessary, and the pace of life prior to the pandemic is gradually resuming. However, considering the disparity in vaccination rates and masking policies in many areas of the United States, it now seems likely that COVID-19 will continue to be an endemic disease. It is something that we will have to live with for years to come, and there is no doubt that the world has been irrevocably changed by the pandemic and hopefully some lessons have been learned. Chief among them is that hopefully policymakers, officials, researchers, and most regular citizens will be far more vigilant about taking precautionary steps when another novel virus emerges. As we have learned time and time again, the longer we wait to mount a response to a threat, the worse it becomes.

We have enjoyed a long period of epidemiological tranquility that is outside of the norm of human history, and it seems as though the peace is about to be disturbed more regularly as wildlife habitats are increasingly encroached upon by humans throughout the world due to land-use changes such as deforestation. As a result, more contact between humans and wild animals—particularly in areas with a high biodiversity of mammals and birds—and increases in zoonotic spillovers will become inevitable, and, in fact, this is already happening.[11] Since 1980, new infectious diseases have emerged at a rate of about one every 8 months.[12] When this is combined with local health systems' inability to detect or monitor novel disease outbreaks and the increasing connectedness of the globalized world, it becomes clear that another pandemic might be on the horizon before we even know it.

Given these three factors (increasing animal-human interface through encroachment, poor local health systems, and ease of international transit), a team led by Michael Walsh, an epidemiologist at the University of Sydney's School of Public Health, has found that the zones with the highest potential for a spillover event are predominantly in sub-Saharan Africa, South Asia, and Southeast Asia.[11] To prevent high-impact spillovers, we need to improve conservation efforts, disincentivize the destruction of existing ecosystems, and invest in better health care and surveillance systems in these regions. These are, of course, long-term goals and will require coordination on an international level, but this is the only way to ensure that outbreaks are recognized early and contained before they can reach epidemic or pandemic levels.

Beyond this kind of monitoring, we need to remember that masking, social distancing, hand hygiene, and other recommendations do work to prevent the transmission of airborne pathogens like SARS-CoV-2. In some cases, these methods may help prevent the spread of a specific pathogen, such as influenza. As mentioned earlier (see Chapter 7, specifically

Individual Ethical Duties), the preventative measures that were taken to flatten the curve for COVID-19 disrupted the 2020 to 2021 flu season. Fewer than 2000 laboratory-confirmed cases (down from around 200,000 in an average year) were reported during that time.[13] Meanwhile, an estimated 600[i] Americans died of influenza during that flu season, down from an estimated average of 38,750.[14,15]

However, not every pathogen follows the same route of transmission, and different types of pathogens will require different preventative measures should the need arise. To mount an effective response against these pathogens, we will need to rely on public health directives which depend on improved and efficient communication to foster trust among the general population.

Restoring Trust

Primum non nocere: "first do no harm." Every physician holds the Hippocratic oath deeply inside their core and intends to practice based on that principle. The foundation of medical treatment is inherently built on trust. It goes without saying that people tend to trust their medical providers and make treatment decisions based on the assumption that clinicians are there to offer them the best available information that is objective, unbiased, and free of any slant influenced by affiliation with a political party or other group. We have been operating under this premise for generations. The important question to ask is what changed during this pandemic that led to the loss and breach of this trust.

One hypothesis to entertain is that the preventive and treatment guidelines for COVID-19 were stated as mandates rather than as suggestions or recommendations, which is antithetical to the physician-patient relationship where recommendations do not feel like demands, information is freely shared, and courses of action are subject to discussion that ultimately allow the individual to make the final decision after hearing all the facts. The mandates about masks and social distancing measures seemed to violate this two-way conversation, and instead, the information was perceived as being delivered in an authoritarian manner. Why some of the public came to believe opportunist pundits and others who claimed that these mandates were based on some ulterior motives or political

---

[i] As noted in footnotes in Chapters 1 and 7, the Centers for Disease Control and Prevention (CDC) estimates the number of influenza deaths each year and tends to add significant padding to that figure, and then revise it when a more accurate count is available later. It is also important to remember that the CDC's flu numbers also include pneumonia deaths. In other words, the figure of 600 deaths is an inflated estimate. Conversely, the figure 2000 refers to lab-confirmed cases. There were certainly a lot of cases that were not reported.

affiliations will be debated for a long time to come and are beyond the scope of this book. However, what is clear is that the general public did not trust these guidelines despite ample evidence of COVID-19's pathology, route of transmission, and the dangers associated with the illness. Public health officials must devise more effective ways of delivering information about safety measures during a public health crisis, especially when it is being rapidly updated, as was the case in the early days of the pandemic and even into fall 2021. Poor messaging can result in members of the public feeling frustrated and left in the dark, which can erode public trust in medical authorities and significantly hinder an effective response.

As much as one can sympathize with the public's skepticism, it is exceptionally dangerous in the time when coordinated action is needed. When we cannot trust one another or officials, it is almost like refusing to believe what our senses tell us, and this leaves us in a treacherous situation. More importantly, mounting a public health response on a larger scale—especially in big organizations, hospitals, or other complex systems—becomes impossible, as this kind of strategy (or nonstrategy) cannot succeed without an all-hands-on-deck approach.

How we restore faith in institutions like the Centers for Disease Control and Prevention (CDC), which was once renowned for their impartiality, medical expertise, and ability to solve seemingly insurmountable logistical problems, is a question I cannot answer.[16] How we restore trust in medicine and science is an even larger question that, once again, I oftentimes feel is too complex and laden with political land mines. However, for mental health professionals, clinicians of all types, and even people who have suddenly found it difficult to have a candid discussion with a friend or family member without it turning into a screaming match, what I can say is that a certain sense of stoicism is vital in these instances, and that one should make every effort to leave their politics at the door when discussing issues of medicine, risk analysis, and how one ought to behave during a pandemic. Our core objective should be to search out the truth and to present it as best and as thoroughly as we can when called upon to do so. Trying to put a thumb on the scale, even with the best of intentions, will ultimately erode trust and undermine whatever policies we believe should be implemented.

Improving Our Indoor Environments

We do not know how the next pandemic will spread, but regularly cleaning surfaces is certainly not a bad idea since it can prevent the spread of a host of common pathogens that may be viral, bacterial, or fungal and can discourage vectors (rodents and insects) from invading our spaces. However, rigorously scrubbing down surfaces has largely been an example of what one might call Hygiene Theater; meaning that it has been almost an entirely performative act that does little to flatten the curve and prevent COVID-19. As of April 2021, the CDC estimates that the risk of being infected with SARS-CoV-2 via fomite transmission is less than 1 in 10,000.[17] However, if the objective is to prevent the spread of SARS-CoV-2 or another virus that follows similar transmission dynamics, there are far more productive means of doing so. One of those ways is to improve the air quality within indoor spaces.

While indoor air quality may not seem germane to a discussion of pandemics, the health of one's indoor environment plays an enormous role in determining levels of respiratory and overall fitness simply because we spend so much time indoors. As Joseph G. Allen and John D. Macomber note in their book *Healthy Buildings*, the average person living in the United States spends upward of 90% of their life indoors. This means that the average 40-year-old American has spent 36 years of their life in an indoor environment.[18] Rich Corsi, an engineering and computer science expert at Portland State University, provides a far more colorful way of digesting this datum: "Americans spend more time inside buildings than some whale species spend underwater."[18]

The analysis performed by Allen and Macomber focuses on how exposure to poor indoor air quality consisting of various particles, environmental toxins, and pathogens (mold and fungi) that are not whisked away by proper ventilation systems can seep into our living spaces and adversely affect cognitive performance and make us more susceptible to certain kinds of chronic illnesses. Similar principles apply to viral pathogens, as well. As discussed earlier (see *Chapter 2: Transmission of SARS-CoV-2*), evidence strongly indicates that SARS-CoV-2 and other respiratory viruses, including influenza, are most certainly spread by short-range, large-droplet transmission but that they may also spread via airborne transmission when specific conditions are met.[19]

There is some but not a great deal of evidence of apartment-to-apartment transfer. Of note, toilet flushing has been implicated in the aerosolization of the pathogen via fecal matter.[20] As many apartment lavatories, particularly in older multifamily structures, use communal ducts for ventilation, this could be an infrequent, but possible route of transmission. An outbreak involving apartment-to-apartment transmission via one such natural ventilation shaft was reported in Seoul, South Korea.[21] Similarly, models dating back before the COVID Era have shown a significant amount of air transfer between apartments in multiunit residential buildings (the study in question was examining the behavior of cigarette smoke between units). The amount of air in one apartment that can be traced back to a neighboring unit has been found to range from 2.1% inside a newer condominium building to as high as 35.3% in a 1930s duplex.[22]

The good news is that the technology already exists to resolve this problem and will require installing sensors capable of monitoring air quality, improving ventilation, and enhancing air filtration systems. Multifamily owners will likely be reluctant to make these improvements in rental units unless required by legislation and incentivized with tax abatements or measures that pass at least part of the cost onto taxpayers since making these kinds of improvements to our indoor environments will not be cheap. However, the economic losses of even an average flu season cost the United States $11.2 billion (due primarily to reductions in productivity and absenteeism). The monthly global cost of COVID-19 has been estimated to be $1 trillion.[23] Factor in the loss of life and turmoil caused by the pandemic, and it becomes clear that the cost of taking preventative steps is not only the most ethical option; it is the more economically prudent one.

Corporations may be willing to cover part of these costs, particularly in office buildings. As Allen and Macomber contend in *Healthy Buildings*, the effect of reduced indoor air quality on cognitive function and alertness is well documented. In fact, most people have experienced it firsthand since just about everyone has been in a poorly ventilated space at least once in their lifetimes. One of the most notable issues in these environments is that levels of carbon dioxide can increase significantly. While these levels do not come anywhere close to life-threatening, they can reduce one's executive functioning and ability to focus. Poorly ventilated rooms can also make occupants feel drowsy. If you walked onto an airplane prior to the pandemic and suddenly felt the urge to sleep while waiting for the plane to start taxiing to the runway, the reason was because many planes did not turn on their ventilation systems until pulling away from the gate. In other words, you went from a relatively well-ventilated environment (the airport) to an environment with significantly higher levels of carbon dioxide (the stationary airplane). A similar phenomenon occurs when you sit in any poorly ventilated space for long periods of time.[18] Consequently, should there be additional urban air pollutants in high enough concentrations, they may also contribute to the kinds of chronic and mild inflammatory responses discussed in Chapter 5 (see *Environmental and Dietary Stressors*).[24] As a result, just by making improvements to air quality that cost employers a fraction of their total utility costs, employers can expect to see both a productivity boost and reduced absenteeism, which means increases to bottom-line net income.[18]

Studies that have examined the effects of improved air quality in schools have found similar results. Children show improved cognitive performance in better-ventilated areas.[25] They also report fewer instances of illness-related absenteeism.[26] While spending billions of dollars to retrofit every classroom in the United States may not be feasible, plug-in air filters that typically cost around $700 per unit appear more than capable of reducing up to 90% airborne pollutants and can even reduce the level of virus-containing aerosol particles.[27]

While these kinds of recommendations certainly sit outside of my technical expertise, it seems as though improving indoor air quality and ventilation may help reduce the severity of the next pandemic or possibly even avoid the kind of shutdowns that have characterized the COVID Era, while also improving the cognitive performance of workers and students. It seems like a win-win situation.

Improving Our Habits

As explored in Chapter 5 (see *Environmental and Dietary Stressors*), stress, excessive substance use, and poor diet may also contribute to inflammation, which can lead to dysregulation of innate and adaptive immune responses. Consequently, this may mean a worse prognosis for either COVID-19 or another pathogen.

Individuals can minimize these risks by adhering to healthy lifestyle changes such as a diet that incorporates more fresh produce, whole grains, and less processed foods. In addition, other elements that may help include reducing in the use of tobacco, alcohol, and other substances, as well as incorporating relaxation techniques such as breathing exercises, yoga, and meditation. These lifestyle changes are an individual's responsibility, but organizations can play a vital role in encouraging healthier routines by creating an environment that discourages employees from overworking because there is a clear correlation between job strain and working overtime on the one hand, and an unhealthy diet, a lack of exercise, obesity, cigarette smoking, and heavy alcohol use, on the other.[28] All of this is associated with the constant engagement of the sympathetic nervous system that was discussed in Chapter 5 (see *Stress*), but it is also just a matter of simple math. If you are forced to work 14 hours per day or are expected to stay up until 3 AM in the morning working on a project and to be ready to go at 9 AM, then you simply cannot get a good night of sleep and will not have time to exercise because you feel exhausted. Similarly, if you do not have time to eat a healthy meal, you will likely eat something on the run, which will almost certainly be heavily processed and loaded with sugar, fat, and calories.

Moreover, you could develop a vitamin D deficiency because you spend all your time indoors in front of a computer instead of outside in the sun.

There are reports that more people appear to be extricating themselves from these deeply unhealthy working conditions,[29] which are positive signs, but I believe employers should take steps to discourage this kind of unhealthy behavior, too. For one, they should clamp down on managers who send unnecessary emails, especially to employees when they are not on the clock. Even if you are not expecting a response, it takes up a serious amount of mental real estate and triggers what is known as the Zeigarnik effect, which is really just a description of the sense of frustration and anxiousness that unfinished business evokes in all of us. It is the nagging thought of maybe I should get on this task that may keep some employees up at night.

Separately, organizations can also create platforms or a space that will allow people to form bonds and support networks. Lifestyle changes are not easily made alone and being part of a larger network can help keep you motivated or help with a high-stress job. Furthermore, being part of a larger group can help fight feelings of loneliness, even if these are virtual networks.

Reducing Loneliness

Minimizing loneliness can also help individuals prepare for the next pandemic or any stressful situation. As noted in Chapter 8 (see *Loneliness*), loneliness is associated with depression and anxiety, as well as cardiovascular diseases, stroke, and pain disorders like fibromyalgia.[30-32] People who are lonely may also be far worse at coping with trauma than those who perceive themselves as being connected to a social network.[33,34] Reaching out to family and support networks in the wake of the pandemic and afterward is going to be necessary to avoid a public health crisis, and it may not require the expansion of telemedicine to a significant degree.

One relatively easy way to do this is to simply call people who sign up to receive phone calls. A study conducted by Dr. Maninder Kahlon at the University of Texas and published in February 2021 found that clients of Meals on Wheels Central Texas who received regular phone calls reported lower levels of loneliness, anxiety, and depression than controls.[35] This study was conducted in July and August 2020 to better understand how the Meals on Wheels clients had responded to reductions in contact with others. Those who received the calls were predominately female (79%), living alone (56%), and had seen a decrease in the frequency of contact they were accustomed to due to COVID (66%). The racial breakdown of the participants in the study was 22% Hispanic, 38% African American, and 43% White, with a median age of 69.4 years. A total of 107 participants were able to complete the 5-week study.

The study design was planned in a manner so that phone calls were scheduled at a time that was requested by participants. These calls were targeted to be around 10 minutes in length but were allowed to go longer depending on the participant's preference. During the first week of the study, the participants received five calls, and then were given the opportunity to choose the frequency of the calls between the range of two and five per week, and to no surprise, the majority opted for five calls per week.

What is interesting about this study is that those who called the participants were just volunteers and not credentialed physicians or therapists. They had essentially no training beyond being taught empathetic conversational techniques (defined as "prioritizing listening and eliciting conversation from the participant on topics of their choice") during one 2-hour session.[35] The 16 callers received a $200 stipend at the end of the study.

What is unique and important about this program is that it can be replicated and deployed elsewhere at very little cost. Furthermore, it employs a technology that the vast majority of seniors and individuals with disabilities are capable of using. This study also highlights how we can reach potentially vulnerable individuals without being intrusive and circles back to the issue of restoring trust. Simply put, by partnering with groups like Meals on Wheels or houses of worship who provide vital services to the community, one can have their representatives introduce the program to such clients. The take-home message of this study is that if the participants hear about such services from a trusted source, rather than a stranger, it is far more likely that they will be willing to take part in the program.

These phone calls can serve as an outreach to get the ball rolling for those who are struggling with mental health issues but are reluctant to seek help. Risk of embarrassment and internalized stigma are obstacles to seeking help from mental health professionals but similar hesitancies may not apply when receiving a phone call from a volunteer. If these calls make the participant feel not only less lonely but also less anxious or less depressed, they may realize the utility of talk therapy, which may encourage additional help-seeking behaviors.

Improving How We Talk About Mental Health

As the expression goes, people tend to wear their stress on their sleeve. To run with this metaphor, many see their high-stress job as a badge of honor. If you can handle the stress, then it legitimizes your success, it justifies your salary, it makes you feel as though you are an exceptional person who can do what others cannot. There is a certain amount of glamor in the idea of the researcher spending night after night rifling through data just waiting to connect the dots and come to a brilliant discovery or the academic digging through dusty archives in search of some arcane nugget of wisdom.

As discussed in Chapter 11 (*Clinicians and Mental Health Services*), this work ethic is an admirable quality in a person, but it needs to be balanced with the recognition that we cannot be these things all the time. As erosion grinds down the largest mountains over the millennia, so too do the stresses of always being "on" wear down the mental fortitude of even the most seasoned soldiers, workers, and clinicians. Not only do we need to recognize our own limitations; we also need to acknowledge just how difficult this pandemic has been on each one of us and our colleagues and that pathologies that arise out of these traumatic experiences do not come from a place of weakness.

This kind of thinking needs to be universally extended and accepted. While it is a stretch to say that every American worker needs some kind of critical-incident stress debriefing, it is safe to say that we need to become more comfortable talking about our mental health without fear of being mocked or having our careers suffer. The COVID Era has placed an immense amount of stress on individuals from all age groups and walks of life. For those who worked on the frontlines, the stress often stemmed from the fear of interacting with the sick individuals and contracting the virus. For those who worked at home, the stress often stemmed from the anxiety and fear associated with social isolation. Talking about these anxieties and fears helps us process them and may ultimately allow us to emerge from the COVID Era happier, healthier, and less stressed-out.

Conclusion

We have the opportunity to use the lessons that we learned from the COVID-19 pandemic to improve how we respond to the next pandemic and to improve some of the social, economic, and psychosocial factors that negatively impact individuals' mental health, as well as their ability to potentially ward off the disease, but none of us can do this alone. We need to be able to ask for help when we need it, to work together to solve major problems, and to embrace an ethos of trust and cooperation.

We need to recognize more than just shared humanity, but the fact that we can only become human through culture and that community is essential for culture. This core concept that has been celebrated by many individual thinkers, as well as in many cultures and religions throughout the world, but is perhaps most succinctly expressed in the Bantu philosophy of humanity or "Ubuntu" (to use the Zulu word), which translates into "I am because we are." It is the acknowledgment that we suffer when the community suffers, that we thrive when the community thrives. This level of cooperation will require not just an international effort but also an interdisciplinary one. Medical professionals and public health officials oftentimes think solely in terms of saving lives, and, consequently, may fail to take into account the importance of economic, social, and psychological impacts of given policies. Conversely, those who focus on the economic, social, or psychosocial effects on things like mental health or financial independence may develop policies through a lens that does not adequately prioritize public health or the fact that hospitals have limited resources and cannot be indefinitely stretched to their breaking points. In different ways, these are all myopic positions, which is why sober planning and compromise can provide the best opportunity to achieve the most comprehensive and balanced response. As we prepare for the next pandemic, we should not only take precautionary steps like those highlighted above but encourage a dialogue among people from a diverse set of academic disciplines and backgrounds rather than siloing expertise and creating echo chambers among practitioners within individual fields.

To return to the words of Parmet and Rothstein and their article on the 1918 influenza pandemic from 2018: "Today, three of the leading threats to global public health are attitudinal: hubris, isolationism, and distrust."[36] They stand in direct opposition to the concept of Ubuntu noted above, and it is these three threats that we need to resolve if we are to prevent the next pandemic. If we are to solve the world's biggest problems, we need to approach them together with humility, compassion, and in good faith.

REFERENCES

1. The National Academies of Sciences, Engineering, and Medicine. *Social Isolation and Loneliness in Older Adults: Opportunities for the Health Care System*. The National Academies Press; 2020.
2. *Household Pulse Survey*. Centers for Disease Control and Prevention website. Accessed April 6, 2021. https://www.cdc.gov/nchs/covid19/pulse/mental-health.htm
3. *Suicide*. National Institute of Mental Health website. Accessed April 5, 2021. https://www.nimh.nih.gov/health/statistics/suicide.shtml
4. Hedegaard H, Miniño AM, Warner M. *Drug Overdose Deaths in the United States, 1999-2019*. NCHS Data Brief No. 394, December 2020. Accessed April 5, 2021. https://www.cdc.gov/nchs/products/databriefs/db394.htm
5. Bower B. 'Deaths of despair' are rising. It's time to define despair. *Science News*. Published November 2, 2020. Accessed June 29, 2021. https://www.sciencenews.org/article/deaths-of-despair-depression-mental-health-covid-19-pandemic
6. Carroll L. U.S. life expectancy declining due to more deaths in middle age. *Reuters*. Published November 26, 2019. Accessed June 29, 2021. https://www.reuters.com/article/us-health-life-expectancy/u-s-life-expectancy-declining-due-to-more-deaths-in-middle-age-idUSKBN1Y02C7

7. Boersma P, Black LI, Ward BW. Prevalence of multiple chronic conditions among US adults, 2018. *Prev Chronic Dis*. 2020;17:e106. doi:10.5888/pcd17.200130

8. Lagu T, Werner R, Artenstein AW. Why don't hospitals have enough masks. Because coronavirus broke the market. *Washington Post*. Published May 21, 2020. Accessed June 29, 2021. https://www.washingtonpost.com/outlook/2020/05/21/why-dont-hospitals-have-enough-masks-because-coronavirus-broke-market/

9. Shih WC. Global supply chains in a post-pandemic world: companies need to make their networks more resilient. Here's how. *Harv Bus Rev*. Published September-October 2020. Accessed February 18, 2021. https://hbr.org/2020/09/global-supply-chains-in-a-post-pandemic-world

10. Goodman PS, Bradsher K. The world is still short of everything. Get used to it. *New York Times*. Published August 30, 2021. Accessed September 12, 2021. https://www.nytimes.com/2021/08/30/business/supply-chain-shortages.html

11. Walsh MG, Sawleshwarkar S, Hossain S, Mor SM. Whence the next pandemic? The intersecting global geography of the animal-human interface, poor health systems and air transit centrality reveals conduits of high-impact spillover. *One Health*. 2020;11:100177. doi:10.1016/j.onehlt.2020.100177

12. Karesh WB, Cook RA, Bennett EL, Newcomb J. Wildlife trade and global disease emergence. *Emerg Infect Dis*. 2005;11(7):1000-1002. doi:10.3201/eid1107.050194

13. Dunn L. After year with virtually no flu, scientists worry the next season could be a bad one. *NBC News*. Published May 9, 2021. Accessed June 19, 2021. https://www.nbcnews.com/health/health-news/after-year-virtually-no-flu-scientists-worry-next-season-could-n1266534

14. McCarthy N. How many Americans die from the flu each year? [Infographic]. *Forbes*. Published October 7, 2020. Accessed June 19, 2021. https://www.forbes.com/sites/niallmccarthy/2020/10/07/how-many-americans-die-from-the-flu-each-year-infographic/?sh=7ba6ee5913ea

15. Faust JS. Comparing COVID-19 deaths to flu deaths is like comparing apples to oranges. *Scientific American*. Published April 28, 2020. Accessed June 19, 2021. https://blogs.scientificamerican.com/observations/comparing-covid-19-deaths-to-flu-deaths-is-like-comparing-apples-to-oranges/

16. Interlandi J. Can the C.D.C. be fixed? *New York Times*. Published June 16, 2021. Accessed June 20, 2021. https://www.nytimes.com/2021/06/16/magazine/cdc-covid-response.html

17. *Science Brief: SARS-CoV-2 and Surface (Fomite) Transmission for Indoor Community Environments*. CDC website. Updated April 5, 2021. Accessed May 18, 2021. https://www.cdc.gov/coronavirus/2019-ncov/more/science-and-research/surface-transmission.html

18. Allen JG, Macomber JD. *Healthy Buildings: How Indoor Spaces Drive Performance and Productivity*. Harvard University Press; 2020.

19. Tellier R, Li Y, Cowling BJ, Tang JW. Recognition of aerosol transmission of infectious agents: a commentary. *BMC Infect Dis*. 2019;19(101):1-9. doi:10.1186/s12879-019-3707-y

20. Tang S, Mao Y, Jones RM, et al. Aerosol transmission of SARS-CoV-2? Evidence, prevention and control. *Environ Int*. 2020;144:106039. doi:10.1016/j.envint.2020.106039

21. Hwang SE, Chang JH, Oh B, Heo J. Possible aerosol transmission of COVID-19 associated with an outbreak in an apartment in Seoul, South Korea, 2020. *Int J Infect Dis*. 2021;104:73-76. doi:10.1016/j.ijid.2020.12.035

22. Bohac DL, Hewett MJ, Hammond SK, Grimsrud DT. Secondhand smoke transfer and reduction by air sealing and ventilation in multiunit buildings: PET and nicotine verification. *Indoor Air*. 2011;21(1):36-44. doi:10.1111/j.1600-0668.2010.00680.x

23. Saey TH. Cleaning indoor air may prevent COVID-19's spread. But it's harder than it looks. *Science News*. Published May 18, 2021. Accessed May 18, 2021. https://www.sciencenews.org/article/coronavirus-covid-air-spread-indoor-clean-ventilation-filtration

24. Schmidt S. Brain fog: does air pollution make us less productive? *Environ Health Perspect*. 2019;127(5):52001. doi:10.1289/EHP4869

25. Marcotte DE. Something in the air? Air quality and children's educational outcomes. *Econ Educ Rev*. 2017;56:141-151. doi:10.1016/j.econedurev.2016.12.003

26. Mendell MJ, Eliseeva EA, Davies MM, et al. Association of classroom ventilation with reduced illness absence: a prospective study in California elementary schools. *Indoor Air.* 2013;23(6):515-528. doi:10.1111/ina.12042

27. Gilraine M. The importance of clean air in classrooms—during the pandemic and beyond. *Brookings.* Accessed June 29, 2021. Published October 28, 2020. https://www.brookings.edu/blog/brown-center-chalkboard/2020/10/28/the-importance-of-clean-air-in-classrooms-during-the-pandemic-and-beyond/

28. Siegrist J, Rödel A. Work stress and health risk behavior. *Scand J Work Environ Health.* 2006;32(6):473-481. doi:10.5271/sjweh.1052

29. Youn S. America's workers are exhausted and burned out—and some employers are taking notice. *Washington Post.* Published June 29, 2021. Accessed June 29, 2021. https://www.washingtonpost.com/business/2021/06/28/employee-burnout-corporate-america/

30. Banerjee D, Rai M. Social isolation in COVID-19: the impact of loneliness. *Int J Soc Psychiatry.* 2020;66(6):525-527. doi:10.1177/0020764020922269

31. Valtorta NK, Kanaan M, Gilbody S, Ronzi S, Hanratty B. Loneliness and social isolation as risk factors for coronary disease and stroke: systematic review and meta-analysis of longitudinal observational studies. *Heart.* 2016;102(13):1009-1016. doi:10.1136/heartjnl-2015-308790

32. Wolf LD, Davis MC. Loneliness, daily pain, and perceptions of interpersonal events in adults with fibromyalgia. *Health Psychol.* 2014;33(9):929-937.

33. Feder A, Ahmad S, Lee EJ, et al. Coping and PTSD symptoms in Pakistani earthquake survivors: purpose in life, religious coping and social support. *J Affect Disord.* 2013;147(1-3):156-163. doi:10.1016/j.jad.2012.10.027

34. Lee JS. Perceived social support functions as a resilience in buffering the impact of trauma exposure on PTSD symptoms via intrusive rumination and entrapment in firefighters. *PLoS One.* 2019;14(8):e0220454. doi:10.1371/journal.pone.0220454

35. Kahlon MK, Aksan N, Aubrey R, et al. Effect of layperson-delivered, empathy-focused program of telephone calls on loneliness, depression, and anxiety among adults during the COVID-19 pandemic. *JAMA Psychiatry.* 2021;78:616-622. doi:10.1001/jamapsychiatry.2021.0113

36. Parmet WE, Rothstein MA. The 1918 influenza pandemic: lessons learned and not—introduction to the special section. *Am J Public Health.* 2018;108(11):1435-1436. doi:10.2105/AJPH.2018.304695

APPENDIX

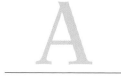

A

As of September 15, 2021, there have been over 225 million confirmed cases of COVID-19 globally. An estimated 4.65 million people have died. Vaccine rates are rising steadily. Globally, 42.4% of individuals have been at least partially vaccinated, while 30.25% of individuals are now fully vaccinated. This appendix shows how the pandemic affected individual countries using the most recent data, as of September 15, 2021, from Our World in Data (https://ourworldindata.org/coronavirus), which has been a phenomenal resource since the earliest days of the pandemic. I have also noted the estimated prevalence of the Delta variant in countries when that information is available since it has emerged as a troubling sign that SARS-CoV-2 may be more protean than we feared. The information about individual states comes from the *New York Times'* COVID-19 page (https://www.nytimes.com/interactive/2021/us/covid-cases.html) and is recent as of September 15, 2021.

Cases per 100,000	Total Fatalities	Fatalities per 100,000	At Least One Dose (%)	Full Vaccination (%)	Estimated Prevalence of Delta Variant (%)
2867.554	4.65 million	59.041	42.4	30.25	N/A
387.042	7171	18.002	0.02	1.08	N/A
5514.606	2553	88.864	31.36	24.69	N/A
449.447	5614	12.583	13.03	9.36	N/A
19,519.353	130	168.059	66.71	54.08	N/A
150.432	1358	4.002	4.45	2.82	6.67
2333.685	48	48.618	44.24	36.17	N/A

Cases per 100,000	Total Fatalities	Fatalities per 100,000	At Least One Dose (%)	Full Vaccination (%)	Estimated Prevalence of Delta Variant (%)
11,467.501	113,816	249.565	63.06	40.53	37.25
8416.18	5034	169.602	7.25	4.06	N/A
N/A	N/A	N/A	75.03	68.26	100
304.573	1116	4.328	55.17	34.33	100
7887.463	10,849	119.97	62.16	58.77	100
4532.04	6167	60.323	44.31	30.81	N/A
4938.349	463	116.65	26.64	16.61	N/A
15,667.608	1388	79.392	66.24	62.95	95.83
922.675	27,007	16.24	12.71	8.45	100
2103.869	52	18.074	42.28	33.54	N/A
5364.801	3941	41.735	17.92	14.75	N/A
10,420.144	25,477	219.019	73.11	71.16	100
4437.228	383	94.588	43.53	20.06	N/A
172.275	146	1.173	1.23	0.34	N/A
N/A	N/A	N/A	69.86	68.51	N/A
332.863	3	0.385	72.72	61.3	N/A
4188.411	18,603	157.214	34.88	25.09	N/A
6831.004	10,099	309.457	19.43	13.06	N/A
6909.78	2337	97.487	14.82	9.11	99.18
9822.651	587,797	274.68	67.17	35.26	44.58
1003.551	21	4.756	53.54	32.2	N/A
6891.732	19,744	286.284	15.79	18.12	97.86
64.934	171	0.796	0.77	0.48	N/A
115.777	38	0.31	N/A	N/A	N/A
594.756	2058	12.144	67.8	57.61	41.05

(*Continued*)

(Continued)

Cases per 100,000	Total Fatalities	Fatalities per 100,000	At Least One Dose (%)	Full Vaccination (%)	Estimated Prevalence of Delta Variant (%)
309.32	1357	4.984	1.34	0.3	N/A
4106.196	27,315	71.753	74.73	68.66	97.56
6530.332	323	57.483	48.5	16.91	N/A
229.858	100	2.032	2.09	0.2	N/A
29.672	174	1.029	0.47	0.11	N/A
8561.321	37,253	193.901	75.56	72.5	27.91
6.611	4636	0.321	75.82	67.15	100
9622.388	125,713	245.218	47.79	30.71	20
461.475	147	16.546	19.67	17.96	N/A
242.195	183	3.235	3.52	1.96	N/A
9665.905	5851	113.854	61.19	33.61	70.91
215.224	534	1.974	4.41	1.01	N/A
9433.816	8456	207.171	43.19	40.49	98.59
6724.631	6449	56.983	62.13	38.04	N/A
13,118.62	534	60.135	66.15	60.51	N/A
15,700.44	30,416	283.611	56.11	54.65	99.17
60.853	1068	1.156	0.09	0.03	N/A
6098.272	2616	45	76.3	74.09	99.95
1187.092	157	15.666	3.85	2.6	N/A
3649.615	8	11.085	31.77	28.35	N/A
3230.749	4020	36.7	54.08	43.54	N/A
2824.601	32,448	181.39	59.81	53.78	36.67
281.945	16,895	16.205	7.16	4.73	N/A
1529.508	3043	46.682	59.23	48.32	N/A

Cases per 100,000	Total Fatalities	Fatalities per 100,000	At Least One Dose (%)	Full Vaccination (%)	Estimated Prevalence of Delta Variant (%)
724.054	131	9.035	14.33	10.97	N/A
184.953	40	1.111	N/A	N/A	N/A
11,119.705	1313	99.08	56.06	43.43	94.81
3845.547	1186	101.163	15.41	14.76	N/A
276.034	5001	4.243	1.98	0.85	N/A
5453.988	539	59.697	63.13	37.9	N/A
2420.625	1052	18.961	73.57	56.83	99.74
10,371.514	116,454	172.36	73.35	63.26	96.77
1180.563	173	7.592	3.7	2.73	N/A
395.989	328	13.189	7.23	6.67	98.55
14,700.235	8287	208.228	22.97	15.58	N/A
4889.427	92,776	110.579	66.11	61.86	100
390.374	1098	3.46	2.73	1.28	94.55
5981.777	14,268	137.579	60.75	56.61	90.08
2341.282	35	30.969	25.23	17.37	N/A
2826.081	12,795	70.11	21.19	10.05	65.15
222.897	368	2.727	7.01	3.18	N/A
299.232	127	6.301	1.39	0.15	N/A
3572.436	692	87.559	42.64	22.15	N/A
184.297	596	5.164	0.32	0.12	N/A
3514.272	9370	93.113	29.29	16.79	N/A
8468.313	30,102	312.451	60.69	57.64	N/A
3293.045	33	9.611	81.75	78.43	100
2391.025	443,497	31.828	41.03	12.99	95.88
1510.417	139,415	50.447	26.87	15.4	100

(*Continued*)

(Continued)

Cases per 100,000	Total Fatalities	Fatalities per 100,000	At Least One Dose (%)	Full Vaccination (%)	Estimated Prevalence of Delta Variant (%)
6281	115,167	135.445	26.98	14.24	N/A
4758.135	21,596	52.444	8.95	4.99	N/A
7399.54	5155	103.454	75.06	71.32	99.49
13,592.872	7438	84.621	68.88	63.29	98.18
7641.887	130,027	215.393	72.76	64.51	100
2589.137	1736	58.383	16.34	5.94	N/A
1310.887	16,919	13.422	64.7	52.39	97.37
7882.377	10,568	102.912	35.03	30.42	N/A
4850.971	15,031	79.132	37.52	31.3	N/A
444.443	4928	8.962	4.13	1.51	100
1.648	0	0	18.8	5.23	N/A
8155.015	2833	146.577	36.11	19.09	N/A
9492.803	2434	56.231	61.64	21.33	98.46
2674.996	2576	38.863	11.3	8.15	N/A
239.614	16	0.217	35.92	25.21	N/A
7916.081	2621	140.391	47.32	42.51	N/A
9080.725	8210	121.286	21.61	17.35	100
666.723	403	18.666	3.32	1.49	N/A
110.555	245	4.73	2.02	0.53	N/A
4690.209	4457	64.051	17.27	1.73	N/A
8861.818	60	156.846	61.6	54.74	N/A
11,519.364	4721	175.511	63.52	58.71	100
12,112.839	834	131.377	65.68	5.96	80.93
150.904	958	3.37	0.74	0.3	N/A

Cases per 100,000	Total Fatalities	Fatalities per 100,000	At Least One Dose (%)	Full Vaccination (%)	Estimated Prevalence of Delta Variant (%)
311.339	2244	11.421	3.69	2.35	97.87
6136.893	21587	65.862	66.06	53.86	98.94
15,280.895	227	41.757	71.66	59.54	100
71.879	543	2.604	1.36	0.41	98.33
7160.042	449	87.258	81.11	80.95	N/A
6.709	0	0	38	32	N/A
733.847	760	15.916	5.97	0.45	N/A
1082.276	45	3.534	65.03	59.94	N/A
2709.129	267,969	206.519	46.96	30.59	99.42
0.86	0	0	38	33	N/A
6876.225	6548	162.723	14.24	18.35	N/A
8309.717	33	83.502	66.93	57.72	N/A
7830.788	1056	31.719	67.5	63.59	N/A
19,604.936	1813	288.671	35.55	31.52	89.83
2432.331	13,683	36.64	53.25	43.88	N/A
464.757	1895	5.892	5.11	2.37	100
796.495	16,693	30.458	8.13	3.28	N/A
4886.478	3437	132.839	8.62	5.02	N/A
N/A	N/A	N/A	70.01	66.69	N/A
2626.77	10,984	37.014	19.8	17.67	97.44
11,713.504	18,469	107.546	70.16	63.46	99.84
81.923	27	0.555	60.44	30.99	100
194.334	202	3.014	7.11	3.86	N/A
23.604	201	0.8	1.61	0.35	N/A
94.634	2637	1.247	1.9	0.8	93.41

(Continued)

(Continued)

Cases per 100,000	Total Fatalities	Fatalities per 100,000	At Least One Dose (%)	Full Vaccination (%)	Estimated Prevalence of Delta Variant (%)
N/A	N/A	N/A	N/A	N/A	N/A
8848.151	6307	302.834	36.57	30.55	N/A
3265.516	829	15.168	72.81	63.55	100
5805.115	4090	78.302	49.63	27.64	N/A
538.548	26,938	11.962	23.45	10.16	100
11.005	0	0	97	83	N/A
7175.675	3837	73.467	22.69	9.36	N/A
10,554.336	7141	162.978	65.57	47.52	N/A
203.334	204	2.237	1.13	0.35	N/A
6363.073	16,114	223.197	33.78	25.38	N/A
6481.81	198,840	596.054	36.61	26.59	34.02
2046.038	35,529	31.995	16.84	15.62	N/A
7657.896	75,433	199.574	51.76	50.65	99.23
10,396.42	17,872	175.768	86.95	81.54	100
8015.461	604	20.611	80.54	75.7	74.14
5889.771	35,132	183.67	27.83	27.26	100
4847.322	190,793	130.759	31.64	27.35	98.77
704.756	1180	8.888	13.72	7.54	76.6
2820.005	8	14.94	46.32	40.93	N/A
5407.238	132	71.583	19.93	15.06	N/A
2265.681	13	11.683	17.54	11.36	N/A
1.499	0	0	48.48	22.75	N/A
15,874.743	90	264.628	71.53	71.53	N/A
1288.032	42	18.803	20.19	5.4	N/A

Cases per 100,000	Total Fatalities	Fatalities per 100,000	At Least One Dose (%)	Full Vaccination (%)	Estimated Prevalence of Delta Variant (%)
1544.478	8610	24.363	64.76	48.52	N/A
427.493	1837	10.683	6.86	3.29	N/A
12,210.629	7601	111.704	43.82	41.84	N/A
20,819.937	106	107.168	75.54	71.68	N/A
78.439	121	1.486	2.22	0.49	N/A
1240.206	58	0.984	78.78	75.97	100
7310.713	12,562	230.043	44.09	40.51	100
13,366.524	4473	215.18	50.21	45.43	99.83
2.841	0	0	9.6	3.05	N/A
113.5	1032	6.308	1.37	0.71	N/A
4770.884	85,302	142.071	18.38	12.45	99.48
541.834	2380	4.639	67.4	40.37	98.75
103.283	121	1.063	0.48	0.1	N/A
10,521.989	85,548	183.009	79.67	75.76	97.27
2283.807	11,567	53.807	63.05	49.65	98.99
84.506	2873	6.397	1.44	0.76	N/A
5852.842	773	130.619	36.17	26.43	16
11,236.763	14,729	144.968	69.27	61.23	99.94
9363.898	10,974	125.914	59.63	52.24	99.75
163.085	2090	11.436	1.1	1.1	N/A
67.483	839	3.517	47.97	4.45	N/A
179.33	125	1.282	22.24	13.11	N/A
2.223	50	0.081	0.57	0.57	N/A
2010.758	14,621	20.902	39.03	17.67	83.54
1392.615	98	7.292	29.71	16.09	N/A

(*Continued*)

(Continued)

Cases per 100,000	Total Fatalities	Fatalities per 100,000	At Least One Dose (%)	Full Vaccination (%)	Estimated Prevalence of Delta Variant (%)
282.452	208	2.453	4.89	2.8	100
N/A	N/A	N/A	38.53	25.55	N/A
3374.938	1386	98.762	39.1	31.98	4.08
5826.238	24,274	203.372	38.33	25.57	N/A
7890.899	60,393	71.015	61.12	48.12	99.85
N/A	N/A	N/A	N/A	N/A	N/A
N/A	N/A	N/A	51.71	37.95	N/A
258.081	3103	6.585	2.19	0.78	94.23
5577.624	57,913	133.235	13.87	11.41	N/A
7307.866	2066	20.678	89.88	78.8	N/A
10,727.519	134,774	197.595	71.05	64.67	100
12,425.139	663,929	199.429	62.43	53.31	100
11,105.054	6044	173.421	77.81	73.18	N/A
487.453	1164	3.43	28.84	8.5	N/A
1.272	1	0.318	12.51	3.59	N/A
3325.123	0	0	N/A	N/A	N/A
1215.376	4214	14.68	23.77	14.88	N/A
646.901	15,936	16.233	25.19	5.73	N/A
27.884	1608	5.274	1.01	0.05	N/A
1099.587	3635	19.212	1.87	1.56	100
840.283	4550	30.148	19.04	12.77	100

State	Total Confirmed Cases	Cases Per 100,000	Total Fatalities	Fatalities per 100,000	At Least One Dose (%)	Full Vaccination (%)
Alabama	754,242	15,383	12,718	259	51	40
Alaska	96,567	25,345	449	61	56	48
Arizona	1,053,487	14,474	19,304	265	58	50
Arkansas	477,191	15,813	7334	243	55	44
California	4,608,094	11,662	67,422	171	70	57
Colorado	645,719	11,213	7498	130	65	58
Connecticut	381,331	10,696	8446	237	75	67
Delaware	125,798	12,919	1902	195	65	56
Florida	3,442,090	16,026	49,251	229	66	55
Georgia	1,474,572	13,828	23,242	218	53	43
Hawaii	70,504	4980	657	46	76	56
Idaho	237,056	13,265	2508	140	46	40
Illinois	1,582,811	12,491	27,008	213	67	52
Indiana	916,901	13,620	14,940	222	51	47
Iowa	421,168	13,349	6337	201	57	53
Kansas	391,113	13,425	5794	199	59	50
Kentucky	638,168	14,284	8167	183	59	50
Louisiana	719,424	15,475	13,241	285	51	43
Maine	81,177	6039	969	72	73	67
Maryland	512,966	8485	10,205	169	69	63
Massachusetts	783,750	11,371	18,393	267	76	67
Michigan	1,093,419	10,949	21,841	219	56	51
Minnesota	673,867	11,949	8008	142	63	57
Mississippi	466,145	15,663	9061	304	49	41
Missouri	806,899	13,147	11,690	190	54	46
Montana	136,304	12,753	1847	173	54	47

(*Continued*)

(Continued)

State	Total Confirmed Cases	Cases Per 100,000	Total Fatalities	Fatalities per 100,000	At Least One Dose (%)	Full Vaccination (%)
Nebraska	254,850	13,175	2613	135	58	53
Nevada	406,212	13,188	6763	220	59	49
New Hampshire	112,747	8292	1448	106	68	61
New Jersey	1,121,089	12,622	27,101	305	71	63
New Mexico	242,399	11,560	4633	221	71	61
New York	2,340,930	12,033	54,317	279	69	62
North Carolina	1,310,185	12,492	15,322	146	58	48
North Dakota	123,136	16,158	1608	211	50	43
Ohio	1,311,518	11,220	21,265	182	53	49
Oklahoma	585,721	14,802	8208	207	55	46
Oregon	303,532	7197	3495	83	65	59
Pennsylvania	1,354,451	10,580	28,651	224	71	56
Rhode Island	167,245	15,787	2808	265	73	66
South Carolina	806,597	15,666	11,349	220	54	45
South Dakota	138,292	15,632	2092	236	58	50
Tennessee	1,133,200	16,594	14,020	205	51	44
Texas	3,857,592	13,304	60,790	210	59	49
Utah	485,554	15,145	2753	86	58	49
Vermont	30,376	4868	291	47	77	69
Virginia	814,738	9545	12,118	142	67	59
Washington	612,176	8039	7095	93	70	62
West Virginia	213,179	11,895	3261	182	48	40
Wisconsin	760,485	13,061	8646	148	60	55

State	Total Confirmed Cases	Cases Per 100,000	Total Fatalities	Fatalities per 100,000	At Least One Dose (%)	Full Vaccination (%)
Wyoming	82,463	14,248	918	159	47	40
American Samoa	0	0	0	0	66	54
Guam	13,741	8156	171	101	73	63
Northern Mariana Islands	258	479	2	4	66	62
Puerto Rico	211,075	6232	3044	90	73	63
U.S. Virgin Islands	6298	5928	66	62	50	42
Washington, DC	58,440	8281	1167	165	69	59

Index

Note: Page numbers followed by "f" indicate figures, "t" indicate tables and "b" indicate boxes.

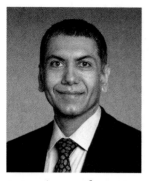

Samoon Ahmad, MD, is a Clinical Professor of Psychiatry at NYU Grossman School of Medicine. A graduate of Allama Iqbal Medical College in Lahore, Pakistan, where he trained in Internal Medicine, General Surgery, and Cardiology, Dr. Ahmad completed his psychiatric training at Bellevue Hospital/NYU Medical Center, serving as chief resident in his final year. Upon completion, he became an Attending at Bellevue and joined the faculty of the NYU School of Medicine. Dr. Ahmad supervises and mentors trainees and lectures globally on various topics, including antipsychotics, obesity, metabolic disorders, and medical marijuana. He is a Diplomate of the American Board of Psychiatry and Neurology, a Distinguished Fellow of the American Psychiatric Association, and an International Associate member of the Royal College of Psychiatrists.

During his tenure, Dr. Ahmad has served as Director of the Division of Continuing Medical Education (CME), on the board of Governors of Bellevue Psychiatric Society, and on various committees including Grand Rounds, CME Advisory, CME Task Force, Educational Steering, Bellevue Collaboration Council, and Bellevue Psychiatry's Oversight Committee. He developed Bellevue Hospital Psychiatry Department's Integrated Systems Conference, based on the morbidity and mortality conference in medicine, to better coordinate services and treatment in the department. He was recognized for 25 years of distinguished service at Bellevue and was named Bellevue's Physician of the Year in Psychiatry (2014) for his continued pursuit of clinical excellence, leadership, and dedication at the institution.

Dr. Ahmad's research has focused primarily on the prevalence of metabolic abnormalities in the chronically mentally ill, specifically the association of psychiatric medications, diet, physical activity, and obesity. He has conducted other research on the role of faith, religion, and resilience in disasters. His documentary *"The Wrath of God: A Faith Based Survival Paradigm"* about the aftermath of the earthquake in Pakistan was awarded "The Frank Ochberg Award for Media and Trauma" by the International Society for Traumatic Stress Studies.

Dr. Ahmad specializes in the psychopharmacological treatment of psychotic, mood, anxiety, and substance use disorders. He is the founder of Integrative Center for Wellness in New York City. He is an author, contributor, and consulting editor for several medical textbooks, most recently coauthoring *Medical Marijuana: A Clinical Handbook*. He lives in New York City with his wife and son and enjoys photography, travel, classic cars, and vinyl records in his spare time.